NARRATIVE MEDICINE
Honoring the Stories of Illness

For George in memory
and
Bernard in the present and future

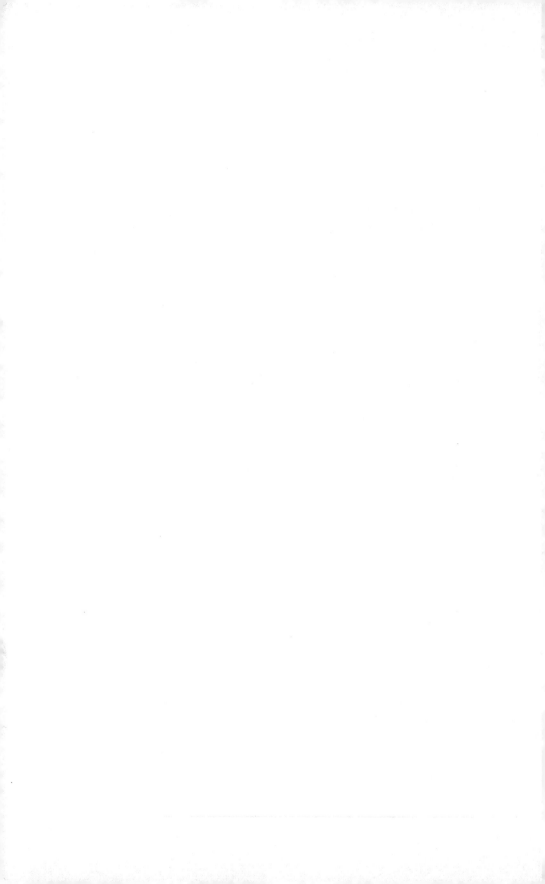

▣ PREFACE

I invite readers to look with my colleagues and me at this form of clinical practice we have come to call narrative medicine, defined as medicine practiced with the narrative competence to recognize, absorb, interpret, and be moved by the stories of illness. When we human beings want to understand or describe singular people in particular situations that unfold over time, we reach naturally for narrative, or storytelling, to do so. When we try to understand why things happen, we put events in temporal order, making decisions about beginnings, middles, and ends or causes and effects by virtue of imposing plots on otherwise chaotic events. We hail our relations with other human beings over time by receiving and alluding to stories told by others—in myths, legends, histories, novels, and sacred texts. We seek connections among things through metaphor and other forms of figural language. By telling stories to ourselves and others—in dreams, in diaries, in friendships, in marriages, in therapy sessions—we grow slowly not only to know who we are but also to become who we are. Such fundamental aspects of living as recognizing self and other, connecting with traditions, finding meaning in events, celebrating relationships, and maintaining contact with others are accomplished with the benefit of narrative. A medicine practiced with narrative competence will more ably recognize patients and diseases, convey knowledge and regard, join humbly with colleagues, and accompany patients and their families through the ordeals of illness. These capacities will lead to more humane, more ethical, and perhaps more effective care.

The field of narrative medicine has emerged gradually from a confluence of sources—humanities and medicine, primary care medicine, contemporary narratology, and the study of effective doctor-patient relationships. A clinical cousin of literature-and-medicine and a literary cousin of relationship-centered care, narrative medicine provides health care professionals with practical wisdom in comprehending what patients endure in illness and what they themselves undergo in the care of the sick. As I was working on a paper tentatively entitled "The Narrative Hemisphere of Medicine" some time ago, I realized suddenly that there is little in the practice of medicine that does not have narrative features, because the clinical practice, the teaching, and the research are all indelibly stamped with the telling or receiving or creating of stories. The phrase "narrative medicine" came to me as a unifying designation to signify a clinical practice informed by the theory and practice of reading, writing, telling, and receiving of stories. The name appealed to me because, as a nominal phrase, it points to a "thing" and not an idea (fulfilling William Carlos Williams's dictum that there are no ideas but in things) and connotes a kind of practice along with a set of conceptual relations in which it nests. The notion would not have been compelling to me had it been either an atheoretical tinkering with how we do things or an abstract but pointless set of ideas. Neither atheoretical nor pointless, the practice of narrative medicine has already shown its proliferative salience to individual practice, clinical education, health professional standards, national policy, and global health concerns.

What do narrative and medicine have in common? What might this field of narrative medicine know that is news to both fields? The enthusiastic and grateful responses of clinicians, students, literary scholars, writers, and patients to early work in narrative medicine have encouraged me to think that we are developing useful approaches to medicine, to literature, and to suffering. Even more powerfully, what this field brings to both clinical practice and narrative theory seem to be exactly what each field needs. On the one hand, medicine, nursing, social work, and other health care professions need proven means to singularize the care of patients, to recognize professionals' ethical and personal duties toward the sick, and to bring about healing relationships with patients, among practitioners, and with the public. Strengthening our narrative capacities can, I suggest in this book, help in all these efforts. My hypothesis in this work is that what medicine *lacks* today—in singularity, humility, accountability, empathy—can, in part, be provided through intensive narrative training. Literary studies and narrative theory, on the other hand, seek practical ways to transduce their conceptual knowledge into palpable influence in the world, and a connection with health care can do that.

Much has changed fundamentally of late within the health care system for patients and for health care professionals, making the habits and ideas included in this book particularly timely. We all lament the incursion of corporate and bureaucratic concerns into clinical practice. Office hours have been sped up. "Hospitalists" who are strangers to patients are replacing doctors who know patients well in caring for the most acutely ill. The passivity of health care professionals in the face of the commodification of health care that began with the marketplace intrusion into health care in the 1980s continues to stun and trouble us. We still do not have a national health insurance plan in this country, and the numbers of uninsured mount. The gap between rich and poor widens and with it widens the gap of health. Corruption and fraud and corporate greed are present in health-related industries as they are throughout the U.S. business landscape. We see more and more clearly how health care decisions are made not by or even for patients but by and for shareholders and corporate executives. Questions of health care policy, in this country anyway, are cynically politicized and prey to ideological power thrusts. Global health is marred by unconscionable and unjust inequities. Aware of our losses, we often feel empty-handed of prospects for more effective systems of care.

In the face of these discouraging developments, there is impressive vitality and creativity in health care. The movements for quality improvement in health care are beginning to be felt in palpable and measurable ways. We are making meaningful progress in understanding and teaching communication skills, professionalism, cultural competence, team-building, and patient-centered care. Patients have found new allies in their search for health, notably among one another in advocacy groups and support groups, in the readership of published and electronic "telling" of illness stories, and in increasingly influential legislative and governmental roles. Health care may be in the process of becoming safer and more effective, and issues of equity and dignity are at least beginning to be recognized.

Optimistic developments are surfacing in how we care for the ill. Doctors, nurses, and social workers practice in new ways today as compared to their routines of even a few years ago. Taking a narrative life history is slowly entering clinical practice, for example, and the notion that nurses and doctors and therapists bear witness to patients' suffering is beginning to be heard and considered. We health care professionals are seeking more and more urgently for means to establish our trustworthiness and to be faithful to our own professional oaths. We and our patients know that time must be devoted to developing knowledge of one another in practice, that eight-minute visits do not suffice to expose all that must be said, and that longitudinal fidelity is critical in safeguarding health or responding to illness. More and more insistently, we are refusing to practice according to someone else's bottom line, knowing that short-term saving of a few minutes here and there cannot make up for the chronic damage done to clinical relationships starved of time, dignity, and regard. Such movements as relationship-centered care, spirituality and medicine, and the ethics of virtue and care signal deep commitment to bettering the tattered state of doctor-patient relationships and to improving the outcomes of our medicine.

I have been humbled and impressed of late to meet with large and diverse groups of health care professionals and patients in this country and abroad who are fired up with yearnings for a medicine that makes sense, that takes care of people—both patients and caregivers—and that replenishes and respects all who are marked by it. To offer narrative medicine as a corrective to some of these failings, a support to these emerging strengths, and response to these widespread yearnings serves to unify and cohere divergent aspects of sickness and health care. If, that is, we can provide what patients long for, we will at the same time provide what health care professionals seek—a form of health care that recognizes suffering, provides comfort, and honors the stories of illness.

Achieving narrative competence, however, is not a trivial goal. Although everyone grows up listening to and telling stories, sophisticated knowledge of how stories work is not attained without considerable effort and commitment. Narrative theory is not easy to master—perhaps no easier to master than the science that we absorb on our way to health care professional competence. Close reading takes practice, skill, and long experience with many texts. The designation of practitioner of narrative medicine must be earned by rigorous and disciplined study over time, mastering new concepts, language, and practices in a longitudinal and demanding schooling. Happily, narrative schooling carries the replenishing dividends of creativity, self-knowledge, understanding of others, and deep aesthetic pleasures.

As we design narrative training programs for health care professionals and as we develop narrative interventions in our clinical practices, we have to be cognizant of what we are asking of our learners. "Hearing the patient's story" has become, sometimes, a catchphrase, as if to do so is a quick corrective to be applied to an existing system of care. As we spell out the implications of narrative medicine for practice and education, we see the radical challenges thrown up by the decision to infuse medicine with narrative competence. Becoming competent in narrative skills *opens up* practice. It does not simply shift some habits or routines. It changes what we do with patients, with colleagues, with students, and with the self. Its implications reach to the health care professional-patient relationship, health professions training, programs for professionalism and humanism in health care, and the practice of narrative bioethics, as well as the structural aspects of routine medical practice, the economics of care, the means to support health care equitably, and the imperative to improve the safety and effectiveness of the American health care system. The circles of influence widen all the way out to global issues of justice and equity in health care. Slowly, we realize that we are no longer doing what we used to do in the office or on the ward or in the professions. We find that we have annexed powers to our work as nurses, doctors, social workers, and therapists that transform our practice.

Narrative training encompasses a constellation of learning. We teach our students fundamental skills of close reading and disciplined and considered reflective writing. We equip them with the skills to receive and critique respectfully and honestly what colleagues write. We introduce them to great literary texts and give them the tools to make authentic contact with works of fiction, poetry, and drama. We present complex theory from literary studies and the narrative disciplines. In settings as diverse as ward medicine attending rounds, staff meetings on the adult oncology in-patient service, the AIDS clinic, and home visit programs, we meet with health care professionals to read and to write, to attend to and to represent all that occurs in these lives led among the sick. As a result, we deepen our students' capacity to hear what their patients tell them.

I have tried to accomplish a number of discrete tasks in this book. I have tried to write a primer for this new field of narrative medicine, detailing the theoretical bases for its practice from literary studies, narrative theory, general internal medicine, and bioethics without getting either arcane or unduly simplified. I have tried to write a manual for teachers of reading and writing in the medical context. My colleagues and I have been learning slow and cumulative lessons about how to teach such narrative skills as close reading, reflective writing, and bearing witness in courses for health care professionals and students, lessons that have been refined in many settings and over many uses. Although I have presented these ideas and procedures at countless workshops and conferences over the years, it made sense to me to collect the guidelines that inform my teaching practices in one more or less coherent statement. I understand that readers with many kinds of proficiency may be joining me in this text, and I beg indulgence of all readers who will find some sections naively condensed and others impenetrably obscure.

I offer several taxonomies in the course of this book—the four types of divides between patients and health care professionals, the five narrative features of medicine, and the five elements in my close reading drill. I hope it will be clear that these taxonomies speak to one another and support one another—the narrative features of medicine "answer," broadly speaking, the divides we find within health care, and the reading drill helps to mobilize attention to all five narrative features of medicine. These taxonomies culminate in the triad of attention, representation, and affiliation that I came to call the three movements of narrative medicine.

Throughout these chapters, I return to several ideas and themes. Were I a poet, I could present these recurring concepts or images with the simultaneity with which they come to me. I want for them to appear to my readers all at once, not serially or sequentially but there, together, always mutually informing the thinking and actions represented in this work. The awareness of the divides between the sick and the well needs to be present as we contemplate patients' and families' experiences with illness. The narrative features of medicine like temporality and ethicality do not take their turns in influencing illness or care but, in practice, must be apprehended all at once. To grow in our understanding of how patients tell of themselves and their bodies seems a pivotal and enduring effort in our willingness and ability to care for the sick. The skills of close reading are applied in all areas and all at once in our professional lives—reading charts, listening to patients, mentoring students, and writing and comprehending our own reflections on care. Our duties toward the sick and toward their bodies are illuminated and fulfilled by developing the capacity for attention and representation. When we turn the corner toward affiliation and contact, we know that our narrative competence has yielded its most valuable dividends in enabling us to bear witness to suffering and, by that act, to ease it.

As I asked myself by what warrant I was writing this book, I realized that it came from all the stories in my file cabinets—written by medical students, doctors, patients, nurses, and social workers over the years. I would sit at my cherry writing table and function as the medium, the amanuensis for all these voices telling of illness and the efforts to care for the sick. Linguistic research projects in ageism in the clinical encounter, early efforts to develop the Parallel Chart, stories from practice that friends and strangers sent to me, final exams for my medical students in the medical interviewing curriculum, my father's medical charts from his solo practice—all these texts spoke to me, sometimes rather eerily, from my records kept faithfully over time. These are the primary texts for this book. These are the texts that have inspired me and goaded me to think and think again about why this matters, what this says, how this changes being sick and caring for the sick.

I have obtained permission from all writers who are identifiable—students, health care professionals, and colleagues from afar—to reproduce their texts. I have decided to publish them, on the whole, anonymously, in part because they "stand for" so many others I might have chosen to print. I have noted throughout the text when descriptions of patients have been changed for the sake of confidentiality. When I was unable to show patients what was written about them so as to obtain their consent for publication, I altered the details of the text to render the patients unrecognizable, even to themselves. There are several times (noted in the endnotes) when I have combined aspects of several patients into one description. This was always done in order to preserve confidentiality.

Writing this book has electrified my own practice of general internal medicine by giving me things to try, ways to improve my routines, new curiosities about patients' experiences of their bodies and their health. I surrender to patients in a different way these days. I think I lend myself to them in new and clinically useful ways. I write a great deal more about my patients than even I ever did before, confirming over and over the truth that writing reveals things to us that we know but didn't know we knew. I show patients what I have written about them as a matter of routine, and I now explicitly encourage writing from patients in the course of routine care. I could go on, but the traces of all these lessons are in the chapters themselves and need no detailed preview.

As I think of what we do with patients and colleagues, I see how complex and fraught and yet *hopeful* are these encounters. So much needs to be said, yet suffering sometimes cannot be asserted but can only be fitfully intimated by another. Sometimes, it is as if doctor and patient were alien planets, aware of one another's trajectories only by traces of stray light and strange matter. "We catch a glimpse of something, from time to time," writes William Carlos Williams, "which shows us that a presence has just brushed past us, some rare thing—just when the smiling little Italian woman has left us. For a moment we are dazzled. What was that?"[1] We can feel like valuable but inscrutable objects of admiration for one another, each trying to penetrate the other's secrets. With what pregnant wonder we meet, trying to take in all that is being emitted by the other, sometimes without the emitter's knowledge. Does the trilobite *know* what truths are transposed on its stony ridges? Do the Pleiades realize what they transmit to earth? Does the dancer whose body is represented on the funerary vase buried with the Egyptian king understand the yield of her gestures? We sit in one another's presence, silenced by the other's mystery, its plenitude, its alterity, in suspense, waiting.

We stay in the presence of this freight of meaning, not only filled with gratitude that we can, now, see it but also filled with satisfaction that we have helped its meaning to be apprehended. Knowing something about the body grants us the license to near another. It grants us admission to a proximity to the self of the other and, by reflection, of ourselves. The images that course through the pages of this book—my amphora, James's great empty cup of attention, Joyce's snow general all over Ireland, the edifices built by form, the spirals of attention and representation that culminate in affiliation—all these images are illustrations of our presence with one another, whether patient or colleague or student.

Perhaps an oncology nurse reads what she has written about the fragility of everyday life. Perhaps a 38-year-old new patient tells with shy pride that she runs 20 miles a week. Perhaps a medical student reveals his rage at the unfairness of disease or its treatment. Perhaps family members gather at the bedside of their mother, who is dying of widespread ovarian cancer. We are at the same time *alone* and *with,* strange and similar. The presence of the other is both mystery and identity. We are simultaneously outside the obscurity and within the familiarity of another's being. Like planets in a solar system, we revolve around and are warmed by a common sun while hosting lives of absolute distinction. In the end, we live with one another as best we can, trying, as health care professionals, to receive what our patients emit and trying, as patients, to convey these all but unutterable thoughts and feelings and fears. Indeed, we are revolving bodies, attracted to one another and held aloft in orbit by the gravity of our common tasks.

I invite you to share this experience with me and to join in developing these ideas and practices. I hope that this frame of narrative medicine can gather new combinations of us—from the humanities, from all the health professions, from the lay world, the business world, the political world—and make new relations among us, so as to look with refreshed eyes at what it means to be sick and to help others get well. Henry James says somewhere that the combinations are, in the end, inexhaustible and, in the preface to *Roderick Hudson,* that "[r]eally, universally, relations stop nowhere."[2] Let us revel in the inexhaustibility of our combinations and the universality of our relations, our affiliations, our common burdens and gifts as we do our best to heal.

NOTES

1. William Carlos Willliams, *The Autobiography of William Carlos Williams,* 360.
2. Henry James, *New York Edition,* 1:vii.

▣ Acknowledgments

I thank the many teachers, friends, colleagues, students, and patients who have nurtured my thinking and writing throughout this project. I was inspired and directed in my studies of literature and of medicine by Harvey Chertok, Elliot Mishler, Joanne Trautmann Banks, and Steven Marcus, whose wisdom and example illuminated my way from the start. I have been fortunate to spend my academic and medical career at Columbia University, whose Departments of Medicine and English shared my time and cross-fertilized one another's imprint on narrative medicine. The dedication to patient care and willingness to come with me into literary exploration exemplified by Gwen Nichols, Steven Shea, Ronald Drusin, Edith Langner, Aaron Manson, and Steve Albert has been of lasting importance in this work. The freedom that has been accorded me at Columbia to try new things in my teaching, research, scholarship, and patient care has been deeply appreciated.

I profess my enduring indebtedness to my colleagues in the National Endowment for the Humanities Exemplary Education Project that has convened regularly from 2003 to 2005 to study the consequences of narrative training in medicine: Sayantani DasGupta, Rebecca Garden, Craig Irvine, Eric Marcus, Tara McGann, David Plante, Maura Spiegel, and Patricia Stanley. Their thinking and insight permeate this text. As an early teacher of English and current coeditor in chief of *Literature and Medicine*, Maura Spiegel deserves particular and happy gratitude. Special thanks go to Tara McGann for keeping many projects and programs afloat during the completion of this book. I am most grateful to Benjamin Everett and Cara Rabin for their careful attention to my bibliographic references.

Far-flung colleagues in literature-and-medicine, including members of the editorial board of *Literature and Medicine*, have over the years shaped and inspired my thinking and helped me to know what to do with my house officer's intuition that there was something for doctors to learn from stories. Humble thanks go to Kathryn Montgomery, Suzanne Poirier, Anne Hudson Jones, Anne Hunsaker Hawkins, Martha Montello, Julie Connelly, Charles Anderson, and David Morris and, in wider circles engaged in this work, to Arthur Frank, Eric Cassell, Jerome Bruner, Shlomith Rimmon-Kenan, Michael Ondaatje, and the late Susan Sontag. My medical colleagues, especially through the good work of the Association of American Medical Colleges, have kept me honest through my literary growth, enabling the transformation of erstwhile marginal interests in humanities and medicine into mainstream commitments in medical education. Many of these colleagues from literary studies and medicine read early versions of these chapters and helped me understand what I was trying to say. Many audiences at Grand Rounds and seminars throughout the country were perhaps the unwitting trial listeners to much of this book in its early stages, listeners whose honest and challenging responses helped me to fashion this work along the way, and I thank them for their attention.

I acknowledge pivotal support from the Fan Fox and Leslie R. Samuels Foundation, which funded the outcomes research on the Parallel Chart. I thank the Rockefeller Foundation for a residence at the Bellagio Study Center in spring of 2001 when the very beginning frame for this work emerged. A Guggenheim Fellowship during 2002 and 2003 enabled me to devote a full year to writing, and the book could not have been completed without this support. The National Endowment for the Humanities has underwritten my and my colleagues' time in our most generative study project during the past two years. I thank Oxford University Press for its steadfast commitment to this project and acknowledge with deep gratitude the insight and pivotal direction given me by editors Jeffrey House and Peter Ohlin.

I thank the patients and students and colleagues who have powered this work by their writing and telling and who have given me generous permission to reproduce their stories and texts in these pages. I recognize my debt to Henry James, who is ever-present in my life as a companion and model, and whose thinking and language have transformed my own.

An early version of chapter 10 appeared as "The Ethicality of Narrative Medicine" in *Narrative Research in Health and Illness* edited by Brian Hurwitz, Trish Greenhalgh, and Vieda Skultans (23–36) and published by BMJ Books of London in 2005. I acknowledge the editors' and publishers' permission to reprint parts of that work.

Finally, I thank Mary Marshall Clark, Nancy Dubler, Richard Frankel, Mary Gordon, Angela Klopstech, Donald Moss, and David Plante for their enduring presence and contact through this period. My husband, Bernard, as always, is behind everything I do.

▣ Contents

PART I

What Is Narrative Medicine?

I ▣ The Sources of Narrative Medicine

Medicine has grown significantly in its ability to diagnose and treat biological disease. Doctors can be proud of their ability to eradicate once fatal infections, prevent heart attacks, cure childhood leukemias, and transplant failing organs. But despite such impressive technical progress, doctors often lack the human capacities to recognize the plights of their patients, to extend empathy toward those who suffer, and to join honestly and courageously with patients in their struggles toward recovery, with chronic illness, or in facing death. Patients lament that their doctors don't listen to them or that they seem indifferent to their suffering. Fidelity and constancy seem to have become casualties of the cost-conscious bureaucratic marketplace. Instead of being accompanied through the uncertainties and indignities of illness by a trusted guide who knows them, patients find that they are referred from one specialist and one procedure to another, perhaps receiving technically adequate care but being abandoned with the consequences and the dread of illness.[1]

A scientifically competent medicine alone cannot help a patient grapple with the loss of health and find meaning in illness and dying. Along with their growing scientific expertise, doctors need the expertise to listen to their patients, to understand as best they can the ordeals of illness, to honor the meanings of their patients' narratives of illness, and to be moved by what they behold so that they can act on their patients' behalf. Nurses and social workers have mastered these skills more fully than have physicians, but all can join in strengthening these capacities in health care.

Doctors, nurses, and social workers began turning for help in these areas to people who know about narratives, which can be defined as stories with a teller, a listener, a time course, a plot, and a point. Teachers of literature, novelists, storytellers, and patients who have written about their illnesses have become collaborators at our medical centers in teaching health professionals the skills needed to listen to narratives of illness, to understand what they mean, to attain rich and accurate interpretations of these stories, and to grasp the plights of patients in all their complexity.[2] These are narrative skills, for they enable one person to receive and understand the stories told by another. Only when the doctor understands to some extent what his or her patient goes through can medical care proceed with humility, trustworthiness, and respect. I use the term *narrative medicine* to mean medicine practiced with these narrative skills of recognizing, absorbing, interpreting, and being moved by the stories of illness. As a new frame for health care, narrative medicine offers the hope that our health care system, now broken in many ways, can become more effective than it has been in treating disease by recognizing and respecting those afflicted with it and in nourishing those who care for the sick.

Years ago when I was just out of internal medicine residency training, I would sit in a little clinic room in Presbyterian Hospital, getting to know relative strangers who were to become my patients for more than 20 years. Most were poor, sick, elderly women of color—from the Dominican Republic, Puerto Rico, Central America, and the American South—who now lived in Manhattan's Washington Heights or Harlem. I realized slowly that my task as an internist was to develop the skills required to absorb my patients' multiple, often contradictory, stories of illness. I came to understand that what my patients paid me to do was to listen expertly and attentively to extraordinarily complicated narratives—told in words, gestures, silences, tracings, images, laboratory test results, and changes in the body—and to cohere all these stories into something that made provisional sense, enough sense, that is, on which to act. These narratives had many tellers—the patient herself or himself, as well as family members, friends, nurses in the emergency room, interns dictating hospital discharge summaries, social workers, therapists, and all the other doctors who wrote in the medical chart. What I was listening for and reading for were diagnostic clues to help identify a biological or emotional source of the patient's symptoms, autobiographical background to help me understand who it was who bore these symptoms, and grounds for personal connections between the two of us sitting in that little room.

In order to do all these things at once, I had to do what all doctors—ideally—do, whether they realize it or not. I had to follow the patient's narrative thread, identify the metaphors or images used in the telling, tolerate ambiguity and uncertainty as the story unfolded, identify the unspoken subtexts, and hear one story in light of others told by this teller. Like the reader of a novel or the witness of a drama—who naturally do all these things seamlessly—I also had to be aware of my own response to what I heard, allowing myself to be personally moved to action on behalf of the patient. I was the interpreter of these accounts of events of illness that are, by definition, unruly and elusive. I saw that, while I had very demanding "listening" tasks, the patient's "telling" tasks were even more demanding, because pain, suffering, worry, anguish, and the sense of something not being right are conditions very difficult, if not impossible, to put into words.

Around that time, the movement called "literature-and-medicine" was just starting to grow, and I was fortunate to be included in a National Endowment in the Humanities Seminar on Literature and Clinical Imagination in 1982. Joanne Trautmann Banks, editor of Virginia Woolf's letters and the first literary critic to be appointed to a medical school faculty, directed a monthlong intensive training program in literary theory, texts, and methods salient to medicine. Part of the training was encouragement to write, in ordinary narrative prose, about our clinical practice. I chose to write about a patient I had just seen the week before the seminar started, because I was unhappy about how I had behaved toward her and it nagged at me that I had acted brusquely and dismissively without knowing her situation. So I wrote a story about this incident, filling in with fiction the gaps there were in fact.

I was picking up some papers from my office, in a hurry, and was stopped by a young woman patient who had dropped in to ask me to sign a disability form for her. I had seen her a couple of times in the office for the evaluation of headaches, headaches that I had not considered terribly worrisome and for which I had prescribed acetaminophen. I remember being irritated, not only that she thought she deserved disability on such slim clinical grounds but that she would appear, without an appointment, and expect me to make time to fill out the form. But I was late for a meeting and did not have the time to inquire about the situation, so, without even putting down the stack of papers in my arms, I quickly scrawled a diagnosis and signed the form, no doubt conveying my displeasure at the patient's request.

In my story, the patient—I called her Luz—had a chance at achieving her dream of becoming a fashion model. Her aunt in Manhattan had met a contact at a big agency and urged Luz to move in with her from Yonkers while preparing for auditions. The disability payments, in my story, would give Luz a needed income while she got a portfolio together and tried to make her dream come true. I wrote the story from Luz's point of view, and the story ends with Luz musing about how hurried her doctor was and how scornful she seemed to be.

When I next saw the patient in the office soon after the seminar concluded, I had been thinking about her a great deal and trying to inhabit her point of view. I had tried, in my imagination, to make sense of her unexplained behavior while realizing what my own behavior must have connoted. And so I asked her with great interest and regard about the situation, apologizing for having brushed her off so quickly the last time.

The stakes were much, much higher in fact than in my imagined fiction. Indeed, Luz *did* need the disability payments to tide her over for an emergency move to Manhattan. But it was not in search of a career in fashion. Luz was the oldest of five daughters, all of whom were being tormented by their father and uncle in their crowded apartment in Yonkers. My patient had been sexually abused since she was twelve, and now she refused to stand by and allow the same thing to happen to her younger sisters. She felt, at age twenty-one, that she could set up a safe house in Manhattan to protect herself and her sisters.

Once I learned all this, the social worker in the domestic violence project and I introduced Luz and her sisters to emergency shelters and support groups and gave them needed resources in facing the violence in her family. They did move to Manhattan, taking their mother, too, away from the abusive male relatives. Over the years, I have taken care of three of the five sisters and their mother. When the father became terminally ill, the women in the family asked me to be his internist too.

Luz taught me about the power of the clinical imagination. Although I did not know what had preceded her visit that day, I had wordlessly registered her urgency and need to leave home. Until my impressions were expressed in language, I did not know what, in fact, I *knew* about the patient. My hypothesis about the modeling career was all wrong—in my story, Luz was running *toward* something, when, in fact, she was running *away*—and yet my acts of guessing at the patient's situation and trying, imaginatively, to make sense of her behavior had some profound dividends. The hypothesis acted like a prosthetic device or a tool with which to get to the truth, like a crowbar or a periscope will enable you to see under a rock or over a wall. Also, this narrative act helped me to get closer to the patient. My writing exercise *invested* me in learning of her true plight instead of blaming her or suspecting her of malingering. The effort, required by my storytelling, to reach for and visualize Luz's point of view helped me take care of the patient by bringing me to her side, seeking to understand her behavior, taking seriously her situation, and gaining access to the unsaid knowledge I had already developed of her strengths and desire.

In the ensuing years, I have come to realize that these narrative skills are deployed not only in the encounter between an individual patient and doctor but throughout the enterprise of medical practice: teaching, doing research, understanding and diagnosing disease, reflecting on one's life in medicine, interacting with professional colleagues, and fulfilling the public responsibilities of medicine.

▣ The Narrative Road to Effective Medicine

Health professionals and patients are at a crossroads. Together, we have to discover means of sustaining the tremendous capabilities of our biomedical sciences while trying to ease the suffering and loss occasioned by serious illness. The price for a technologically sophisticated medicine seems to be impersonal, calculating treatment from revolving sets of specialists who, because they are consumed with the scientific elements in health care, seem divided from the ordinary human experiences that surround pain, suffering, and dying. Whether to protect themselves from the sadness of taking care of very sick people or to guarantee the objectivity of their clinical judgment, doctors seem to operate at a remove from the immediacy of sick and dying patients, divided from sick people by deep differences in how they conceptualize illness, what they think causes it, how they choose to treat it, and how they respond emotionally to its presence. Patients long for doctors who comprehend what they go through and who, as a result, stay the course with them through their illnesses. A medicine practiced without a genuine and obligating awareness of what patients go through may fulfill its technical goals, but it is an empty medicine, or, at best, half a medicine.[3]

Although they may not show it, doctors, too, long for a medicine different from the current fragmented bureaucracy that health care has become. Everywhere—in high-powered academic medical centers, in small-town hospitals, and in rural communities—clinicians seek out means by which to reflect on their practice, to talk to one another seriously and intimately about their lives around sickness, and to grasp with as much accuracy and emotional clarity as they can what their patients undergo in serious illness.[4] On my many visits to distant medical centers, doctors, nurses, and social workers attend workshops where they can write about their lives with patients, ruminate together about their feelings and failures, and review with joy their triumphs. What the participants in my workshops understand urgently (although perhaps preverbally) is that the self is the caregiver's most powerful therapeutic instrument and that effective health care professionals have to find means toward self-knowledge, forgiving self-criticism, and inner nourishment.[5]

Doctors with long lives in medicine behind them know what has been disrupted by the recent economically driven changes. They join primary care physicians and proponents of patient-centered health care in their belief that doctors should grow with their patients, getting to know their bodies and their lives through decades.[6] They know how the knowledge doctors accrue about their patients' families, fears, and hopes and the trust they earn through dutiful attention are critical to their providing their patients with effective health care.[7] Not only the personal dimensions of disease but its biological dimensions become clear only over time: to understand what disease a patient might have requires schooled longitudinal curiosity about that person's state of health. Sicknesses declare themselves over time, not in one visit to the consultant. The doctor who has accompanied a patient over a prolonged period of time will have the bank of biological knowledge about that individual necessary for timely and accurate diagnostic vision along with the muscular therapeutic alliance necessary to engage the patient in effective care.[8]

If doctors seem divided from their patients and from themselves, they also seem divided from their students, from one another, from other health professionals, and from the society they are meant to serve. The personal mentorship and role modeling that was once the hallmark of medical education have been eroded by time and money pressures. The competitive—and deficit—environment of most teaching hospitals leaves little room for the dutiful raising of young professionals or the nurturing of those in full career.[9] Instead of committing themselves to the professional development of their members, professional medical organizations more often indulge in legislative lobbying or market positioning. Turf battles threaten to undermine respectful alliances with nurses, physician assistants, social workers, therapists, and psychologists, leaving many health professionals feeling isolated, distrusted, and struggling against one another instead of working together on behalf of the patient. The threat of malpractice litigation leaves doctors feeling they must practice a rigid, suspicious medicine. And, as medicine has had to round up on itself defensively, it is less equipped to initiate honest and consequential dialogue with the public about such grave issues as equity in health care, the limits of medical power, and the ideals of health care envisioned—and invested in—by this country.

Medical schools, residency training programs, and professional societies have, in the past two or three decades, responded to the need to humanize medicine. In addition to equipping students and doctors with sophisticated technical knowledge and skills, medical educators are working hard to enable physicians to practice with empathy, trustworthiness, and sensitivity toward individual patients. Such developments as biopsychosocial medicine, primary care medicine, bioethics, and professionalism in medicine have arisen since the 1960s to widen doctors' narrow focus on biological disease and to encourage them to take stock of patients' emotional, social, and familial needs.[10] These movements have led to several major advances: training in communication skills in medical schools, research and teaching in the social and emotional dimensions of health and illness, awareness of ethical aspects of health care, and attention to doctors' own well-being and personal awareness.[11]

Until recently, however, these efforts have not had much impact, because no one knew very well how to describe the traits lacking in medicine nor how to teach them. Most agree that medical schools and training programs cannot train adults to be empathetic, respectful, altruistic, and ethically responsible, for such traits are developed and nurtured from infancy onward. Indeed, it is charged that doctors' innate empathy, respect for the suffering of others, and ethical discernment *diminish* in the course of medical training and that doctors become hardened against the suffering they witness through their education.[12] How, then, are we to advance beyond the uncomfortable state of knowing what the matter is but being unable to fix it?

Even if medical educators cannot require a student to respond to a patient's suffering with compassion, they might be able to equip students with compassion's *prerequisites:* the ability to perceive the suffering, to bring interpretive rigor to what they perceive, to handle the inevitable oscillations between identification and detachment, to see events of illness from multiple points of view, to envision the ramifications of illness, and to be moved by it to action. Those who espouse professionalism have learned already that, however highly medicine might prize altruism and accountability, doctors cannot be forced to practice with these traits unless they are helped to develop the antecedent skills required to reflect on their work, to recognize the duties incurred on them by virtue of being doctors, to feel rewarded by the humble intimacy afforded by trustworthy medicine, and to unite with their colleagues in swearing to uphold medicine's ideals. And, however urgent seems the national need for frank discourse and consensual decisions about our health care system, one cannot expect doctors and other health professionals to take the lead in opening the complex and risky discussions that must take place without providing them with the skills of respecting multiple perspectives, hearing and mediating competing voices, and recognizing and paying heed to a multitude of contradictory sources of authority.

To provide to medicine what it lacks today, we have to conceptualize the problems in terms global enough to envision the whole and practical enough to suggest workable solutions. I think it helps us to see that many of the failures of contemporary medicine are concentrically widening consequences of the same set of fundamental problems. Whether enacted in the situation between an individual doctor and patient, within the doctor himself or herself, among medical and nonmedical colleagues in the health professions, or in dialogue with the larger society, medical practitioners often seem isolated from authentic engagement, unused to recognizing others' perspectives and thereby unable to develop empathy, and at a loss to understand or to honor the meanings of all that they witness.

To know what patients endure at the hands of illness and therefore to be of clinical help requires that doctors *enter* the worlds of their patients, if only imaginatively, and to see and interpret these worlds from the patients' point of view. To reach accurate diagnoses calls for the kind of lived-in, tacit knowledge of disease and health available only through immersion in the natural history of diseases and scrutiny of the changes in individual patients' bodies over long periods of time. To take stock of the costs and rewards of a life lived around sick and dying people entails reflection and self-examination, while to make oneself available to patients as a therapeutic instrument demands risky self-knowledge and personal awareness. To fulfill one's duties toward colleagues and students, to admit mistakes and to lessen the chance of their occurrence, and to commit oneself to medicine's ideals flows from one's fidelity to an affirming yet disciplined (and potentially disciplinary) professional community. And to bring about meaningful decisions with the public regarding matters of health requires the sophisticated communication powers to open fear-laden discussions without triggering defensive anger and to illuminate, despite multiple clashing perspectives, common goals and shared desires.

To accomplish all these goals—empathic and effective care of individual patients, candid reflection, professional idealism, and responsible societal discourse about health policy—requires a unified set of skills. To do all these things requires what psychologists and literary scholars call narrative knowledge, that is, the kind of knowledge that Luz taught me years ago. If narratives are stories that have a teller, a listener, a time course, a plot, and a point, then narrative knowledge is what we naturally use to make sense of them. Narrative knowledge provides one person with a rich, resonant grasp of another person's situation as it unfolds in time, whether in such texts as novels, newspaper stories, movies, and scripture or in such life settings as courtrooms, battlefields, marriages, and illnesses. As the literary critic R. W. B. Lewis writes, "Narrative deals with experiences, not with propositions."[13] Unlike scientific knowledge or epidemiological knowledge, which tries to discover things about the natural world that are universally true or at least appear true to any observer, narrative knowledge enables one individual to understand particular events befalling another individual not as an instance of something that is universally true but as a singular and meaningful situation. Nonnarrative knowledge attempts to illuminate the universal by transcending the particular; narrative knowledge, by looking closely at individual human beings grappling with the conditions of life, attempts to illuminate the universals of the human condition by revealing the particular.[14]

Medicine can benefit from learning that which literary scholars and psychologists and anthropologists and storytellers have known for some time—that is, what narratives are, how they are built, how they convey their knowledge about the world, what happens when stories are told and listened to, how narratives organize life, and how they let those who live life recognize what it means. Using narrative knowledge enables a person understand the plight of another by participating in his or her story with complex skills of imagination, interpretation, and recognition. With such knowledge, we enter others' narrative worlds and accept them—at least provisionally—as true. Our genuine curiosity and commitment toward the truth enable us to peer through the twilight of another's story as we try to see the whole picture and as we reflect on what it might mean. We recognize what parts we play in one another's lives and how entailed we are in our shared creation of meaning. We get to know ourselves as a result of the vision of others, and we are able to donate ourselves as instruments of others' learning.[15]

This form of knowing about the world that makes sense of the told predicaments of others—risky, demanding, self-defining, horizon-opening—seems to be at least part of what medicine today is lacking. Narrative medicine—or medicine practiced with narrative competence—is at once attuned to the individual patient, replenishing for the individual professional, dutiful in generating and imparting medicine's knowledge, and cognizant of the responsibilities incurred by the public trust in medicine.[16] Narrative medicine can help answer many of the urgent charges against medical practice and training—its impersonality, its fragmentation, its coldness, its self-interestedness, its lack of social conscience.

Narrative medicine not only describes an ideal of health care but also provides practical methods to develop the skills needed to reach that ideal. Narrative medicine recognizes that some of the skills currently missing from medicine are, in fact, narrative skills, that we know what narrative skills are, and that we know how to teach them. Literature departments, creative writing courses, anthropology and ethnography departments, and psychotherapy training programs, among many others, have developed well-tested methods of teaching students how to read, write, and interpret texts; how to systematically adopt others' points of view; how to recognize and honor the particular along with the universal; how to identify the meaning of individuals' words, silences, and behaviors; how, as a reader or a listener, to enter authentic relation with a writer or a teller or a text; and how to bring one's own thoughts and sensations to achieving the status of language. We know how to educate students in these skills. We just have not been doing it in medical schools or nursing schools. By recognizing these skills as fundamentally narrative competencies, medicine is beginning to know how to provide them.

HOW NARRATIVE COMPETENCE ENTERS MEDICINE

An 85-year-old woman with bad asthma comes in to see me. I've know her for almost 20 years. We have managed to decrease her hospitalizations and emergency room visits dramatically over the years, and so she is grateful and I am proud. Today she sits and weeps. I know that her 28-year-old grandson just last week drowned in the ocean off Miami. I know that her son, this dead man's father, was shot to death on the streets of Harlem at the age of 36. She sits next to me and she weeps. Her English and my Spanish enable us to reach one another. Her pain is unbearable. Suffering again the loss of her son by virtue of the loss of her grandson, she is overwhelmed by her grief. Yes, she prays to a God she still feels near; yes, she is comforted by the presence of her daughter; yes, she allows herself to talk about her two lost men. She knows that time will heal her pain, and she knows to wait. I weep with her, unable to fathom her agony but able to honor her bereft state. I listen as she tells of her anguish, knowing that her telling of it is therapeutic. I will see her next week, and the week after that, not to fix anything but simply to watch with her, to listen to her, to behold, in awe, her faith and power and love.

Medicine is joining other disciplines such as anthropology, history, psychology, social science, law, and even mathematics in recognizing the elemental and irreplaceable nature of narrative knowledge.[17] A narrative shift has taken place across these many fields of human learning, challenging scholars and practitioners from religious studies to psychoanalysis to police work to concentrate on not just the facts but the situations in which these facts are told.[18] Although narrative is defined somewhat differently by literary scholars, psychologists, autobiographers, and historians, each of these narrative-users shares fundamental ideas—that narrative knowledge and practice are what human beings use to communicate to one another about events or states of affairs and are, as such, a major source of both identity and community. The narrativist turn that has overtaken many fields exposes the centrality of storytelling in many human activities from teaching kindergarten to enacting religious faith. Telling stories, listening to them, being moved by them to act are recognized to be at the heart of many of our efforts to find, make, and honor meaning in our lives and the lives of others.

Narrative is a magnet and a bridge, attracting and uniting diverse fields of human learning. The Ozark storyteller knows something that helps the lawyer in the courtroom. The police officer interviewing the crime victim adopts methods developed by the anthropologist in the field. The richness and exhilaration of narrative studies today, whether in the social sciences or in journalism or in a class on Henry James, arise from our recognition of our common concerns and shared goals. In an age of specialization and fragmentation, how satisfying to discover the deep, nourishing bonds that hold us together—storytellers all, bearing witness to one another's ordeals, celebrating our common heritage as listeners around the campfire, creating our identities in the stories we tell.

As an enterprise in which one human being extends help to and shares knowledge with another, medicine has never been without narrative concerns. Like narrative acts, clinical practice requires the engagement of one person with another person and realizes that authentic engagement is transformative for all participants. Narrative competence permits caregivers to fathom what their patients go through, to attain that illuminated grasp of another's experience that provides them with diagnostic accuracy and therapeutic direction. And, as has more recently come into view, this same narrative competence increases the power of all health professionals to come to grips, through reflection, with what being a caregiver means in their own lives and the lives of their families. It makes them all better teachers, better researchers, better colleagues with all other health professionals. It equips them to more effectively enter serious conversations with the public about the choices medicine forces upon us and gives us the privilege to consider those choices.

By no means a replacement for scientific competence, narrative competence allows all that a professional knows to be placed at the service—now—of this patient who suffers from asthma and grief. It allows the doctor or nurse or social worker to provide care that strengthens and does not belittle, care that deepens and does not blunt the patient's search for meaning in the face of illness. Most important, medicine practiced with narrative competence can bridge some of the divides between the sick and the well, enabling all to recognize their common journey. Using narrative competence, caregivers can do what anyone who witnesses suffering does—in a family, among friends, in the news, on the stage, in fiction, on the street, in the hospital—one knows, one feels, one responds, and one *joins with* the one who suffers.[19] It is as if the heads of the teller and listener are bowed over the suffering that happened in the attempt to interpret and understand it.

A young man came in to see me, referred by his wife who had been my patient for some time. She said that he had been enduring bothersome symptoms for years but had not wanted to subject himself to a medical evaluation. The patient, a muscular man of serious demeanor and stiff carriage, described severe abdominal pain, terrible difficulty with digestion, and bowel symptoms that interfered dramatically with his work performance and his leisure time. I wondered at his stoic acceptance of these intrusive symptoms for many years, and I noticed the pressure with which he held himself in during our conversation.

It was then time for the physical examination. Instead of changing into the cotton gown as I had asked him to, my patient stood hunched over the stainless steel sink near the examining table, fists clenched, head bowed, his back to me, motionless. I knew not what was happening, but I knew not to move. I sat at my desk, quarter-turned away from him, gaze slanted down, arrested by the force field of his stillness. We were part of a tableau, wordlessly enacting what, it came to me, must be an old truth.

When he spoke, it was to say, "It's because of what happened the last time I was at the hospital." And so I knew to use great caution, slowness, and gentleness in touching him, so that performing the physical examination could be not an assault but an effort to help.

To call this medicine narrative medicine brings to health professionals and patients critical knowledge and practice from many other fields of human learning and actions. What Luz and I did in marshaling the clinical imagination forms a part of what has become an international movement toward incorporating narrative studies into medical education and practice. By now, medicine is beginning to acknowledge the requirement for narrative knowledge and skills in the care of the sick. In the same way that medicine can do more today by virtue of all that it has learned from the scientific disciplines, medicine can do more today by virtue of all that has been learned from the narrative disciplines.

Narrative medicine has come to understand that patients and caregivers enter whole—with their bodies, lives, families, beliefs, values, histories, hopes for the future—into sickness and healing, and their efforts to get better or to help others get better cannot be fragmented away from the deepest parts of their lives. In part, this wholeness is reflected in—if not produced by—the simple and complicated stories they tell to one another, whether in medical interviews, late-night emergency telephone calls, or the wordless rituals of the physical exam. Without narrative acts, the patient cannot convey to anyone else what he or she is going through. More radically and perhaps equally true, without narrative acts, the patient cannot himself or herself grasp what the events of illness mean. And without telling about or writing about the care of a patient in a complex narrative form, the caregiver might not *see* the patient's illness in its full, textured, emotionally powerful, consequential narrative form. It remains to be proven— although it appears a most compelling hypothesis—that such narrative vision is required in order to offer compassionate and effective care to the sick.

Not so much a new specialty as a new frame for clinical work, narrative medicine gives doctors, nurses, and social workers the skills, traditions, and texts to provide nuanced, respectful, and singularly fitting clinical care to the sick while also achieving genuine contact with their own and their colleagues' hopes and ideals as health professionals. As a result, the health care they practice is focused on the fully envisioned plight of each patient, of each caregiver, of each institution of health care, and of the whole society that suffers and that tries to heal.

NOTES

1. See Norman Cousins, *Anatomy of an Illness as Perceived by the Patient;* Anatole Broyard, *Intoxicated by My Illness;* Anne Fadiman, *The Spirit Catches You and You Fall Down;* and Simone de Beauvoir, *A Very Easy Death* for clear statements, by patients, families, and their allies, of the health care system's failures to care.

2. Joanne Trautmann, *Healing Arts in Dialogue,* and Delese Wear, Martin Kohn, Susan Stocker, eds., *Literature and Medicine: A Claim for a Discipline* document the beginnings of these practices.

3. Many of the pathographies written by patients or their families about their illnesses document these problems. See William Styron, *Darkness Visible;* Reynolds Price, *A Whole New Life;* or Nancy Mairs, *Waist-high in the World: A Life among the Nondisabled.* Health professionals, too, are deeply troubled by the emptiness of contemporary medicine. See Melvin Konner, *Medicine at the Crossroads;* Arthur Kleinman, *The Illness Narratives;* Rachel Remen, *Kitchen Table Wisdom;* and Bernard Lown, *The Lost Art of Healing.*

4. See the regular features entitled "A Piece of My Mind" in the *Journal of the American Medical Association,* "On Doctoring" in the *Annals of Internal Medicine,* or "Narrative Matters" in *Health Affairs* for examples of reflective writing, published in professional medical journals, that testify to doctors' growing desire and need to tell of their lives in medicine and to struggle to understand what their patients go through.

5. The British psychoanalyst Michael Balint made the observation that the self is the most powerful therapeutic instrument in his 1957 book, *The Doctor, His Patient, and the Illness.* Dennis Novack et al., "Calibrating the Physician: Personal Awareness and Effective Patient Care," survey and summarize recent work done in the field of reflection in health care. Diane Meier and Anthony Beck apply these concerns to individual clinical decision-making in "The Inner Life of Physicians and the Care of the Seriously Ill."

6. See Christine Laine and Frank Davidoff, "Patient-Centered Medicine: A Profes-

sional Evolution"; William Branch, *Office Practice of Medicine*; Thomas Delbanco, "Enriching the Doctor-Patient Relationship by Inviting the Patient's Perspective"; Eric Cassell, *Doctoring: The Nature of Primary Care Medicine*; and Laurence Savett, *The Human Side of Medicine*, 163–71.

7. Recent examples include William T. Close, *A Doctor's Life*; Jerome Groopman, *The Measure of Our Days*; and John Stone, *In the Country of Hearts*. See review of evidence-based studies of the consequences of continuity of care in Richelle Koopman et al., "Continuity of Care and Recognition of Diabetes, Hypertension, and Hypercholesterolemia."

8. I thank Peter Watkins for helping me to understand this fundamental point.

9. Kenneth Ludmerer, *Time to Heal*.

10. George Engel, "The Need for a New Medical Model: A Challenge for Biomedicine"; John Stoeckle, ed., *Encounters between Patients and Doctors*; Albert Jonsen, *The Birth of Bioethics*; and P. Reynolds, "Reaffirming Professionalism through the Education Community." The transformations in these areas within medical education and practice are, indeed, most startling and impressive, even as they seem not to have had very much impact on the routine medical care that patients experience. For summary overviews of the developments in humanistic medicine, see Moira Stewart et al., *Patient-Centered Medicine*; Jeremiah Barondess, "Medicine and Professionalism"; Eric Cassell, *The Nature of Suffering and the Goals of Medicine*; and Rachel Remen, *My Grandfather's Blessings*.

11. Mack Lipkin Jr., Samuel Putnam, and Aaron Lazare, eds., *The Medical Interview: Clinical Care, Education, and Research*; David Mechanic, *Medical Sociology*; Tom L. Beauchamp and James F. Childress, *The Principles of Biomedical Ethics*; C. P. Tresolini and the Pew-Fetzer Task Force, *Health Professions Education and Relationship-Centered Care*; and Ronald A. Carson, Chester R. Burns, and Thomas R. Cole, eds., *Practicing the Medical Humanities*.

12. Jodi Halpern, *From Detached Concern to Empathy*; Susan Phillips and Patricia Benner, eds., *The Crisis of Care: Affirming and Restoring Caring Practices in the Helping Professions*; and Fred Hafferty, "Beyond Curriculum Reform: Confronting Medicine's Hidden Curriculum."

13. R. W. B. Lewis, *The American Adam*, 3.

14. For useful and nontechnical descriptions of narrative knowledge, see Jerome Bruner, *Actual Minds, Possible Worlds* and *Making Stories: Law, Literature, Life*. See also such seminal works written by literary scholars and narratologists as Seymour Chatman, *Story and Discourse*; Shlomith Rimmon-Kenan, *Narrative Fiction: Contemporary Poetics*; W. J. T. Mitchell, ed., *On Narrative*; Paul John Eakin, *How Our Lives Become Stories: Making Selves*; and Wallace Martin, *Recent Theories of Narrative*.

15. See the recent works by physicians and nurses that endorse the use of narrative in their practices. Trish Greenhalgh and Brian Hurwitz, eds., *Narrative Based Medicine*; Kathryn Montgomery Hunter, *Doctors' Stories: The Narrative Structure of Medical Knowledge*; Rita Charon, "The Narrative Road to Empathy"; Melinda Swenson and Sharon Sims, "Toward a Narrative-centered Curriculum for Nurse Practitioners"; and C. Skott, "Caring Narratives and the Strategy of Presence: Narrative Communication in Nursing Practice and Research."

16. Rita Charon, "Narrative Medicine: A Model for Empathy, Reflection, Profession, and Trust."

17. For narrative's influence in psychology, see Theodore Sarbin, ed., *Narrative Psychology*; Jerome Bruner, *Acts of Meaning*; and Karen Seeley, *Cultural Psychotherapy*. John Paulos describes the relationship between statistics and stories in *Once upon a Number: The Hidden Mathematical Logic of Stories*. Hayden White outlines history's reliance on narrative processes in *The Tropics of Discourse*. Alasdair MacIntyre recognizes the narra-

tive nature of ethical thought in *After Virtue*. There are just a few examples of this very widespread intellectual current toward narrative modes of thought and practice.

18. See Martin Kreiswirth detailing what he has called the narrativist turn in the social sciences and the humanities in "Trusting the Tale."

19. Eric Cassell, "The Nature of Suffering and the Goals of Medicine"; Charles Aring, "Sympathy and Empathy"; Patricia Benner and J. Wrubel, *The Primacy of Caring;* and Louise Rosenblatt, *Literature as Exploration.*

2 ▣ Bridging Health Care's Divides

Narrative medicine is a very practical undertaking. It arises from the day-in, day-out events of the doctor's or nurses' office—right there off the crowded waiting room, the desk drawers filled with prescription blanks and rubber hammers, the gauze and the scalpels and the needles and the betadine, the telephones ringing and the computer screens filled with lab test results. Or it arises in the anonymous hospital room, strangers overhearing, through the green cloth curtain, a doctor telling a patient bad news, sad news, news of defeat, and sometimes—though it seems rarely—news of success and cure. Here, relative strangers meet—one prepared to deploy clinical knowledge and the other prepared for the worst.

In addition to needing expert diagnosis and treatment, seriously ill people simultaneously need those caring for them to recognize that something of value has abandoned them, that a deep and nameless sadness has settled in at home. It would seem that those entrusted with the care of the sick should by nature extend great reserves of comfort, of hope, of tenderness, and of strength toward those struggling through the pain of disease, the discomfort of treatment, and the toll of all the losses.

In *Devotions upon Emergent Occasions,* John Donne writes, "As Sicknesse is the greatest misery, so the greatest misery of sicknesse is *solitude.*"[1] A doctor who recognizes the patient in the face of the sickness, who respects the patient's strength despite the fear, who accompanies the patient through the territory of illness that the doctor knows well, and who honors the meaning of the patient's suffering provides not just knowledge of diseases but knowledge of the direction toward either health or the ability to live authentically without health. Such a doctor provides *company* to combat the isolation and with it an animating belief in the patient's ability to endure whatever will come.

The 2000 Pulitzer Prize in drama went to a young author unknown until she published the play *Wit.*[2] Margaret Edson captured the attention of theater audiences and the culture at large by her depiction of literary scholar Vivian Bearing in her ordeal with ovarian cancer. The play enacts the divides between this patient and all the health professionals who attempt to provide medical care for her—the arrogant senior oncologist who lies to her, the young physician-scientist so intent on getting data for his research project that he is blind to his patient's suffering, the nurse who cannot mobilize her awareness of Vivian's pain into effective action. Professor Bearing is a scholar of the work of John Donne, an expert on Donne's courageous sonnets about death. *Wit* unfolds with Donne as backdrop, and all that happens to Vivian is underscored by the immense power of Donne's poetic vision about death.[3]

When the play opened at a Union Square theater in New York, the producers had to hire psychologists to facilitate after-theater discussions of the play: playgoers refused to leave the house! Many came time and time again to view the play, and then they stayed in their seats, some weeping, needing to talk together about what they had witnessed. Clearly, this depiction of routine health care was recognized as true—or at least recognized as feared—by New Yorkers.

I hated the play the several times I saw it. I felt attacked by what I considered to be a crude and one-dimensional caricature of doctors and nurses. I felt defensive in the face of the wholesale blaming of medicine as a cruel enterprise. I could not assess the play's literary merits, for I felt deeply hurt by its assault. Many of my colleagues in health care were more humbly accepting of Edson's message, hosting readings or productions of the play in their hospitals and medical schools, and assigning the play as required reading to their medical students.

I have come to realize that Edson has done a great service to medicine by offering, in her creative synthesis, the portrait of a complex woman, crushed by an incurable disease, who learns of her own failings as a teacher and scholar by virtue of the failings of her doctors. Here, she recalls a session with her eminent professor of Donne, E. M. Ashford, discussing Holy Sonnet Ten:

> E.M.: The sonnet begins with a valiant struggle with death, calling on all the forces of intellect and drama to vanquish the enemy. But it is ultimately about overcoming the seemingly insuperable barriers separating life, death, and eternal life. . . .
>
> In the edition you chose, this profoundly simple meaning is sacrificed to hysterical punctuation:
> And Death—*capital D*—shall be no more—*semicolon!*
> Death—*capital* D—*comma*—thou shalt die—*exclamation point!*
> Gardner's edition of the Holy Sonnets . . . reads:
> And death shall be no more, *comma*, Death thou shalt die.
> (*As she recites this line, she makes a little gesture at the comma.*)
> Nothing but a breath—a comma—separates life from life everlasting. It is very simple really. With the original punctuation restored, death is no longer something to act out on a stage, with exclamation points. It's a comma, a pause.
>
> This way, the *uncompromising* way, one learns something from this poem, wouldn't you say? Life, death. Soul, God. Past, present. Not insuperable barriers, not semicolons, just a comma.
> VIVIAN: Life, death . . . I see. It's a metaphysical conceit. It's wit! . . .
> E.M.: It is *not wit*, Miss Bearing. It is truth. (14–15)

The truth of the situation is not a metaphysical conceit. The truth of disease is pain, isolation, and hopelessness, in which even those appointed to care for Vivian—including the oncology fellow Jason—become hazards, their presence only exposing her aloneness:

> VIVIAN: (*To audience*) In isolation, I am isolated. For once I can use a term literally. The chemotherapeutic agents eradicating my cancer have also eradicated my immune system. In my present condition, every living thing is a health hazard to me. . . .
> (JASON *comes in to check the intake-and-output.*)
> JASON: (*Complaining to himself*) I really have not got time for this . . .
> VIVIAN: . . . particularly health-care professionals. (46–47)

And later, when she is very close to death, a death accelerated by the aggressive chemotherapy research protocol, her oncologist, Dr. Kelekian, and Jason display how aggressively barricaded they are against her condition:

> KELEKIAN: Dr. Bearing, are you in pain? (KELEKIAN *holds out his hand for chart;* JASON *hands it to him. They read.*)
> VIVIAN: (*Sitting up, unnoticed by the staff*) Am I in pain? I don't believe this. Yes, I'm in goddamn pain. (*Furious*) I have a fever of 101 spiking to 104. And I have bone metastases in my pelvis and both femurs. (*Screaming*) There is cancer eating away at my goddamn bones, and I did not know there could be such pain on this earth.
> (*She flops back on the bed and cries audibly to them.*) Oh, God. (71)

Patients and their families seeing performances of *Wit* felt recognized or even vindicated by the play's savage portrayal of contemporary health care because, I suspect, such inhumane and therefore ineffective care is enacted every day in hospitals everywhere. Health professionals do not understand what patients go through unless they themselves are ill, and so patients feel unbridgeable chasms between themselves and those who are supposed to take care of them. The isolation of each is arresting—the patient isolated by fear of disease, the professional isolated by knowledge of it. There are dangerous divides also, for example, between nurses and doctors, between surgeons and physical therapists, between social workers and psychiatrists, and between home care nurses and hospital nurses. These divides prevent them all from doing their best.

Health care professionals may be knowledgeable about disease but are often ignorant of the abyss at which patients routinely stand. They have no idea, most of the time, of the depth and the hold of the fear and the rage that illness brings. They have no idea how fundamentally everything changes when one's husband or mother or child is seriously ill. That which once seemed important—mortgage payments, getting the promotion, the Dow Jones, the Middle East—shrivels in comparison to the baby's white blood cell count or the result of Mom's head CT. The wife weeps in the shower, asking herself, "Why didn't I make him go to the doctor when he first had trouble breathing? Why didn't I make him stop smoking? Why did I keep cooking steaks?" as her husband lies, alone, miles away, without her, in his narrow bed in the coronary care unit. All is as if lost. Her view of life narrows to her husband's pale wrist encircled by a plastic hospital name tag, his pale forearm taped up with intravenous tubing.

Later, the cardiologist makes his rounds in the CCU and tells the wife, "He's got a severe blockage in two of his coronary arteries, and we feel we need to do an emergency bypass operation right away." What does this mean? Will he live? Will he die? They will open her husband's heart like a bruised fruit; he will bleed into the gloved hands of strangers. But will he be well? Will he live? Will he die?

Pale and tired-looking, the wife tightens her grasp on her husband's wrist— she better not dislodge that intravenous line, thinks the cardiologist, the nurses had trouble getting it started. The patient's wife stutters something about her husband's allergy to anesthesia and getting a second opinion at Cornell. Doesn't she realize how sick her husband is? Sending him across town for a second opinion is too risky. He might not survive the ambulance ride. She doesn't trust me to be her husband's doctor, the cardiologist thinks with a sinking heart. How can I do the right thing in the face of her suspicion?

This doctor, this patient, and this family are at a loss. They are unable to deploy the powers of medicine to help them unless they can reach one another. Unless they find ways to grasp one another's perspective, they are doomed. The husband's heart disease will claim him while his cardiologist and his wife argue about proper treatment, separated by differentials of language and knowledge, divided by mistrust and fear.

We are beginning to understand what is *missing* in this imaginary scenario. In a repetition of the scenario enacted in *Wit*, what is missing is the health professional's ability to comprehend the plight of this patient and this wife. This doctor is not equipped with the imagination, the ability to see from another's point of view, the knowledge of human fears and hopes, and the ear for language and silence necessary to grasp fully the predicament of his patient and his patient's wife. If only the doctor would, as a matter of routine, be prepared for the jarring, jolting, inarticulate presence of dread; if only he would be attuned to the inevitable and exorbitant terrors that illness brings. Of *course* the wife thinks she has been slowly killing her husband. Of *course* she is already imagining her life as a widow, her children as part orphans. This is the nature of illness, that it transports ordinary people to imagine extraordinary losses.

THE DIVIDES

As a doctor, I can speak with some experience about what I have observed to occur between doctors and patients. I believe that the relationships patients have with nurses, social workers, and therapists are less troubled than the relationships they have with doctors, due in part to issues of power, gender, class, clinical training, and patients' expectations of the different professions.[4] Although the barriers described here no doubt exist in clinical situations with all health care professionals, I cannot speak to their consequences with professionals other than physicians. I suspect that the divides between nurses or social workers and their patients are less formidable than those of doctors; in an ideal world—perhaps in a narrative health care world—doctors will learn from nurses and social workers about how to lessen these gulfs and how to bridge the inevitable divides among us all.

Despite the complexity and consequences of the events that unfold in the doctor's office, the participants are often ill prepared for their meeting. They speak different languages, hold different beliefs about the material world, operate according to different unspoken codes of conduct, and are ready to blame one another should things go badly. Many patients feel abandoned by their doctors, dismissed in their suffering, disbelieved when they describe their symptoms, or objectified by impersonal care.[5] As personified in part by *Wit's* Dr. Kelekian, the intellectual ambition, scientific competition, professional privilege, and greed of many doctors too often overshadow the primary service goals of medicine. Sadly, patients have come to reconcile themselves to a forced choice between attentiveness and competence, between sympathy and science.[6] At the same time, many doctors feel aggrieved by the extravagant hopes patients have come to hold for the powers of medicine. They feel unable to measure up to patients' inflated expectations and demands that medical treatment will reverse the results of unhealthy behaviors, poor health choices, or random and unfair bad luck. Realizing how "slow" are their true fixes, doctors prepare to disappoint patients or to be sued for not being as effective as everyone seems to think they are.

What is enacted in these medical offices is the divide between the sick and the well, or, in Susan Sontag's words, the realization that "illness is the nightside of life, a more onerous citizenship."[7] Unlike other divides—gender, race, class, place, age, time—that separate one human being from another, the divide between the sick and the well is capricious, unpredictable, sometimes reversible but in the end irrevocable. It spares no one. One hurtles with the speed of a fall down a mountain from one side of the divide to the other; one is turned by years-long, silent, cell-by-cell malignant change into a person with cancer. The world is transformed after the diagnosis of a serious disease, not only in the corporeal aspects of everyday life—now with pain, now with pills, now with slippers, now with a wheelchair—but in the deepest wells of meaning—now with limits, regrets, forced separations, final plans.

These divides between the sick and the well are unspeakably wide. Levered open by shame, rage, loss, and fear, these chasms can be unbridgeable. And yet, to get better, the patient needs to feel included among those who are not ill. The sick person needs to continue to be, somehow, the self he or she was before illness struck. For the sick patient to accept the care of well strangers, those strangers have to form a link, a passage between the sick and the healthy who tender care.

We need to see the chasms clearly if we want to bridge them. Here, I describe four different types of divides that contribute to the divisions between doctor and patient. They seem to me the most urgent among the many divides that separate us. Each reflects a peculiar dimension of the difference between the sick and the well:

> *The relation to mortality:* Doctors and patients differ fundamentally in their natural understanding of mortality. Doctors, who know materially about death, accept an actual, present awareness that we are mortal and we will die, while patients, depending on their own personal experiences with illness and death, usually have not developed such concrete realizations. Doctors may look upon death as a technical defeat, whereas patients may see death as both unthinkable and inevitable.
>
> *The contexts of illness:* Doctors tend to consider the events of sickness rather narrowly as biological phenomena requiring medical or behavioral intervention while patients tend to see illness within the frame and scope of their entire lives. The doctor's concept of a sickness can be incommensurable with the patient's concept of the same sickness. They deal with two different things.
>
> *Beliefs about disease causality:* Health care professionals and patients can have deeply conflicting ideas about the causes of symptoms and diseases and fundamentally different ways of thinking about those causes. Because beliefs about causality dictate action and ascribe meaning to the illness, the treatment, and the ill person, these conflicts can rend care.
>
> *The emotions of shame, blame, and fear:* These emotions, among others, saturate illness and add immeasurably to the suffering it causes. Unless explicitly acknowledged and examined, these emotions and the suffering they cause can irrevocably separate doctor from patient, therefore preventing effective care.

▣ THE RELATION TO MORTALITY

Leo Tolstoy writes, in the magnificent story "The Death of Ivan Ilych," about a St. Petersburg lawyer who becomes seriously ill. Although written in the mid-nineteenth century, there has perhaps not been a more eloquent, accurate, and brave depiction of terminal illness and dying conveyed in literature. When the doctor pays a house call on the now wasted and terminally ill Ivan Ilych, Ivan finds the doctor's health offensive:

> And Ivan Ilych began to wash. With pauses for rest, he washed his hands and then his face, cleaned his teeth, brushed his hair, and looked in the glass. He was terrified by what he saw, especially by the limp way in which his hair clung to his pallid forehead. . . .
>
> Always the same. Now a spark of hope flashes up, then a sea of despair rages, and always pain; always pain, always despair, and always the same. . . . "I will

tell him, the doctor, that he must think of something else. It's impossible, impossible, to go on like this." . . .

There is a ring at the door bell. Perhaps it's the doctor? It is. He comes in fresh, hearty, plump, and cheerful with that look on his face that seems to say: "There now, you're in a panic about something, but we'll arrange it all for you directly!' " . . .

The doctor rubs his hands vigorously and reassuringly. . . .

"Well now, how are you?" . . .

Ivan Ilych looks at him as much as to say: "Are you really never ashamed of lying?" But the doctor does not wish to understand this question, and Ivan Ilych says: "Just as terrible as ever. The pain never leaves me and never subsides. If only something . . ."

"Yes, you sick people are always like that."[8]

What seems unbearable to Ivan is the contrast between his terrifyingly wasted body and the doctor's hearty, plump, and cheerful one. Whoever occupies the role of the doctor—no matter what his or her actual physical health status—will stand for health to the person diagnosed with sickness. What distinguishes them, fundamentally, is that Ivan is dying and the doctor is not.

Like Ivan, the newly sick person looks across the desk or examining table to see the not-sick, exemplified for the time being by the doctor peering at the chart, summing up the numbers, assessing the patient's chances, oblivious to the patient's horror at his or her change in status, seemingly smug in his or her own freedom from illness. The presence of health in the office can be galling, taunting, jeering. "What gods intervened on your behalf," the patient might silently ask, "that you were spared this AIDS that I got, this lung cancer that I got, this diabetes that I got? What gods failed to intervene on my behalf to spare my sight, my kidney function, my mind?" This awareness of mortality, so different for patient and for doctor, pinpoints one's present position in the trajectory of life, calculating what portion of life has been lived and what portion remains.

An old man was dying. He had had a large stroke, leaving him partially paralyzed and with the ability to say only one word, the name of his wife, "Sarah." Over and over, he called out, "Sarah, Sarah." His rhythmic one-word lament told me, an inexperienced third-year medical student, all that he could not put into words. His lament conveyed to me that he was lost, that he felt alone, that he wanted to be with those who could recognize him, even in his altered state. Over the time that I helped to take care of him, I grew to know his body very well. I examined him and drew his blood as tenderly as I could, slowly coming to know how not to hurt him. I think he came to recognize me, or at least my hands on his body.

Sarah and her daughter were usually in his room, staunch in the face of their suffering, bereft even before his death by the loss of him. They, too, lamented, their full vocabularies no more eloquent than his one word.

The night he died, I remember I was on call and was often in his room. I remember very specifically how he was lying on his side and that he would wave his thin arms in front of his face and then curl them palms outward as if to shield himself from some unwanted visitor. In retrospect, I wondered if he had seen death coming for him, if he had known before the rest of us did that he was being taken away. I always wonder what he must have suffered, having known.

I remember that the next day our whole team had to go his autopsy. The pathologist displayed my patient's organs in rectangular stainless steel pans—his shrunken kidneys, his baggy heart. I tried to hide my tears from my intern and resident, but how I wept to see him now so finally dead, so finally not alive, this man I had tried to care for, this man I had watched decline.

The day after he died, his wife and daughter came to get his belongings from the hospital. His daughter gave me a gift to thank me for taking care of her father, a little scarf, that I have kept through many moves over the intervening decades. I behold it as a reminder of him and all that he and his family taught me about grief and about death and about love.

Thinking of this man and his family helps me to dwell on the gravity of what we do every day. This moment changed their lives—for his daughter, there is before Daddy died and after Daddy died. For his wife, there is now widowhood. For him, of course, we cannot know. For me as an inexperienced medical student witnessing her first death, there was a grave and sad and frightening realization that I had given myself over to mystery, to irrevocable loss, to irremediable sadness. It was also the beginning of my experiencing these tragic human events within the capsule of pathology, of technical duty, and of the inevitable guilt over medicine's powerlessness.

As a result of these routine elements of medical training, doctors suffer two conflicting delusions about their own mortality. On the one hand, the ordeals of training during which they are awash in other people's sickness and other people's deaths can convey the irrational belief that such intimate contact with disease and death confers immunity. The intern's consolation for the unbearable months of forty-hours-at-a-stretch training is the irrational belief that he or she will never die. But equally powerful are the opposing candid realizations that all must die, that no one escapes death, and that death is never easy. When I wrote a former medical student to get his permission to reproduce in this book a description of a death he had witnessed and written about, he wrote back about his life as a general surgery resident on a busy trauma service: "Strange to remember a single passing at this point in residency when the dead of West Harlem seem to have blown between my feet like so many autumn leaves."

Patients suffer their own delusions about death. Depending on one's own contact with death—in the military, as a hospitalized patient, with family losses, through personal experiences of political violence or natural trauma—a patient might feel death a personal enemy or a distant abstraction. Some patients feel they have forestalled death many times and, catlike, will continue to find more and more lives within themselves. Others—perhaps for religious reasons or psychological ones—sense their own portion running out or their own desserts coming to an end. As Susan Sontag reminds us, the constant media exposure of the violence of war and repression and natural disaster simultaneously shocks the viewer and inures the viewer against repeated, unspeakable destruction of human beings.[9] If the Vietnam War was fought as if in our living rooms and the Iraq invasion was accomplished as if in a video game, the contemporary layperson's relation with death is highly detailed by virtue of the global web of pictures and information that now bombard us, leaving us familiar with dying but certain that it occurs only far away. And yet, in part because today's health care system insulates people from death by moving it from home to hospitals, people have little concrete idea of what really happens as death nears, what is that passage from the living to the dead.[10]

Awareness of mortality, although very different for doctor and patient, need not separate them. What would happen if doctors asked, as a matter of course, about each patient's assessment of his or her current health status or how close to the end a patient feels? Doctors may want to know something about each patient's frank appraisal of his or her state of health, including survivorship as well as frailty, hope as well as resignation.[11] And perhaps doctors could share some of their realism about death with patients. Instead of seeming to gloat about their own freedom from evident disease, doctors might reach to attain an equilibrium between their two deluded beliefs about death and then help patients achieve a balanced perception of their own relation to their ends.

Doctors may look at death with the worry that they have caused it—purposefully, passively, through negligence or error—and patients may look at death as something that they fear or defy or desire. Death divides not only doctors from patients but also all the sick from all the well and the living self from the dying self. And yet, if death seems often to divide, it also unites as the universalizing, ultimately humanizing element of life. Gabriel muses in the final scene of James Joyce's magnificent story "The Dead" as he comes to grips with the knowledge of his wife's long-dead lover Michael Furey and the future deaths he can so easily envision:

> [S]now was general all over Ireland. It was falling on every part of the dark central plain, on the treeless hills, falling softly upon the Bog of Allen and, farther westward, softly falling into the dark mutinous Shannon waves. It was falling, too, upon every part of the lonely churchyard on the hill where Michael Furey lay buried. It lay thickly drifted on the crooked crosses and headstones, on the spears of the little gate, on the barren thorns. His soul swooned slowly as he heard the snow falling faintly through the universe and faintly falling, like the descent of their last end, upon all the living and the dead.[12]

Charon is a grave name for a doctor, recalling Charon the boatman in Greek mythology who ferries the dead across the River Styx to Hades. My grandfather Dr. Ernest Charon, my father Dr. George Charon, and I are all marked by this mournful name. The first time a patient recognized my name was on the hospital wards when I was a third-year medical student. A 26-year-old man was dying of a hepatocellular carcinoma, widely metastasized. On the first day that I joined the ward team, he read my red student name tag and said, "So this is it?" He died two days later of pulmonary hemorrhage. Aghast at having perhaps added to this unfortunate young man's suffering, I thought I should change my name. I did not, however, slowly coming to realize that Charon's task is ours—to know as best we can how to navigate that journey, how to recognize that shore.

▦ The Contexts of Illness

Any phenomenon has to be contextualized in order to be understood. We locate events in space and historicize them in time, registering their contiguity with related events while divorcing them from distracting ones. The efforts to make sense of anything—the Battle of Gettysburg or *The Wings of the Dove*—require fundamental decisions about the spheres within which to consider them. Differences of interpretation proceed, in large part, from differences in how we contextualize the matter at hand.[13]

The context of events of illness can be drawn narrowly, for example, around the left anterior descending artery in our ICU patient's chest or broadly around the lives of this patient, his wife, and their family's experience of the past and hopes for the future. The psychiatrist George Engel propounded what he called the "biopsychosocial" framework for medicine years ago, suggesting that medicine had to take into account not only biological changes of illness but also the familial, community, and societal consequences of disease.[14] Engel's work was influential in challenging medical practice and medical schools to look beyond pathophysiology toward social and cultural factors that permit disease, that alter patients' behavior in the face of disease, or that influence the effectiveness of medical treatment for it. A robust research enterprise in medical sociology, behavioral medicine, and cultural studies of health and illness continues to widen medicine's knowledge about what, in the end, constitutes health and what signifies an effective response to it.[15]

The sociolinguist Elliott Mishler best describes the contexts that clash in the doctor's office. He examined tape-recorded and transcribed routine medical interviews and distinguished between the stretches of talk originating in what he calls the World of Medicine and those originating in the Lifeworld. In his pivotal 1986 study, *The Discourse of Medicine: Dialectics of Medical Interviews*, Mishler traces the course of conversations that veer between one end of meaning and the other. As the doctor interviews a woman patient with abdominal pain, he learns of her considerable alcohol intake:

"How long have you been drinking so heavily?"
"Since my husband died."
"How long ago was that?"[16]

A chasm opens up between the doctor placing the patient's symptoms in chronological order and allowing them, perhaps, to make biological sense and the patient offering her symptoms in the unfolding order of her life allowing them, perhaps, to make personal sense.

A horrified patient reported how a doctor insulted her gravely during her very first visit to him. "He asked me whether my two daughters had the same father! What could he possibly think of me?" While the patient felt that she had been taken for a loose woman, the doctor, no doubt, was going through his first-visit routine, starting with the history of present illness, past medical history, and social history. When he got to the so-called family history, he perhaps tried to save time by drawing the family tree at the same time that he collected the information about the new patient's family illnesses. One doesn't know where to draw the symbol for each child without knowing the identity of both parents, and so the doctor's question about the father of the daughters was simply a formal one from the World of Medicine, while the patient took it as a question of meaning from the Lifeworld.

This clash of contexts pits the doctor's impulse to reduce against the patient's impulse to multiply. Medicine's reductionism narrows its gaze, eliminating that which proliferates around the biological phenomena of sickness in a patient's always generative and teeming life. It is as if medicine were ametaphoric. What is at stake in this conflict is the singularity of the patient's life. What, the doctor should learn to ask, is *different* about this disease as it manifests itself in this particular patient? What, he or she should ask at the same time, is unique about this patient as a host of this disease? Clinical medicine is only beginning to tailor therapeutic approaches to disease to the particular patient. Only recently have clinical researchers distinguished between how men and women experience symptoms of a disease and how they respond to treatments for them.[17] Only recently have we begun to understand, at the genetic and molecular level, why some diseases occur more frequently or act more aggressively in some races than in others.

The recent growth in patient-centered care is a response to the narrowness of medicine's contextualization.[18] Patient-centered care is a conceptual and clinical movement, arising both in the United States and the UK, that emphasizes the patient's perspectives and desires throughout all aspects of health care. Such care respects patients' preferences, attends to patients' needs for information and education, involves family and friends, assures continuity and coordination of care, and addresses the emotional aspects of illness. One of the leaders of the movement, Moira Stewart, notes that "[p]atients want patient centred care which . . . seeks an integrated understanding of the patients' world—that is, their whole person, emotional needs, and life issues; finds common ground on what the problem is and mutually agrees on management; . . . and enhances the continuing relationship between the patient and the doctor."[19] Patient-centered care is, in effect, health care without the divides.[20]

As medicine matures, perhaps its practitioners will develop the skill to register the singular contexts that donate meaning to each clinical situation and will take upon themselves the responsibility to learn about singular aspects of their patients' lives. Such efforts are bound to enhance clinical effectiveness, not only by guiding choices of treatment interventions but also by alerting doctors to all considerations that might help or hinder patients from following medical recommendations and becoming true partners in achieving and maintaining the best health within their reach. Even more fundamentally, such partnerships can help to equalize the ground on which we all stand as sick and well, contributing to our efforts to see clearly our bodies and lives in time, in relation, and in meaning.

BELIEFS ABOUT DISEASE CAUSALITY

The *causes* of illness can be understood in divergent and even contradictory ways, often leading to baffling and damaging differences between doctors and patients. Doctors may be convinced that autoimmune cellular reactions in the joints, probably of viral and genetic origin, cause the symptoms of rheumatoid arthritis. What happens when the patient is convinced that the pain in her hands is caused by all the housework she's done over the decades? Western doctors may ascribe seizure disorders to abnormal foci of electrical activity in the neural tissue in the brain, while the Hmong parents of a little girl with epilepsy ascribe the seizures to their family ancestral spirits' inability to settle down.[21] Prescribing methotrexate for the arthritis or diphenylhydantoin for the seizures is not likely to work, not only because the pills will probably not be swallowed but also because the other causes—biological or not—will continue to exert their power over the patients' behavior and expectations and sensations. Matters of belief as well as fact, ideas about the causes and cures of disease run deep in one's culture, religion, and family, and discrepancies between the causal ideas of doctor and patient are inveterately difficult to mediate.

Beliefs about the cause of disease—or etiology—recapitulate one's very deeply held ideas about how the universe is put together. (I remember once being at a seminar in which the presenter was talking about the etiology of tuberculosis. I followed all he said with great interest, learning only at the close of the seminar that the word he was saying was not "etiology" but "ideology," pronounced with the short "i." The whole discussion made sense either way.) Doctors might be convinced about the cause of a disease only by replicable scientific evidence, while patients may be swayed in their beliefs about etiology by faith, culture, family lore, and mythic/magical notions of human biology. Doctors' beliefs about etiology are revised every time new knowledge or data become available. Their insistence on the truth of a causal fact is matched only by their certainty in the truth of a more compelling competing claim. That is to say, the grounds on which scientifically trained people subscribe to a causal belief are both rigid and revisable, while the grounds for a lay belief in disease causality might be based less on up-to-the-minute findings and more on an enduring and meaningful sense of the workings of the world. And so, when the cardiologist and the patient's wife meet in the coronary care unit, not only the need for open-heart surgery is at issue: their entire way of making sense of the universe is in conflict as they survey the future for this patient and husband.

Clashes over etiology pit the general against the particular.[22] Doctors, as a rule, offer explanations for disease that "apply" to more than one person, and a finding or theory or method must be generalizable if it is to be clinically useful. Patients, on the other hand, are usually not troubled if what is true of their disease is true *only* of theirs. More: they realize the value of recognizing what is true only of their disease, hoping that their caregivers too will recognize the importance of these unique phenomena. What is true only of their disease is true only of them, and so the experience of being sick—be it a small consolation—at least reveals something enduring about the self.

One can trace the development of Western medicine's beliefs about disease from its Hippocratic and Galenic roots to the present by attending to the tensions between the general and the particular.[23] The anticontagionists of the 1840s in England, for example, understood cholera to be caused by miasmatic or global or religious forces that exerted themselves in the environment with little regard for the specific behaviors of the charwoman or the harness-maker, whereas the contagionists believed cholera to be caused by specific occurrences within the bodies and proximities of individual stricken patients.[24] Today, the "quantitative researchers" are pitted acrimoniously against the "qualitative researchers" in performing studies of health and illness, one group accepting only findings that are replicable and generalizable and the other group addressing those aspects of illness that are singular and, well, narrative.[25]

A bracing critique of Western medicine's slant on the nature of disease was published in 1923 by Dr. F. G. Crookshank as a supplement in *The Meaning of Meaning*, written and edited by the eminent literary scholars and aesthetic theorists I. A. Richards and C. K. Ogden. Crookshank exposed the mistaken and dangerous notion that a disease is a thing. He reminded his readers that people make up diseases so as to have conceptual means of attending to symptoms and accountable ways of treating them. And yet, entreats Crookshank, diseases are not countable things in the universe. Instead, they are manners of speech:

> It is a vulgar medical error to speak, write, and ultimately to think, as if these *diseases* we name, theses *general references* we *symbolize,* were single things with external existences. . . . Nevertheless, in hospital jargon, "diseases" are "morbid entities," and medical students fondly believe that these "entities" somehow exist *in rebus Naturae* and were discovered by their teachers much as was America by Columbus.[26]

Calling the notion of diseases as entities an "inheritance from Galen," Crookshank concludes this section:

> That our grouping of like cases as cases of the same disease is purely a matter of justification and convenience, liable at any moment to supersession or adjustment, is nowhere admitted; and the hope is held out that one day we shall know all the diseases that there "are," and all about them that is to be known.

Although the search for the diagnosis is *always* part of an effort to cure it or to at least relieve its symptoms, the search for diagnosis can eclipse or even replace the attempt to relieve suffering. In Eric Cassell's words:

> [W]hen a patient has a widespread cancer whose primary (place of origin) is unknown, physicians will often go to considerable lengths to find the place of origin even though it may cause the patient great discomfort without offering *any* benefit. They do this because disease theory (the concept that when people are sick a disease can always be discovered whose constant characteristics provide a rational basis for the illness and for the action of doctors) dictates the importance of making a diagnosis—knowing the disease. . . . [T]he need to know the disease conflicts with the more fundamental dictum, "Above all, do no harm."[27]

The effort, in the end, to assign causality to symptoms is an effort to *know* and, therefore, to control. Whether a psychiatrist chooses a number to the second decimal point from the DSM-IV to signify the condition of a mentally ill patient or a patient asserts that her headaches come from thunderstorms, all who suffer or try to relieve suffering strive to banish the unknown from their ills and to replace it with the known. Even if, in retrospect, the hypothesis of causality is wrong—miasma does not cause cholera, the *Vibrio cholera* toxin does—the hypothesis has functioned to limit uncertainty temporarily, giving at least the impression of purposeful action in the face of the disease and some help in tolerating the uncertainty that remains.

After his hearty, cheerful doctor leaves Ivan Ilych, having lied to him, the specialist arrives:

> At half-past eleven the celebrated specialist arrived. Again the sounding began and the significant conversations in his presence and in another room, about the kidneys and the appendix, and the questions and answers, with such an air of importance that again, instead of the real question of life and death which now alone confronted him, the question arose of the kidney and appendix which were not behaving as they ought to and would now be attacked by Michael Danilovich and the specialist and forced to amend their ways. (143)

Ivan dies alone, doubly injured by his disease and the deceit of his doctors and family who have not the courage to face with him the unknown, "the real question of life and death." Nothing will ease patients' uncertainty in the face of illness, but perhaps their doctors can help them to articulate the uncertainty and thereby live less painfully with it. Our clashes, in the end, over the causes of disease signify the desperate need for answers, for knowing, for certainty about why disease comes and how to remedy it. The bridge over this chasm may come not from more knowledge or shared epistemologies but from the bravery to face the contingencies of health and illness and death.

THE EMOTIONS OF SHAME, BLAME, AND FEAR

The emotions of shame, blame, and fear erect the most unbreachable divides between doctors and patients. I start with shame. Much of what goes on inside the body is, to some people, shameful to discuss. Patients often do not feel comfortable talking with physicians—especially of the opposite gender—about their sexual practices, bowel habits, substance abuse, or emotional problems. Questions about these matters are often left unasked because of embarrassment or humiliation.[28] If patients feel ashamed to talk about such symptoms, doctors are embarrassed to hear them or cannot find the equanimity to ask about them. Furthermore, some doctors cannot ask about particular aspects of patients' symptoms because they fear giving in to voyeurism or unprofessional curiosity. And so the doctor and the patient collude in their experiences of shame or their gambits to avoid it, all of it truncating attention to important aspects of health and illness.

If shame is the interior experience that one must hide from others what one is, its counterpart, guilt, is the remorseful realization that one has done something wrong. Guilt saturates the lives of patients and health care professionals. Some of the guilt experienced by patients is due—the smoker who develops lung cancer or emphysema *knows* his or her part in having brought it about and, hence, suffers a more complex form of despair than would one who had had no hand in what befell him.[29] The movements to medicalize such conditions as alcoholism, obesity, or drug addiction can be understood, in part, as efforts to absolve sufferers of the full guilty responsibility for their situations and to shift the blame to brain chemistry or genetic propensity. On the other hand, illness seems to induce irrational guilt in patients who search for *something* they may have done to cause their lymphoma or breast cancer or multiple sclerosis, almost as if identifying something concrete in their experience as the proximal cause of an illness is preferable to accepting its random unfairness, even at the cost of assuming some of the responsibility for their illness themselves.[30]

Health care professionals' guilt is a powerful engine for their behavior. We are burdened and also supported by a highly developed sense of personal accountability. When we inevitably err in the course of practice, we must deal with the tremendous pain of guilt. David Hilfiker was perhaps boldest in publishing an account of a really terrible error in the *New England Journal of Medicine*—he had aborted a live fetus on the mistaken belief that fetal death had occurred.[31] Since Hilfiker's brave revelation, there have been many, many such accounts, both in the professional and the lay literatures, confessing serious error and metabolizing the induced guilt. Because we hope that guilt leads to caution and increases safety in the future, we endorse such public displays of personal accountability as mortality and morbidity rounds (professional meetings of a clinical department in which bad clinical outcomes are scrutinized so as to identify fixable sources of error) and the more systems-oriented examinations of error-prone practices endorsed by the Institute of Medicine's *To Err Is Human*.[32] In the face of a more forgiving stance toward medical mistakes, many health care professionals and patients hope to bring about openness in speaking of error, for the sake both of patients and of professionals who suffer from the silence and the concealment induced by guilt.[33]

Blame can block patient and doctor from understanding one another's perspective and achieving good medical treatment. Patients' readiness to blame— and sue—their doctors for bad outcomes leads many doctors to practice defensively and to treat patients with suspicion. (Malpractice litigation is, of course, a most complex phenomenon. Some who study the phenomenon have found that patients sue their doctors when they feel they have not been listened to.[34]) Doctors blame their patients, too, for having caused their own diseases—"What does she expect, she smokes a pack a day for twenty years? What does he want after bacon and eggs every day for breakfast?" Patients are routinely blamed by doctors for the oddest things. "Patient a poor historian," doctors typically say when they cannot follow a complex story of an illness. "Patient noncompliant" says the doctor whose advice to take certain medicines is declined. Such descriptors as "morbidly obese" and "sexually promiscuous" transform a physical or behavioral description into not only a moral judgment of the patient but also an accusation that the patient caused whatever ails her. Interns at a New York City municipal hospital used to refer to it as the "Hospital for Self-Inflicted Diseases." As soon as the patient is identified as having caused the illness, the doctor's responsibility is accordingly shifted from cure to censor. "We cannot be expected to reverse the effects of decades of physical abuse," reassure the doctors to one another and to themselves. Blaming the patient gives the doctor an excuse in failing to cure disease—if only the patient had behaved!

Of all emotional factors that separate the doctor from the patient, the most powerful and important to face is the fear. Patients come into the doctor's office, even for a routine checkup, with fear in their hearts. "What will she tell me now?" wonders the 48-year-old sedentary man whose father died suddenly of a heart attack at age 49. "Is he going to make me get a mammogram?" broods the middle-aged woman who cared for her aunt through a long, slow death from breast cancer. "Can they tell if my baby got it?" thinks the young pregnant woman afflicted with sickle cell disease, hospitalized already 52 times in her short life, looking ahead to strokes, infections, and always in pain, tormented that she may have bequeathed this curse to her yet-to-be-born child.

Unless the doctor has recently been ill or has illness in the family, he or she will not as a matter of routine be attuned to the patient's fear. Doctors know cognitively that patients fear for their health, and they understand abstractly that patients will be apprehensive as they wait to hear a biopsy report or a diagnostic test result. Yet the depth of the anguish cannot be appreciated by the person in health. In the same way that pain is difficult to remember once it is over, fear is difficult to imagine when one is not afraid. The doctor setting about his or her routine, medical chart open, computer screen showing that the 48-year-old man's LDL cholesterol is 167 and that the middle-aged woman's mammogram is overdue cannot enter the patient's state of fear. It is usually a soundless fear. The body tells—in tremor, in nausea, in paleness, in sweat—what the words cannot: I will die and my kids will lose their dad at 14 like I did; I will develop the horrible disease that killed Aunt Bernadette; my baby will suffer as do I.

The doctor, too, undergoes deep and painful emotions in his or her care of the sick. Although the patient's suffering must remain at the heart of medicine, it is undeniable that doctors, too, suffer through the illnesses of their patients. The most moving evidence of such emotional suffering is to be found in the hundreds of memoirs of training written by medical students and physicians.[35] Although the specifics of the suffering may change—paralleling the technological realities of practice—the heart of the suffering remains the same: shame at being powerless, guilt and rage in the face of the blame, and fear of all the dying.

Sadly, though, these dual sufferings are not joined. A metaphor can be taken from child psychology. Before infants develop the intersubjective capacity to respond to one another, they engage in what psychologists call parallel play, in which they play happily alongside one another without true interaction. It is only when infants mature into the capacity for relation that they are able to enjoy collaborative play, that is, playing *with* instead of simply playing *next to*. At this stage, the unique contributions of each "player" are allowed to inflect and give meaning to the activity of the other, heralding the beginning of genuine relation. In like manner, patients and doctors seem to engage in parallel suffering, in which both parties suffer, but they suffer in isolation from one another. Only with the capacity to be open to genuine intersubjectivity can these two participants approach an authentic relation in which the suffering does not separate them but is shared. Once shared, the suffering is lessened.

What power would devolve on our medical care if these two could take stock of one another's emotions and engage fully in their joint suffering. The intersubjective recognition of doctor by patient and patient by doctor would deepen knowledge, steady presence, and prove commitment. Such mutual recognition, transcending parallel suffering, would enable them both to reflect on their common journey and, by virtue of being "together" on it, would lessen one another's suffering. The practical effects of such a change on the delivery of health care would be impressive, leading to more accurate knowledge of the patients' experience of illness and a realistic understanding of the powers of medicine to counter the disease. More of the patient's difficulties would be acknowledged and faced, while care would proceed in full view of the uncertainty and limitations of our science. By recognizing the mutuality of their work together, patient and doctor would call forth the authentic in one another. Together, they would stay the course.

◻ BRIDGES WITHIN OUR REACH

This encounter between health professional and patient lies at the heart of medicine. So many pitfalls are possible—the professional might not be smart enough, patient enough, imaginative enough; the patient might not be trusting enough, brave enough, receptive enough. Yet from this inauspicious meeting between two unlike people proceeds whatever healing medicine might provide. Perhaps caring for routine or trivial or reversible symptoms can be accomplished despite such divides. But when faced with serious, life-threatening illnesses that come randomly, unfairly, and without warning, how can these two people reach toward health?

I remember taking care of a gravely ill elderly man in the hospital. I was an intern—sleep-deprived, unused to my authority, unsure of what to do for this patient. He was irretrievably sick, bed-bound for months, with a large infected craterlike skin wound on his lower back. He had a serious infection in the blood, and his kidneys were failing. Multiple strokes had left him comatose for many months in the nursing home. And yet his wife sat at his bed all day, every day. I remember her tasteful blouses and her pearls. She would ask me every day, "Is he going to be all right?" And I would page the plastic surgeon to come attend to my patient's wound. Eventually I learned to debride the wound myself, for plastics would not come. The surgeons could do nothing to save my patient's life. I did not know he was beyond saving. I was alone with his wife in her pearls, her life that was coming apart, and I couldn't get plastics to come. We were in it, together, we three—this gravely ill man trying so hard to die, his wife bereft by his loss and unable to fathom her life without him, and me, the intern, who wanted like crazy to save him.

All I learned about medicine from trying to take care of my patient was its anguish and isolation and powerlessness in the face of disease and age and time. We had little clinically to offer this man. I did not know, then, that there is no limit to what one can give as a doctor. I did not know that I was allowed, as a doctor, to donate my presence, my attention, my regard. The patient's wife need not have been utterly alone in her ordeal; I could have accompanied her with courage and vision instead of caving in, with her, to the fear of the disease.

What I did not know how to do for my patient and his wife was to get to the heart of their suffering. I knew how to manage the man's fluid status and antibiotics, and I even knew, more or less, when to call a halt to aggressive care, but I did not know how to manage the fact of his dying. I did not know how to manage his wife's fear and loss. Nor did I know what to do with my own suffering in the face of theirs.

What I needed, I now can see in retrospect, was to be able to imagine the plight of my patient's wife and to realize that she required honesty and support and courage from me, her primary doctor. With more sophisticated narrative skills than I had as an intern, I would have been able to articulate my own fear of incompetence and lack of clinical judgment and therefore seek better guidance from my supervisors. I might have been able to identify personally significant memories—of the long, slow death of my own grandmother—stirred up by the patient's ordeal. I might have better imagined the situation of the patient himself, realizing the injustice of continuing to subject him to such painful procedures—if, indeed, he was sensitive to pain—as deep surgical scraping of his sacral wound. And by reflecting critically on my own professional actions and complementing my judgment with that of more experienced doctors, I would have made myself available to this patient and his wife—and his children or siblings or friends, the presence of whom I had not even wondered about—in living through the losses of his terminal illness. By having recognized more accurately the patient's and family's experiences and by having claimed my own fear and horror and sadness, I could have released the natural collective impetus in all of us to extend help toward the frail and injured. As it was, I remained divided from my patient by his nearness to a death that was unacceptable to me, my reduction of the complexity of his full life, the mismatch between his wife's and my calculus of the road we were on, my shame at my own inexperience and uncontrollable emotion, and my paralyzing sadness for us all.

Donne's Holy Sonnet Ten, of course, begins with these lines:

> Death, be not proud, though some have called thee
> Mighty and dreadful, for thou art not so;
> For those whom thou think'st thou dost overthrow
> Die not, poor death, nor yet canst thou kill me.
> From rest and sleep, which yet thy pictures be,
> Much pleasure, then from thee much more, must low
> And soonest our best men with thee do go,
> Rest of their bones and soul's delivery.

Addressing the poem directly to death—and not to God or to Satan as most of the Holy Sonnets are—Donne personifies and *lowers* that which claims us mortals. In stripping poor death of its haughtiness, Donne achieves an expansiveness of life despite its measured end. If "soonest our best men with thee do go," then we who go, including my patient, are also of the best.

The divides between doctor and patient erected by different notions of mortality, causality, context, and emotions can be bridged by doctors and patients who are committed to the health of their clinical relationships. In the following chapters, I outline specifically how narrative methods can help to bridge each of these divides. If with narrative's help, we can grasp our relation with mortality and time, the singular contexts in which illness arises, the central roles of both causality and contingency in health and illness, and the emotional forces that prevent genuine and ethical relation, then patients and doctors can find their way to unite in the shadow of death, to respect that which is unique about each one, to join in authentic regard, and to face the unknown with courage, justice, and hope.

NOTES

1. John Donne, *Devotions upon Emergent Occasions*, 30.

2. Margaret Edson, *Wit*. Page references to this work appear in parentheses in the text.

3. Wayne Booth, "The Ethics of Medicine, as Revealed in Literature," 10–20.

4. See Barbara Ehrenreich and Deirdre English, *Witches, Midwives, and Nurses: A History of Women Healers* and Susan Reverby, *Ordered to Care; The Dilemma of American Nursing, 1850–1945* for explorations of the gender, class, and power situations within medicine and nursing.

5. Many patients have published such accusations about the heartlessness of medical care. In addition to Edson's *Wit*, see Louise DeSalvo, *Breathless*; Kathlyn Conway, *Ordinary Life*; Jay Neugeboren, *Open Heart*.

6. The choice between sympathy and science is enacted in the impressive flight from conventional Western medicine to alternative and complementary care. What masseuses and acupuncturists and holistic healers provide that doctors do not is attention and regard, and their lack of scientific rigor is overlooked for the dividends of their caring. In *Sympathy and Science: Women Physicians in American Medicine*, historian of medicine Regina Morantz-Sanchez writes about medicine's gendered dichotomy between sympathy and science, some early women physicians seeming to choose the first while disdaining the other, or perhaps only lusting after it.

7. Susan Sontag, *Illness as Metaphor*, 3.

8. Leo Tolstoy, "The Death of Ivan Ilych," 140–41.

9. Susan Sontag, *Regarding the Pain of Others*.

10. When the surgeon Sherwin Nuland wrote his *How We Die*, it was to fill this gap in laypersons' knowledge of what really happens to people in the course of dying. The combination of pathological, phenomenological, and lyrical prose in the book testifies to the extraordinarily complex dimensions of these moments at the ends of our lives. The hospice movement, of course, tries to build familiarity with the inevitability of death and the

comfort available to all involved by admitting it into our midst. See Michael Kearney and Timothy Quill for recent publications on the care of the terminally ill.

11. See, for example, ongoing work characterizing the contribution of patient optimism to clinical outcomes of health and recovery. Michael Scheier et al., "Optimism and Rehospitalization after Coronary Artery Bypass Graft Surgery," and Michael Scheier and Charles S. Carver, "Effects of Optimism on Psychological and Physical Well-Being: Theoretical Overview and Empirical Update."

12. James Joyce, "The Dead," 223–24.

13. See W. J. T. Mitchell, ed. *The Politics of Interpretation* for a series of essays examining these fundamental intellectual operations. See E. D. Hirsch, *Validity in Interpretation* for a study of interpretation as an exercise of mastery and Wolfgang Iser who, in *The Range of Interpretation*, suggests that interpretation is a mode of translation.

14. George Engel, "The Need for a New Medical Model: A Challenge for Biomedicine."

15. See David Morris, *Illness and Culture in the Postmodern Age;* Phil Brown, *Perspectives in Medical Sociology;* David Mechanic, *Medical Sociology;* Arthur Kleinman, Veena Das, and Margaret Lock, eds., *Social Suffering* for examples in these vast fields of social commentary on biological illness.

16. Elliott Mishler, *The Discourse of Medicine,* 85.

17. The NIH only in the 1990s insisted that women and members of minority races be enrolled in clinical trials of experimental drugs because of the inability to generalize therapeutic response from one gender to another or one race to another. The recently inaugurated *Journal of Gender-Specific Medicine* reports on findings local to either male or female patients, giving respect to their ineluctable differences throughout the provision of medical care.

18. See the report of the Committee on Quality of Health Care in America, Institute of Medicine, *Crossing the Quality Chasm,* 48–51, for a summary of patient-centered care developments.

19. Moira Stewart, "Towards a Global Definition of Patient Centred Care."

20. See Moira Stewart et al., *Patient-Centered Medicine.* The U.S. Agency for Healthcare Research and Quality provides resources on the web to help patients and providers to arrive at singularly fitting health care decisions—from choosing surgery or watchful waiting for BPH to choosing a health care plan—for patients based on individual symptoms and preferences. UK researchers are investigating the contributions of shared decision-making on outcomes as well and providing patients with guidance through the Centre for Health Information Quality. See Halsted Holman and Kate Lorig, "Patients as Partners in Managing Chronic Disease: Partnership Is a Prerequisite for Effective and Efficient Health Care" and Michael Barry et al., "Patient Reactions to a Program Designed to Facilitate Patient Participation in Treatment Decisions for Benign Prostatic Hyperplasia" as instances of the voluminous literature on the importance of recognizing and respecting patients' preferences in tailoring their health care.

21. Anne Fadiman's brilliant study of the Hmong culture's understanding of disease, *The Spirit Catches You and You Fall Down,* stands as a cautionary tale for all health professionals working with members of other cultures.

22. Rita Charon, "To Build a Case: Medical Histories as Traditions in Conflict."

23. I am indebted to Eric Cassell for his private tutorial in modern medicine's epistemology. I cite heavily here not only from his writings but from his conversation and inspiration. See particularly chapter 1, "Ideas in Conflict: The Rise and Fall of New Views of Disease" in *The Nature of Suffering and the Goals of Medicine,* 3–15.

24. See Arnold Weinstein, ed., "Contagion and Infection," special issue of *Literature and Medicine* for a collection of essays on the nature of contagion and its theories within

the rise of Western medicine. See also Harris Coulter, *Divided Legacy* and Robert Hudson, *Disease and Its Control* for helpful summaries of these developments.

25. An almost laughable outbreak of this clash was published in the *Journal of General Internal Medicine* in 1998. See the essay by Roy Poses and A. M. Isen crankily refuting the findings of qualitative researchers and the deluge of indignant responses.

26. F. G. Crookshank, "The Importance of a Theory of Signs and a Critique of Language in the Study of Medicine," 342.

27. Eric Cassell, *The Nature of Suffering and the Goals of Medicine,* 5.

28. See the psychiatrist Aaron Lazare's landmark study "Shame and Humiliation in the Medical Encounter." Lazare contends that much of the routine procedures and "manners" of the office visit are manifestations of the attempts to manage both the patient's humiliation and the doctor's potential shame. He argues that a medicine attuned to safeguarding the patient from undue shame or humiliation will provide a major improvement in effectiveness.

29. A survey of recently published pathographies fails to identify illness narratives about lung cancer in a smoker. Alice Trillin's prescient "Of Dragons and Garden Peas," published in the *New England Journal of Medicine* in 1981, takes pains to point out that the author/patient was *not* a smoker. Some pathographies about heart disease, for example Jay Neugeboren's *Open Heart,* assert that the author is *not* a smoker, obese, sedentary, or a consumer of a high-fat diet. See William Styron's *Darkness Visible* for one pathography in which the author admits to having contributed to at least one aspect (alcohol intake) of his illness.

30. See Richard Zaner's "Broader's Hill" in *Conversations on the Edge: Narratives of Ethics and Illness,* 89–110, for a discussion of the difficulty of "living in the face of the awful happening of chance events," 101.

31. David Hilfiker, "Facing Our Mistakes." See also his more recent book-length examination of errors in medical practice, *Healing our Wounds.* See also Atul Gawande, *Complications* and Charles Bosk, *Forgive and Remember* for examinations—the first by a surgeon and the second by a sociologist—of the occurrence of error and the medical profession's response to it. In very large part, what must be handled is not only the result of the error itself on the welfare of the patient but also the sequelae of guilt and fear in the practitioner who committed the error.

32. Committee on Quality of Health Care in America, Institute of Medicine, *To Err Is Human.*

33. See Nancy Berlinger, "Broken Stories: Patients, Families, and Clinicians after Medical Error." See also accounts written by patients or their survivors of serious clinical error, including Sandra Gilbert, *Wrongful Death.*

34. Wendy Levinson et al., "Physician-Patient Communication: The Relationship with Malpractice Claims among Primary Care Physicians and Surgeons."

35. See, for example, *The House of God* by Samuel Shem; *Gentle Vengeance* by Charles LeBaron; *A Not Entirely Benign Procedure* by Perri Klass; and *The Desire to Heal* by Rafael Campo.

3 ▣ Narrative Features
of Medicine

The divides in health care need to be bridged in order for effective treatment to proceed. I have proposed that narrative means might help to bridge these chasms, because narrative ways of knowing and experiencing the world and self are held in common by health care professionals and patients. Anterior to our differentiating into doctors, nurses, and patients, that is, we are united *and can be reunited*. Furthermore, the specific divides that separate doctors from patients—beliefs about mortality, the contextualization of illness, understanding of disease etiology, and emotional factors that lead to suffering—have direct correlates in narrative aspects of medicine.

Medicine is itself a more narratively inflected enterprise than it realizes. Its practice is suffused with attention to life's temporal horizons, with the commitment to describe the singular, with the urge to uncover plot (even though much of what occurs in its realm is, sadly, random and plotless), and with an awareness of the intersubjective and ethical nature of healing. I invite you to examine with me five narrative features of medicine—temporality, singularity, causality/contingency, intersubjectivity, and ethicality. All these complex conditions or states are active aspects of routine clinical practice. They are also bedrock aspects of narrative practice. They line up with the divides we have just considered in almost a one-to-one configuration, helping us to examine and perhaps even to bridge each of these complex and deep chasms. *Lancet* editor Richard Horton writes in *Health Wars* that there is "a schism in medical practice that is at the heart of the present challenge to medicine. The solution is to discover a way to reconnect doctor to patient through a bridge of common understanding and shared ways of knowing about disease. We need nothing less than a new philosophy of medical knowledge."[1] I suggest that this new philosophy of medical knowledge is a narrative one, and that learning about and developing competence in these narrative dimensions of medical practice can offer urgently needed help to us all as we try to bridge the divides in health care and improve the effectiveness of our care.

As a living thing, narrative has many dimensions and powers. The novelist values its creative force; the historian relies on its ordering impulses; the autobiographer redeems its link to identity; the anthropologist requires its recognizing specificity. What is clear is that narrative *does* things for us, perhaps things that cannot be done otherwise. Narrative structures such as novels, newspaper articles, and letters to friends enable us to recount events, to depict characters, to suggest causes for events, to represent the passage of time, to use metaphor to convey meanings otherwise elusive. As an instrument for self-knowledge and communion, narrative is an irreplaceable—and often silent or at least transparent—partner to human beings as they make and mark meaning, coping with the contingencies of moral and mortal life.

Those who study narrative are in some agreement about its basic elements. Such texts as Shlomith Rimmon-Kenan's *Narrative Fiction*, Seymour Chatman's *Story and Discourse*, and Gérard Genette's *Narrative Discourse*, originally published between 1978 and 1983, identified central features of narrative that continue to be endorsed by the narrative theorists who follow them.[2] These theorists agree, roughly speaking, on the major features of narrative. Some event happens or state of affairs obtains within a temporal sequence and specified setting to and by characters or agents, and the opening state gives way to an altered state. This situation is represented for the reader or listener by a speaker or register who absorbs and reports the event from a particular point of view. The large objects in the room, if you will, in narrative theory can be distilled into time, characters, narrator, plot, and the relationships that obtain between teller and listener, which accord with the narrative features of medicine we are examining. With these simple components, stories are built, told, undergone, and understood. The branch of literary studies called narratology analyzes how stories are built, how they are told, and how they are received, the better to understand what they mean and how they exert their profound effect on us.

Narratology's evolution began with the Russian formalists Vladimir Propp and Boris Tomashevsky, the phenomenologist Roman Ingarden, and the linguists Frederic Saussure and Emil Benveniste in the 1950s and 1960s, who developed very complex taxonomies to describe a text's narrator, the generic properties of the narrative, a rather limited number of characters (or actants or agents), and a catalog of discrete action elements that could be combined to form plot.[3] These early formalists aspired to a scientific examination of text, that is to say, a reproducible, generalizable system of understanding and of describing the anatomy of a story. By the 1960s and 1970s, these formalist concerns informed what became known as structuralism, a movement powered by the French anthropologists and linguists Claude Lévi-Strauss, A. J. Greimas, Claude Bremond, Roland Barthes, and Gérard Genette. Blending linguistics and anthropology with traditional literary studies, the structuralists paid attention to the semiotic conventions of the works they studied, the linguistic rules and norms that encode meaning, and the social and cultural work accomplished through discourse. These interests contrasted with the other major development in Anglo-American formalism, New Criticism, which came of age around the same time. The New Critical scholars T. S. Eliot, Ronald Crane, Cleanth Brooks, and William Empson studied such intratextual aspects of poetry as irony and ambiguity with restrained interest in the personal or cultural worlds from which the text emerged.[4]

Although by now, in poststructuralist times, we do not believe that a story can be dissected scientifically to reveal the same meaning to more than one observer, literary scholars today owe a great debt of clarity to the work of the structuralists for having recognized that the structures of texts are the sources of their meaning. However, in retrospect, the reversals of the effort are striking. The early structuralists thought they could banish singularity from texts and replace it with measurable, generalizable knowledge (with predictive value!) of paradigm texts and others like it, that they could develop metrics with which to analyze stories' plots and times, and that they could dispense with the reader in favor of the laws of language. They failed at these tasks. Yet their failures have led to the realization of the brilliant singularity of each narrative text and the irreplicability of any narrative situation, so complex and individualized have acts of writing and reading been found to be. The field of study that inspects how stories are built and how they work continues to renew itself. Lately, narratology—or the new formalisms, the pluralism with which narratology often designates itself—is concerned with subjectivity, race, body, and culture in written texts as well as in oral, film, and visual texts. "[T]he concept *narrative* has come to encompass a wide range of semiotic, behavioral, and broadly cultural phenomena; we now speak of narratives of sexuality, for instance, as well as narratives of history, narratives of nationhood, and even, more notoriously, narratives of gravity."[5] In the face of the democratic uses to which narrative theories and practices have been put, its theory has consequently become more pluralistic, populist, and accessible to writers and thinkers along a wide range of interests.[6] Students of narrative today are committed to close examination not of dead texts but of living textuality and discourse, wherever they may erupt, for narrative "*constitutes* a logic in its own right, providing human beings with one of their primary resources for organizing and comprehending experience."[7] They find that a commitment to form, in W. J. T. Mitchell's words, "is also finally a commitment to emancipatory, progressive political practices united with a scrupulous attention to ethical means."[8]

Like lawyers, teachers, historians, and journalists, health care professionals have come to realize that they must understand these building blocks of stories in order to do their work.[9] A symptom or disease is indeed an event befalling a character, sometimes caused by something identifiable, within a specified time and setting that has to be told by one to another from a particular point of view. However, health care professionals often lack the means to recognize explicitly the temporality within which lives and diseases unfold, to grasp and value the singularity of each person or character, to face both the search for causality and the acknowledgment of underlying contingency in life in general and in disease in particular, and to comprehend the intersubjective and ethical demands of telling one's story and receiving the stories of others.

▥ TEMPORALITY

Henry James writes, in the third and last (and unfinished at his death) book of his autobiography, "We are never old, that is we never cease easily to be young, for *all* life at the same time: youth is an army, the whole battalion of our faculties and our freshnesses, our passions and our illusions, on a considerably reluctant march into the enemy's country, the country of the general lost freshness."[10] James's figure of youth invading the enemy territory of the future gives particular sharpness to the stories clinicians hear in their day-in, day-out work. We sit in our offices, hearing patients tell of the defeat—or the fear of such—of their youth and their health, at the hands not necessarily of disease but of time. Degenerative diseases—what most of our patients these days die of—are not so much pathology as they are the consequences of the passage of time.[11]

Human beings take stock of the passage of time through narrative, the only kind of telling that takes account of chronology, duration, and temporal order. In his comprehensive *Time and Narrative,* philosopher Paul Ricoeur asserts that narrative dwells in temporality and that, conversely, time dwells in narrative. "[B]etween the activity of narrating a story and the temporal character of human experience there exists a correlation that is not merely accidental but that presents a transcultural form of necessity. To put it another way, *time becomes human to the extent that it is articulated through a narrative mode, and narrative attains its full meaning when it becomes a condition of temporal existence.*[12] From *One Thousand and One Nights'* power to postpone the sequelae of time, to Proust's masterful reimaginings of the intimate moments of his life, to Joyce's re-creation of a day in the life of Leopold Bloom, a day that contains and recapitulates and contests all we might consider to be of human meaning, narratives provide the traces as well as the sources of our consignment to and our celebration of time.

Narratives teach us where we come from and where we are going, allowing us to understand the meanings of our own lives.[13] Fairy tales, bedtime stories, family myths, and traditional holiday legends contribute to a child's understanding of where he or she is from. Families, towns, nations, and cultures rely on the commonalities donated by shared accounts—Genesis, Columbus's voyage, the Middle Passage, the Holocaust—to identify what it is that binds them as one in the present. The patrimoniacal practice of continuing names along a blood line can be read as a narrative reminder—or even a metaphor—of the familial progression in time. Novels, memoirs, plays, movies, and what we ourselves write are the forms of knowledge that help us to wonder at where we are going or, more savagely, what it is all *for.* By respecting the beginnings, middles, and ends of human events, narratives require, from each reader and writer, adherence to the human's obligatory existence within the flow of—and the buoyancy of—time.

Narrative might be the most important discovery humans have made in order to deal with the problem of time. The philosopher and literary scholar Georg Lukács writes, "We might almost say that the entire inner action of the novel is nothing but a struggle against the power of time."[14] Such scholars and writers as Henri Bergson, Marcel Proust, Gérard Genette, and Fredric Jameson all try, in their turns, to face the twin submission to and mastery of time as it passes, time as it stamps us, time as we waste it and use it and live through and beyond it, and it is through narrative thought—in fiction, in history, in reverie, in dreams—that humans are able to come to at least provisional accord with the relentless and merciful passage of time.[15]

Both writing and reading are activities accomplished within time, and both activities leave tracks of their journey from past to present to future. In the introduction to *The Golden Bowl* written for the 1909 *New York Edition,* James makes explicit his journey as a reader through a text he himself had written some seven years ago. In a breathtaking trope, James figures his act of reading to be like a walk on newly fallen snow, his footsteps marching through a territory he had invented yet creating new tracks through it. "It was, all sensibly, as if the clear matter being still there, even as a shining expanse of snow spread over a plain, my exploring tread, for application to it, had quite unlearned the old pace and found itself naturally falling into another, which might sometimes indeed more or less agree with the original tracks, but might most often, or very nearly, break the surface in other places."[16] *He read a different book from the one he had written,* because his new reading act took place at a new temporal stance.

Not an undifferentiated element of stories, fictional time is distinguished into order, duration, frequency, story-time, and discourse-time. Readers compare the time it takes to read a passage with the time it might have taken for the action of the passage to occur to arrive at the so-called velocity of the text. The order of some stories is chronological, starting at the beginning and moving sequentially through the actions depicted. Often, though, a story is told in flashbacks (narratologists call these analepses) in which the narrator recalls or reports on events of the past. Sometimes, there will be prolepses, or flash-forwards, in which the reader is given access to events of the future. A pivotal distinction was made by the linguists in structuralist times between diachrony and synchrony; roughly speaking, diachrony is the condition of time passing, of being "within" sequence, while synchrony is an epiphanal eternal state of having arrived. Diachrony contains frequency and repetition, while synchrony has no habit or antecedent. Diachrony is longitudinal; synchrony is cross-sectional.

A narrative's reading time, or the literal amount of time it takes to read it, is an oddly powerful determinant of the text's influence. Living within the narrative world of Hans Castorp and his fellow Berghof residents for the time it takes to read *The Magic Mountain* conveys, as the plot alone could not, what Mann means to tell us about time. Wayne Booth argues that reading a novel enables the reader to dwell within its climate and to inhabit the world of its characters for "long enough" to achieve familiarity with the story-space and intimacy with its people. Short stories cannot give the reader this transforming contact, merely as a function of the time one spends in the work.[17]

We see that medicine's accounts of events, too, are "nothing but a struggle against the power of time." Humans struggle to come to terms with the bracketing, in time, of their own existence, engaging in many of the local battles against immortality in the presence of doctors and nurses—in the delivery room, in the emergency room, in the waiting room outside the OR, in hospice. While waiting for the birth of the first grandchild, the older adult feels the pinch of senescence and the grandeur of fecundity. As the daughter reaches the age at which her mother died, she resigns herself to duty or she rages against her doom. And when the doctors offer comfort care, the patient submits to counting days, no matter how brazenly time was snubbed in the healthy past. The temporal fragmentation and rupture seen especially in postmodern narratives are exactly what occur when disease forecloses narrative coherence over time, leaving the patient able to say only, "Now what?"

When the doctor or nurse enters the room to do something—to palpate, to cut, to medicate, to stitch—he or she remains within vectored time, that is, a state of time in which one event leads to another and can even be conceptualized as having caused it while the patient inhabits a timeless enduring. This is not just the difference between passivity and activity but the more unfathomable distinction between living within and outside of time, between diachrony and synchrony. When the pediatrician John Lantos depicts the difference between being a patient and a doctor, he figures it in literary terms, suggesting that patients dwell in modernism's focus on the interior while doctors enact the premodernist choice for acting, causing, derring-do.[18] Not only does the nature of the actions accomplished by the sick and the well differ but also their temporal states of being differ according to their tempo, durability, evanescence, and stillness. T. S. Eliot's "still point of the turning world" indeed refers to the timelessness within the shell of time that, perhaps, best explains the sick person's dwelling in temporality.[19]

Time is medicine's necessary axis—in diagnosis, prevention, palliation, or cure. Time is, as well, the irreplaceable ingredient in the healing relationship: time to listen, time to recognize, time to care. Medicine becomes transformed if it is practiced with a real respect for time and timeliness.[20] Doctors equipped with temporal sense might not make patients wait through a weekend for the result of a biopsy, realizing that the fear of an illness is almost as painful as the reality of it. The skirmish about waiting room time might be taken seriously—we doctors are never on time, and our assumption that patients do not mind being kept waiting is a pervasive and powerful message about differential worth. Some doctors have changed their appointment policies dramatically, vowing to see patients on the day they call, and find that such schedules of immediacy are, as it turns out, easy to manage.

Temporality grounds most diagnostic and therapeutic acts. We need time and continuity to understand what disease afflicts a patient, to let a disease declare itself. And yet, however skilled we get, we will never govern time; no matter how far into the country of the general lost freshness we extend life expectancy, death will come. What, finally, might a practice of medicine become if it were fortified with a real, earthy, lived sense of mortality? Our current health care system assumes that everyone lives forever, turning away from the realization that lives begin and end, on their own trajectories, but within the biological limits for the species. It is we health care professionals, as curators of the body, who should model the bravery to face the shadow of the end, the honesty to desist from false promises, and the humility to remind us of our limited portion on earth.

A third-year medical student described in his Parallel Chart an early lesson about temporality:[21]

A 57-year-old woman with terminal ALS was admitted refusing food, water, and non-palliative treatment. We were to control her pain until she died. Though there were other patients on our service, the resident and I revolved around the patient with this horrible disease like shy comets. She was paralyzed, unable to speak, in tremendous pain, and, worst of all, fully lucent. Every couple of hours she would breathe with loud strider and indicate she was in pain and we would draw up huge boluses of morphine and push it into the line. A minute later she would fall silent and then sleep for a time until she awoke in pain. Then we would go through the routine again.

After a few cycles of this the intern told me that the doses of narcotic we were giving her were enormous and that another bolus that afternoon would probably put her in respiratory failure. I asked what we would do if she were in more pain. He told me we would give her more morphine.

When the pain came again I offered her morphine and her blue eyes accepted it. As the resident prepared the syringe that would end her life, I stood by the bedside, my emotions roiling. Then, at that fateful moment, I sneezed. Her eyes met mine and her lips moved in the last communication they would ever have with another person. They said, "God bless you."

▥ SINGULARITY

What distinguishes narrative knowledge from universal or scientific knowledge is its ability to capture the singular, irreplicable, or incommensurable. Despite the organizing principles donated to literary study by linguistics and semiology—and in the wake of the now dashed hopes of the ancestors of structuralists that the codes of literary works could be "cracked" and their understanding based on replicable processes—the text remains a zone of indeterminacy, of the pleasure of the new, the never seen. As described by Gérard Genette, the French structuralist who christened the field "narratology" in 1969, no story (narratologists call the events or state of affairs to be represented the story, or *l'histoire*) replicates any other story. No representation of that story in words (the narrative, or *le récit*) repeats any other representation. And no act of telling (the narrating, or *le narration*) recurs in any other performance or delivery of that which is being told.[22] In *Narrative Discourse*, itself a book-length comment on Proust's *A la recherche du temps perdu*, Genette writes, "The specificity of Proustian narrative, taken as a whole is *irreducible*, and any extrapolation would be a mistake. . . . [T]he *Recherche* illustrates only itself."[23]

Form confers singularity. Built into each narrative's structure and genesis is its originality and irreproducibility. The Russian narratologist Tvetzan Todorov emphasizes the emergence into view, through narrativization, of that which does not exist prior to its being told: "Meaning does not exist before being articulated and perceived . . . ; there do not exist two utterances of identical meaning if their articulation has followed a different course."[24] The narrating, that is to say, creates that which is seen for the first and only time. The telling does not merely expose or report that which exists prior to the narrating. It produces it.

Writers understand how they watch the paper or the computer screen, in great suspense, to see what will appear next, even if it is their fingers on the pen or the keyboard. Whether writing fiction or autobiography, authors have surrendered to the realization that, however much they might covet control or power or *authority*, they function merely as hosts to the writing impulse.

This idea of telling as creation, however, may threaten those who regard themselves as dutiful observers of reality and careful scribes of what is found. The dermatologist describes a rash as a "2 cm diameter dry, erythematous eruption with silver-scaling periphery." It is a case of psoriasis, identical to many others seen. There is no creativity in that act of describing, merely a transparent rendering of fact. Not so: despite the commitment to describe only what one sees, one's seeing is influenced by prior categories, diagnostic impulses, comparative memory, conventionalized diction, and concurrent clinical facts that suggest this diagnosis instead of that one. As the philosopher Arthur Danto puts it, "observation is (if I may borrow a locution from Derrida) 'always already' permeated by theory to the point that observers with different theories will interpret even retinally indiscriminable observations differently."[25] An experiment could easily be done in which an artist and a dermatologist describe the same rash. The artist and the dermatologist would see and describe different phenomena—the artist responding to color, form, and texture and the dermatologist responding to taxonomy, pathology, and probability.

However, the medical impulse toward replicability and universality has muted doctors' realization of the singularity and creativity of their acts of observation and description. When a dermatologist meets a patient complaining of scaling and itch, he or she is a singular person in that room with the singular patient. That dermatologist *donates* to the situation more than a memorized dermatological atlas. That doctor donates all human powers of thought and emotion, able to categorize the lesion correctly while able to comprehend empathically the patient's plight. These two events happen at the same time because of the singularity of the human instrument.

How can we create as we tell and, at the same time, recognize what we see? Doesn't the singularity cancel out the usefulness of the diagnostician? The diagnostic act entails two contradictory impulses at once: the effort to register the unique features of that which is observed and the simultaneous effort to categorize it so as to make it "readable." The French structuralist Roland Barthes, who initiated and instigated much of what has come to be called both structuralism and poststructuralism, distinguishes between *le lisible* and *le scriptible*, that is, the readerly and the writerly.[26] The readerly text is the dead one, the one that, once written, can only be read in one certain way. The reader cannot contribute to its meaning or form, and the only action open to the reader in the face of such a text is to submit to it. The writerly text, on the other hand, comes into the hands of the reader incomplete, still alive, requiring active creation from each reader it visits. The reader of the writerly text is coauthor of it, not by virtue of observing what its author did but by virtue of performing what the text compels. In reading a readerly text, Barthes says that "reading is nothing more than a *referendum*," while "the writerly text is a perpetual present . . . the writerly text is *ourselves* writing."[27]

And so the rash, to the dermatologist, is simultaneously a readerly text and a writerly text. It is readerly in its recognizability. The doctor has seen psoriasis before. He or she is *cognizant once again* of the silvery scales, the characteristic array of patches on extensor surfaces of the joints, the marks of excoriation surrounding the eruption signifying scratch. Is it too much to ask of the ordinary dermatologist that he or she also apprehend the singularity of this event? Perhaps the patient has just come down with psoriasis and is terrified that it is terminal. Perhaps the patient thought that, with all the tar and UV light, he was cured. Perhaps, like John Updike, the patient feels at war with his skin while feeling its certain distinction, "I was always in danger, with my skin, of forgetting that I was its victim and not its author."[28]

When patients complain that doctors or hospitals treat them like numbers or like items on an assembly line, they lament that their singularity is not valued and that they have been reduced to that level at which they repeat other human bodies. It is in the sphere of narrative that patients, of late, have attempted to take back their singularity, their subjectivity. In explaining the explosion of illness narratives being published by patients in the last few decades, Thomas Couser writes, "As patients seize, or at least claim, more authority over their treatment, they may also be more inclined to narrate their stories, to take their lives literally into their own hands in part to reestablish their subjectivity in the face of objectifying treatment."[29] Proving the assertion that singularity resides in narrative, patients' new authorship of their illnesses may exert a tremendous power on medicine's capacity to recognize the singularity not only of every case of psoriasis but of every patient, every doctor.

Some developments in medical practice speak to a growing respect for singularity in care. Biologically, health care has become more tailored—think of the many regimens for treating hypertension or diabetes or depression—to take into account comorbidities, genetics, and patient preferences. Concurrently, medicine is making room for patients' personal singularity—witness advance directives regarding end-of-life care. House calls are coming back into vogue, in part because seeing a patient in his or her home gives a wealth of knowledge about that singular life, knowledge that can inflect care profoundly.

Along with recognizing patients' singularity, doctors seem more willing to recognize their own. The reflective writing that is growing in medicine for students and for professionals (see chapter 7) testifies to professionals' willingness and skill to examine their own experiences and to make sense of their own journeys, not for solipsistic reasons but for the sake of improving the care they can deliver. That dermatologist who understands that there are two singular people in the room—one with psoriasis and one who can treat it—will accept his or her singularity, not as a risk to objectivity but as a bonus to effective care. Genette continues, as if speaking to our dermatologist, to observe that though "there are no objects except particular ones and no science except of the general" it is the case that "the general is at the heart of the particular, and therefore (contrary to the common preconception) the knowable is at the heart of the mysterious" (23).

A social worker wrote the following text in narrative oncology, a narrative training program in which doctors, nurses, and social workers who staff the in-patient oncology unit at Presbyterian Hospital meet regularly to read to one an-other what they have written about their clinical work.

> My gruff, unpleasant friend, always an insult, "For a short person, you make a lot of noise around here," you say. You interject, correct me when I speak with each of your roommates, so many in these 69 days of captivity. We both know you are my favorite. I savor my end of the day time with you, no chart or pen comes in with me. You take me to the battlefields of W.W. II, to your kitchen table where you and your brothers debate baseball—back in time we fly to-gether, leaving your always darkened room behind. You transform this environ-ment subtly, magically. My access to you, your past, your point of view is a gift to me, Pete. No code on the statistics sheet so honored here captures this.

Here the health professional savors her magical time *outside* the generalized sta-tistic, finding within the highly personalized past of this patient an enlivening, "favorite" mode of being as she listens, in a darkened room, on a flight into the past, to the captivating intersubjective truth of another human being.

Causality/Contingency

By definition, a narrative has a plot; that is, it not only announces a series of separate events or states of affairs, but also asserts meaningful causal relations among them. We remember E. M. Forster's definition of a plot: "'The king died and then the queen died' is a story. 'The king died and then the queen died of grief' is a plot."[30] The engine of narrative is its urge to make *sense* of why things happen, its longing to find or imagine connections among things, either through motive or cause. This might even be true of fragmented postmodern texts that find "sense" by reconciling to the absence of connections among things. Myths, legends, novels, historical accounts, and admission notes in a hospital chart search for reasons for events, their purposes, their antecedents, their conse-quences and encode these reasons in their plots.

Plots are functions of the beholding of events and not a function of the nar-rated events themselves: "[O]ur minds inveterately seek structure, and they will provide it if necessary. . . . The reader 'understands' or supplies it; he infers that the king's death is the cause of the queen's."[31] Causality is always a human in-vention, as we saw in the discussion of patients' and doctors' differing assump-tions about disease causality, whether one thinks that Merton Densher's betrayal in *Wings of the Dove* led to Milly Theale's death or that the tubercle bacillus leads to pulmonary consolidation. Defining plot as "the very organizing line, the thread of design, that makes narrative possible," Peter Brooks finds that "plot is the prin-ciple of interconnectedness and intention which we cannot do without in moving through the discrete elements—incidents, episodes, actions—of a narrative."[32] Whether the cause of an effect has been proven conclusively or is fancifully hypothesized, one expresses their relation by putting them together into a plot, or, as a narratologist would say, through narrative emplotment.

Emplotment is the action not of the tale but of the teller, not Genette's story but his narrative. Any sequence of events or actions can be "told into" different plots. Perhaps vertiginous, the realization hits most listeners and readers that there is not a replicable and governing *story* at all. Depending on the teller's point of view, intention, and stance, the same set of events can be told so as to make many contradictory plots. As Tod Chambers and Kathryn Montgomery write in describing the emplotment of bioethics, "Plot *is* meaning. Plot shapes a story to represent the significance of its events and to reveal their meaning for the teller and (the teller hopes) the listeners."[33]

In fact, we all know that many events are random, unpredictable, unexplainable, and unknowable. Even those who believe that meteor showers or genetic mutations are random, acausal events seek out with great rigor their grounds, the better to feel less victimized by their occurrence. Danger is contained in the unknown, and human astronomy, navigation, exploration, natural science, and medicine evidently emerged as a response to the perilous unknown. The imperative to sail across the unsailed sea, to settle wild frontier lands, or to peer within the human body all emit from the refusal to be frightened in the face of the unknown. The 42-year-old mother of three with Stage 4 breast cancer asks, "Why did this happen to me?" and all know that her question has no answer. Even without a provable answer, she may develop a plot line that posits *some* cause for her ordeal, for "how can we live and make sense of our lives in the face of the awful happenings of chance events?"[34]

The emplotments of epic, myth, and the novel are, like the emplotments of astronomy or genetics, impulses to address the unknown, to tame danger, to conquer fear, to brave, full in the face, any predicament in which a human being finds himself or herself. (Think, for example, of what Joseph Conrad represents in *Heart of Darkness*.) If the future, the great unknown, waits, then what one does while waiting might, in some form of magical thinking, alter the future to come; it will at very least ease the suspense or the anxiety of anticipation. So Columbus probably told tales of East India on the blank blue mid-Atlantic; Sioux hunters enact buffalo dances around the campfire to prepare for the hunt; and prayers like the Hail Mary or the Kaddish await death with some promise of being accompanied into it.

All efforts to find causes—from science to space travel to literary prose—try to bring order, to unearth Genette's "knowable at the heart of the mysterious." Emplotment, whether in an earthly garden or a fictional text, *claims* land or thought as one's own, as possessed, as ordered, as granted form. However, unlike other impulses with which to face the unknown—the expropriative impulse, the imperialistic impulse, the reductionist impulse—the narrative impulse does not excavate the unknown beyond recognition. It does not sanitize it of danger; it does not consign it to sameness with other such predicaments. Nor does it take away from it what makes it itself, or take it apart beyond putting it back together. It celebrates the uniqueness and respects the unity of the event while representing it. Expansive rather than restrictive, multiplying possibilities instead of reducing them, narrative practices enable the observer or the participant to live in the face of contingency without trying to eradicate it. Writing and reading are, in the end, expeditions into the mysterious, potentially dangerous, uncharted continent of the contingent.

Causality and contingency join in the development of plot as the teller arranges the events or states of affairs in hand in order to lead, provisionally anyway, to one of many endings. In both of conclusion's definitions, plot enables us to find meaning and, quite literally, to stop. Frank Kermode, the obligatory literary critic to cite on theories about endings, ends his meditations in *The Sense of an Ending* with these thoughts, "Our geometries, in James's word, are required to measure change, since it is on change, between remote or imaginary origins and ends, that our interests are fixed."[35] It is only when human representers frame events or states of affairs that beginnings, middles, and ends are mapped and measured and that meanings emerge from them. As Verbal Kint's crippled foot straightens out at the end of the movie *The Usual Suspects,* we viewers too ask Slavoj Žižek's question: "Does Keyser Soze . . . exist at all, or is he the fantasmatic invention of the pitiful Kint? . . . Is he the fabricator of his own myth? In a properly dialectical way, the very quilting point (*point de capiton*) that promises to establish the true narrative resolving all inconsistencies, radically undermines our narrative security, throwing us into an abyssal echoing of deceptions."[36]

Clinical practice is consumed with emplotment. Diagnosis itself is the effort to impose a plot onto seemingly disconnected events or states of affairs. We test one diagnostic algorithm after another—and the more seasoned we get, the more automatically and underconsciously this process occurs—in the effort to categorize this set of events, *in the effort to emplot it.* The clinician endowed with the gift of plot—and aware of the abysmal echoing of deceptions possible with illness—will search out with great inventiveness and open-endedness and courage (for tolerating the unknown requires it) multiple possible causal relationships among the disparate symptoms and situations that the patient presents. Improving the effectiveness and range of diagnostic powers, this gift teaches the listening doctor or nurse how many possible plots there might be hidden within a simple recitation, how many motives and antecedents might be at work, how many different points in time might be considered the "beginning" of the story. The plot-strong clinician will not stop with the obvious or the evident story line but will keep looking—generatively, creatively, hopefully in collaboration with the patient—to construct a wide and deep and varied differential diagnosis. This is narrative medicine in practice.

I close this section with an excerpt from a clinician's writing for narrative oncology. The poem is a meditation offered by an oncologist to a patient, trying to fill in what she does not know about how he got to where she found him:

> I know he must be embarrassed, sitting in his ICU bed
> With tears he has no energy to hide
> He knows me so poorly, for only 3 days
> And he feels he has failed in some way.

"How are you holding up emotionally?" I ask
although it is patently obvious the answer is "poorly."

He's in a hospital far from home, with an illness that came on suddenly
And with such an aggressive force to make him a prisoner
To ICU beds, dialysis machines, Tenckhoff catheters.
He has a brother and a sister who appear to be close,
But I know nothing of why he is 50 and alone
Who he is as a man, when he's not incapacitated in a bed
Or whether he'd normally let a woman he barely knows see him cry.

The plots that we encounter and create in medical practice are very practically and irrevocably about their endings. They point to human ends, using their geometries to understand or to imagine the vectors of life, the plottedness of life, the inevitability of death, and the narrative connections among us all.

▣ INTERSUBJECTIVITY

The subject is the self-who-knows, the self-who-acts, and the self-who-observes or, in the philosopher Paul Smith's formulation, the "bearer of a consciousness that will interact with whatever the world is taken to consist in."[37] Intersubjectivity, it follows, is the situation that occurs when two subjects, or two authentic selves, meet. It is in meeting with other selves that the self comes alive. As Charles Taylor writes, "One cannot be a self on one's own. . . . A self exists only within what I call 'webs of interlocution.'"[38] Analytic philosophers consider intersubjectivity in a narrow sense as the triangulation that occurs when two subjects simultaneously observe an object external to both. Starting with Heidegger and Husserl, the phenomenologists deepened philosophy's ideas about intersubjectivity to not only encompass the cognitive acts of perception and interpretation but to include as well the personal transformations incurred by virtue of human relation. Complexly joining cognitive, perceptual, and ontological considerations, Husserl writes, "I *experience* the world (including others)—and, according to its experiential sense, *not* as (so to speak) my *private* synthetic formation but as other than mine alone, as an *intersubjective* world, actually there for everyone, accessible in respect of its Objects to everyone."[39] Their joint being-in-the-world grants fellowship to its cohabitants, in both their mutual regard of its objects and their becoming objects for one another's regard and experience. Emmanuel Lévinas culminates this stream of philosophical exploration by promoting ethics, which he defines as the responsibility that one human harbors toward another human, to become the *cause* of philosophy. Replacing Husserl's problem of knowledge and Heidegger's problem of being, Lévinas proposes the problem of ethics as primary, transforming philosophy into an enterprise committed to intersubjective human responsibility.

Literary scholars are of late greatly interested in the intersubjective events of authorship, readership, interpretation, and influence. They probe the complexity that results when one human being engages with another in transmitting and receiving texts. Like medicine, narrative situations always join one human being with another, and, indeed, one can argue that the joining of one human being with another always requires narrative acts of one kind or another. The literary scholar Barbara Herrnstein Smith defines narrative discourse as "someone telling someone else that something happened," emphasizing narrative's requirement for a teller and a listener, a writer and a reader, a communion of sorts.[40] Much of narratology's early work examined the acts of narrating that occur in works of fiction, discriminating between first-person and third-person narrators, narrators within the action and those outside the action, and the like.[41] Although most of such formal narratology is beyond the scope of our discussion, its focus on the obligatory locatedness of any act of telling reminds us, in medicine, to attend to the consequences of *how* and *from whom* we hear the narratives of patients—the demented woman's unrecognized daughter? the ER face sheet? the note scribbled by the night float at 4 A.M.?

Any act of reading embroils the reader and narrator in an intersubjective situation, because a relation obtains between the person who tells and the person who listens or reads. The narratively skilled reader or listener realizes that the meaning of a narrative—a novel, a textbook, a joke—arises from *and is created by* the meeting between teller and listener. It follows that narrative acts build relationship as they convey information, emotion, and mood. When I read a novel by Henry James, I can be thought of as entering a relationship with him. Even though he has been dead for almost 100 years and I never met him and he does not know who I am, my act of seriously reading him engages the two of us in a powerful and transformative connection.

Serious readers and writers have always known that their literary acts make them who they are by virtue of a baffling communion with one another. The contemporary field of reader-response criticism arose specifically to understand the intersubjective dimensions of reading and writing. Whether described in terms of expressivity, inspiration, or collective cultural wisdom, writing texts and reading them were recognized as powerful, mysterious, interior acts that define the self through contact with the thoughts and productions of others. A confluence of interest from phenomenologists, psychoanalysts, cognitive psychologists, neurobiologists, and literary scholars raised the interpersonal events of reading to visibility. Readers, we realized with great excitement, are fundamentally changed by virtue of their reading acts. Whether by exercising their metaphorical range, intensifying some of their characterological means of coping with uncertainty, or rhetorically remodeling their patterns of thought, reading was identified as transformative.[42]

Now, reading and writing do not generate the kind of personal relationships one finds in, say, families or neighborhoods. My relationship with Henry James cannot be called a friendship, or a sexual union, or a familial bond, but it is a central and very powerful relationship in my life. Those who disagree with me so far in this section will say, "But, Rita, James does not *know* you," or, perhaps, "James does not know *you*." Here is where the mystery starts. James writes for his reader. He may not know exactly who that reader is—in the "now" in which he writes and during the future life of the work. Nonetheless, as he writes, he has forcefully in mind the image of *and the reality of* the person who holds his book to read him. Despite the centuries and the distance, he knows me, as, might I say, I know you.

The dedicated reader finds herself in a delicate pact with her author. Once armed with the knowledge that unlocks the text, the reader owes something to her author. She has entered the world of meaning of an author, perhaps bidden, perhaps not. She has overheard the secrets, has maneuvered around the subterfuge or surface distractions to "get" what the text is about. And so upon her is conferred a duty to honor, to protect, to respond to, and even to expose the true meaning of the work. Old-fashioned notions of authority vested in the person who writes must contend with opposing notions of the creative freedoms of readers able to find their own meanings within any given text, meanings that perhaps the author cannot see. The tensions inherent in this relationship—writer/reader, teller/listener, analyst/analysand, patient/doctor—are exactly the tensions that *produce* the intersubjective connections and duties of the text and that clarify, through contradiction, that which the reader owes the writer or the teller owes the listener.

Writing, or telling, gives a speaker the authority and the opportunity to reveal the self. Writing, or telling, includes within its act the thrust, the penetration into the meaning-making apparatus of another to deposit that which one has to discharge. Reading, or listening, requires an equally perilous and daring ability to acknowledge another self, to open oneself to being penetrated by another. What a remarkable obligation toward another human being is enclosed in the act of reading or listening. Assuming genuineness in the transaction, the speaker is revealing deep and unknown truths, not only by the words chosen but also by the forms, the diction, the metaphors adopted in the course of telling a tale, while the reader is exposing his or her private organ systems of meaning-making for use by another. Within these acts of intimacy and trust arise notions of the erotics of text, championed by Roland Barthes before anyone knew what he meant.[43] Two strangers, the reader and the writer, ultimately surrender themselves into one another's hands. They both experience great peril, insofar as both selves are exposed beyond the ability to call the exposure back.

The relationships that develop in medicine, as it turns out, bear an uncanny resemblance to the relationships between tellers and listeners in general, perhaps more resemblance than they do to other categories sometimes used to describe them—friends, neighbors, adviser/advisee. What literary studies give medicine is the realization that our intimate medical relationships occur in words. Our intimacy with patients is based predominantly on *listening to what they tell us*, and our trustworthiness toward them is demonstrated in the seriousness and duty with which we listen to what they entrust to us. Yes, doctors touch patients and do rather extraordinary physical things to them, but the textuality and not the physicality defines the relation. These therapeutic relationships are not conventional love relationships, nor carnal relationships, nor familial dependency relationships, nor relationships of the marketplace. In fact, we are misled when we try to conceptualize medical relationships as if they were based on love, desire, power, or commerce. They are based on the complex texts that are shared between doctor and patient, texts that encompass words, silences, physical findings, pictures, measurements of substances in the body, and appearances.

If this aspect of the parallel between medicine and literature holds, then literary methods are of tremendous practical use to us in medicine. These methods can help us learn how to be astute receivers of our patients' stories and how to join with them to create meaning. Literature is hardly of interest to medicine only because great books have been written about illness and death. More fundamental by far than the content of *Bleak House* or *King Lear* is the modeling, by literary acts, of deeply transformative intersubjective connections among relative strangers fused and nourished by words. Recognizing that my responsibility toward my patient includes my being a dutiful and skillful reader helps me to understand what skills to develop within my doctorly self.[44]

The following text is transcribed from an interview with a third-year medical student completed as part of the research study on the use of the Parallel Chart in medical training. Although the interviews are reported anonymously, the sentiments of attunement heard by this student are widespread among these young protodoctors. Here, the student describes meeting with a young woman patient, dying of AIDS, who was looking back with great regret at her relationships with her children, two of whom had been taken away from her and raised in foster care.

INTERVIEWER: This AIDS patient, who, you know, you began to talk with. How is that going? Is it easy to talk to her? How do you do it?

STUDENT: Well—I guess today—I mean, I'm very moved by her, because, today we mostly just talked about her sons, she has a $2\frac{1}{2}$ year old son, and, I guess I just really appreciated and, you know, gave her room to appreciate her relationship with him, and I was just kind of marveling, you know, what a gift that she gets to know this kind of love, you know, 'cause she actually had two other kids and they're like, twelve and thirteen but, you know, I don't think [she] was ever their primary care giver, and so, she just talked about what it meant to like, you know, breast feed and to really love him, and just, he's her life, and it's very beautiful, and—I don't—she hasn't raised this with me, but I read from one note with the social worker that she had talked about this being the last birthday of his that she'll see—I know I said $2\frac{1}{2}$ but I think he's turning three, and so, that's . . .

INTERVIEWER: That *she'll* see.

STUDENT: Yeah. That she'll be there for. I guess I—I guess I was appreciating, you know, she's recognizing the end of her life, I think, although we haven't talked about it exclusively, um, about how she's just enjoying these things, enjoying her son and the beauty in their relationship. I think that—I think a lot of times when you're talking to patients is mostly giving them room to talk, and I think that a lot of times, patients don't have that safe space . . . so kind of listening for a minute and giving people, you know, just exploring what they're going through or what they're feeling and—it doesn't always have to be, you know, that she has to explore the fact that she's dying, but that she can explore, you know, what's meaningful to her right now.

We can learn from this sensitive student that the intersubjective meetings that occur in hospitals, between relative strangers, are replete with the occasions of great personal discoveries. These meetings are therapeutic to the extent that they enable one person to tell while the other listens, and to tell and therefore to know of "what's meaningful to her right now."

⊞ ETHICALITY

Now that the intersubjective relations that develop between teller and listener (or writer and reader) have been examined, the ethical relations that develop in narrative can be recognized. Both bioethicsts and literary scholars write about narrative ethics, scaling the disciplinary boundaries between health care and literary studies to contemplate the obligations incurred in narrative acts, the ethical vision afforded by stories, and the ethicality of the very acts of writing and of reading. A branch of literary criticism called ethical criticism has arisen recently to look specifically at these questions. Although muted in today's climate of ironic skepticism toward earnestness of any kind, the voice of the ethical critic gently but gravely reminds us that reading and writing are high-stakes actions with consequences not only in books but in ordinary lives.[45] Adam Zachary Newton in *Narrative Ethics* suggests that "a narrative *is* ethics in the sense of the mediating and authorial role each takes up toward another's story. . . . Storytelling lays claims upon all its participants, those circumscribed within the narrative as well as those . . . witnesses and ethical co-creators from without—its readers."[46]

The receiver of another's narrative owes something to the teller by virtue, now, of knowing it. This is the intersubjective bridge to narrative's ethics. The act of reading or hearing an author's work confers upon the receiver an uncanny intimacy, as if learning a new private language. The learner of such a personal language incurs duties toward the originator of it; once one is fluent in the language of another, one harbors toward him or her a great and sacred trust. Serious literary scholars bend toward their authors a delicacy and honor, even when critiquing the work. Unlike those who expose or expropriate damning facts about a writer's life or demeaning aspects of the work, the serious scholar devoted to an author enacts the same kind of professional demeanor toward the author that an analyst might toward an analysand.

Beyond the intersubjective threshold of narrative ethics, we enter the ethical dimension of stories. "There is a peculiar and unexpected relation between the affirmation of universal moral law and storytelling," writes J. Hillis Miller in *The Ethics of Reading*. "Without storytelling there is no theory of ethics. Narrative, examples, stories . . . are indispensable to thinking about ethics."[47] The philosopher Martha Nussbaum found that she could not *say* what she meant to say in moral philosophy without recourse to Henry James's *Golden Bowl*. It was only the singularity and penetration of James's densely woven narrative context that could represent and enact the moral texture of human life that she wished to probe: "The adventure of the reader of this novel, like the adventure of the intelligent characters inside it, involves valuable aspects of human moral experience that are not tapped by traditional books of moral philosophy. . . . For this novel calls upon and also develops our ability to confront mystery with the cognitive engagement of both thought and feeling."[48] By representing particular events, characters, obligations, rights, and wrongs in language, stories display for readers varieties of ways in which to consider what one "ought" to do or how one might judge the actions of others. "The real problem in life is knowing how to *judge* things," suggests the critic Marshall Gregory, "and this is a problem that, over and over, narratives' ethical visions help us answer."[49]

The ethical vision of a story displays what the *story* itself deems to be the right way to live, while also intimating what the teller or writer deems to be the right way to live. An author achieves an enduring ethical vision, developed or repeated in work after work, that can educate his or her serious reader. Geoffrey Hartman writes that "Shakespeare's plays are certainly pervaded by moral concerns, by questions about public and private life, by concerns about justice, goodness, friendship, fidelity, love. He rouses our sympathy for all these positive qualities, even when he shows their defeat. He makes us think, again and again, 'How should one act in such a world?'"[50] When a reader is claimed by an author as is Hartman by Shakespeare or Nussbaum by James, it is because there is a powerful *channel* between the author's moral vision and the reader's own. "This is how *I* see the world," the amazed recognizing reader says—feeling, of course, recognized in the process. Through such mutual recognition, reading *constitutes* the reader's own moral vision, feeding the reader the proteins and carbohydrates and vitamins that get metabolized into the reader's ethical self.

Narrative ethics exposes the fundamentally moral undertaking of selecting words to represent what before the words were chosen was formless and therefore invisible and unhearable. It is the very act of fitting language to the thoughts and perceptions and sensations within the teller so as to let another "in on it" (that other, the listener or the reader, now bound intersubjectively if, indeed, authentic contact is made) that constitutes the moral act. The telling exposes the moral freight of the story (along with, of course, its aesthetic freight, its psychological freight, its freight of delight) not only to the light of day but also to the lights of others. When James writes in the preface to *The Golden Bowl*, "To put things is very exactly and responsibly and interminably to do them," he nails for us the *fact* that writing is an act, that writing carries the irrevocable moral duty to live up to one's actions of having told.[51] If it is in the "putting" that acts of cognition and art occur, then the ethical response to having known or perceived something requires that the "putting into words" occurs.

The reader is also summoned by the text to act. Miller asserts that "there is a response to the text that is both necessitated, in the sense that it is a response to an irresistible demand, and free, in the sense that I must take responsibility for my response and for the further effects . . . of my act of reading" (43). The compact of reading or listening is that the receiver will try to live up to the reception. "I can take it," claims the reader or listener in the face of the full force of another's telling. In discussing Conrad's *Heart of Darkness* and Wordsworth's "The Ruined Cottage," Geoffrey Hartman focuses on the teller's duties and the reader's response to the telling. He suggests that the narratings in both these works "get through . . . because the incidents are embedded in a responsive human milieu by a structured ethics of narrative. Both authors know that the reception and transmission of traumatic knowledge is like handling fire."[52] Not unlike the kind of telling and listening that go on in Holocaust survivors' testimonies or accounts of September 11 by those who were there, these literary tellings as well as our clinical tellings are like handling fire, for both participants in the narrating acts. If the psychiatrist Dori Laub finds that the interviewer who receives the testimony of the Holocaust survivor is himself or herself traumatized by the listening, then so too might be the nurse or the doctor listening gravely to the patient's complaint (see chapter 9, "Bearing Witness").[53] These different forms of telling—romantic poetry, modernist fiction, trauma testimony, and clinical interviewing—combine the need to know with the duties incurred by virtue of knowing. The trauma studies scholar Cathy Caruth observes that "the shock of traumatic sight reveals at the heart of human subjectivity not so much an epistemological, but rather what can be defined as an *ethical* relation."[54]

There is no need, in the clinical context, to detour through textuality when we have a flesh-and-blood patient in the waiting room who indeed exacts ethical duties from her internist unless the transposition from patient to text has dividends. The dividend is that acts of reading, accomplished with adequate skill, will *develop* the means by which that internist can fulfill his or her ethical duties. These means are in the living through. "Literature," writes Louise Rosenblatt, "provides a *living through,* not simply *knowledge about,*" suggesting that the reader does not remain untouched through the act of reading but rather becomes open to fundamental transformation by virtue of having read.[55] What a reader undergoes in the kind of reading described by Nussbaum or Miller deepens his or her capacity for perception, discrimination, "ability to confront mystery," and freedom.

Such exposure risks exploitation. Readers can get ravished by what they read. It has been an anxiety about literature for millennia that writers could force themselves onto unsuspecting victims, damaging their innocence through artful mastery and influence.[56] Some stories' ethical visions might be dangerous ones, shaping readers into instruments of sadism or destruction (the dark Gothic novels read by some militant fundamentalist groups come to mind.) Subjects can get exploited by those who write about them, especially subjects vulnerable by reason of age or infirmity and exposed in relationships of professional or personal intimacy.[57] On the other hand, readers can wield great power against those they read by *knowing* them so intently. If reading or writing is done without authenticity and good faith, the reader's or writer's power becomes a source of violence. Lévinas says that "if one could possess, grasp, and know the other, it would not be the other. Possessing, knowing, and grasping are synonyms of power."[58] The anxiety about mastery in psychoanalysis rehearses this same issue.[59] Such cautions about the powers of narrative must be raised, not as excuses to turn away from understanding stories but as reminders of the risks as well as the benefits of this potent force.

One key to the risk/benefit analysis of narrative is altruism. The altruistic listener listens to advance the project of the authentic speaker so that, after a while, the speaker says, "Thank you, now I understand what I meant to say." Such clarity would not have come to the speaker or writer without an airing of thoughts, and the airing of thoughts could not have occurred with just any listener or reader. The listener, or reader, is not a passive receptacle. Instead, he or she is shaping, questing, asking, probing, forming hypotheses, trying hypotheses, delving into possible interpretations, looking for clues everywhere, listening for the authentic voice. This is what the good listener does: she listens for the authentic voice. To do this, there must be no preconceptions of the right answer or the good outcome. The listener listens as an instrument of the speaker. The writer writes as an instrument of the reader.

A social worker on the oncology service wrote this description in narrative oncology of a meeting with a patient's daughter and the interior conversation it occasioned:

> I arrive on the floor, rushing to get to support group. A patient's daughter is standing outside the lounge waiting for me. "How is she?" I ask. "She said she's scared," the daughter replies. I look at her and see the cold fear in her eyes. Her mother is dying. The patient knows it, the daughter knows it, and I know it too.
>
> What can I do? What help is the daughter asking for? . . .
>
> Sometimes a dying patient just needs and wants someone there. Company. Human contact. I turn and tell the daughter, "Can you go back inside, sit with her, hold her hand?" "That's easy," she replies and turns on her heels, back to the room.
>
> I think about the patient, a Holocaust survivor, a lung cancer survivor, succumbing now to a different, primary cancer. How can a woman who's been through the greatest atrocities known to humankind still have the capability to feel fear?
>
> I think about myself. Caught like a deer in the headlights. A patient or family member in crisis comes to me for help. At that moment I am gripped by fear. Will I help? Can I help? How long till they see through my flimsy façade of knowledge, experience, school-book learning. I take a deep breath and practice what I preach and put one foot in front of the other and take a wild (hopefully informed) stab in the dark. I enter her room.

This health care professional put into practice her own knowledge about the needs of suffering people, fully realizing that she herself would undergo suffering in the process of receiving the fear and aloneness of her patient. That it was her duty to do so had also been learned.

▦ CODA

An architect made an appointment to see me to discuss medical decisions she had to make. I had been her internist for some years and knew about treatment she had received for a cerebral hemangioma. There had been regrowth of the mass despite embolization, and the patient had to decide between two surgical approaches, one of which might threaten her vision and another of which might threaten her cognition. In her recitation in my office, she reported in great detail the opinions of her neurologist and neurosurgeon. She described the results of magnetic resonance angiography (MRA) scans and the like, but I didn't want to see the studies or read the reports. I did not feel the need to perform a physical examination, not even to check her blood pressure. Instead, we sat together, close to one another, as she told in detail what she was going through and I listened—not taking notes, not filling the hospital chart, but doing my best to absorb her transmission. I wanted to hear her out as she described what she had been through in this ordeal. I wanted to let her *hear* herself tell of what the judgments were, what they meant, which of the several scary things she feared the most. I wondered myself how angry she felt that this thing she thought she had bested had come back.

As we sat in my office, I understood that she wanted both my internist's brain and my narratologist's brain. I understood the pact we had made that, by my hearing her out, she would hear herself out. What this "hearing out" took was a complex combination of all five narrative features of medicine. We appreciated the time-bomb nature of this recurrence, the singular details of her own work situation, and how the possible operative complications would interfere with her work, and attempted to look full in the face at the uncertainties incumbent on any course of action, including doing nothing. We relied on our own inter-subjective history as patient and doctor, realizing that our previous truth-telling and mutual confirmation were now, when she needed it, paying off. Because she felt free to say *fully* what was in her to say, I could take the measure of her fear, her courage, her resilience, her lack of blame, and her tremendously brave awareness of the possibility for grave losses. I, meanwhile, fulfilled my ethical duties toward my new knowledge of her situation by offering to contact a renowned hematologist at another institution whose research might contribute to the patient's decision-making. As we left my office, we both bowed our heads to signify that we had done important, serious, and moving work together, all of it narrative, all of it medical, all of it mutually constitutive of ourselves.

These five features of narrative are not isolated one from the other. Instead, they arise in congress, intertwining, emboldening one another as the reader and the writer try, in unison, to find meaning in the words. You have noticed, I trust, how singularity blends into intersubjectivity, how temporality is required for causality, and how ethicality devolves from the intersubjective acts of writing or reading. Like any organic whole, the narrative is made up of its conceptually separable "organ systems," but in its living whole, the narrative combines these elements, and life is breathed into static words and forms. The story lives, as the reader and writer live through it and through one another. When the tellers and listeners are patients and their caregivers, the stories give them the means to bridge the divides that might otherwise separate them.

In either telling or hearing a story, our participants are gravely and joyously giving and receiving at the same time. Both teller and listener achieve both the bountiful and the compliant stance, as it were, together at once. A dance of confirmation, these narrative acts declare the self, celebrate the other, mark their meeting as a mutual creation of identity.

Notes

1. Richard Horton, *Health Wars*, 58.

2. Shlomith Rimmon-Kenan, *Narrative Fiction: Contemporary Poetics*; Seymour Chatman, *Story and Discourse: Narrative Structure in Fiction and Film*; Gérard Genette, *Narrative Discourse: An Essay in Method* are the classic narratological texts. See also such recently published narratological texts as H. Porter Abbot, *The Cambridge Introduction to Narrative*; Brian Richardson, *Narrative Dynamics*; and Gerald Prince, *A Dictionary of Narratology*.

3. See the first chapter of David Herman's *Narratologies* for a summary of the developments of Russian formalism, French structuralism, and the study of semiotics and linguistics that developed narratology as we know it today. Jonathan Culler's *Structuralist Poetics* is also a fine examination of the development of these ideas.

4. For more background on New Criticism, see Cleanth Brooks, *The Well-Wrought Urn* and William Empson, *Seven Types of Ambiguity*.

5. David Herman, introduction to *Narratologies*, 20. See also Michael Kearns, *Rhetorical Narratology*; Mieke Bal, *Narratology*; and James Phelan, *Narrative as Rhetoric* for recent formulations of contemporary narrative theory.

6. See Monika Fludernik, "The Diachronization of Narratology" and Bruno Latour, "Why Has Critique Run out of Steam? From Matters of Fact to Matters of Concern."

7. David Herman, "Story Logic in Conversational and Literary Narratives," 130. See also David Herman, *Story Logic: Problems and Possibilities of Narrative*.

8. W. J. T. Mitchell, "The Commitment to Form; or, Still Crazy after All These Years," 324.

9. See Martin Kreiswirth, "Trusting the Tale: The Narrativist Turn in the Human Sciences." A recent, well-attended yearlong symposium on storytelling at New York University has displayed and furthered the interest in stories by such groups as law school faculty, psychoanalysts, American historians, performance artists, and medievalists.

10. Henry James, *The Middle Years*, in *Autobiography*, 547.

11. See Rita Charon, "Medicine, the Novel, and the Passage of Time," for a description of medicine's reliance on a nuanced awareness of temporality.

12. Paul Ricoeur, *Time and Narrative*, 1:52. Emphasis in original.

13. See the many general introductions to narrative theory's illumination of human development as it unfolds in time. Jerome Bruner, *Actual Minds, Possible Worlds* and *Making Stories: Law, Literature, Life*; Theodore Sarbin and Karl Scheibe, eds., *Studies in Social Identity*; Paul John Eakin, *How Our Lives Become Stories*.

14. Georg Lukács, *The Theory of the Novel*, 122.

15. Henri Bergson, *Time and Free Will*; Fredric Jameson, "The End of Temporality"; Marcel Proust, *A la recherche du temps perdu*.

16. Henry James, *The Art of the Novel*, 336.

17. Wayne Booth, *The Company We Keep: The Ethics of Fiction*.

18. John Lantos, "Reconsidering Action: Day-to-Day Ethics in the Work of Medicine."

19. T. S. Eliot, "Burnt Norton" in *Four Quartets*, 15.

20. See Kenneth Ludmerer, *Time to Heal: American Medical Education from the Turn of the Century to the Era of Managed Care* for a rigorous examination of contemporary medicine's difficulty making time for the important ingredients of healing. As befits a chapter on the narrativity of these features of clinical practice, I can point to fictions and literary memoirs of physicians as the richest and most accurate representations of the nature of and problems of temporality in practice. See, first, Thomas Mann's *Magic Mountain*. Also, the realist biography *A Fortunate Man* by John Berger and Jean Mohr; Martin Winckler's fictionalized memoir *The Case of Dr. Sachs*; and Franz Kafka's surreal short story "A Country Doctor."

21. The Parallel Chart is a method, developed at Columbia, of encouraging health care professionals and students to write, in nontechnical language, about what they witness about their patients experiences and what they themselves undergo in caring for the sick. They are asked to write that which does not belong in the hospital chart but must be written somewhere. See chapter 8 for a detailed discussion of the method.

22. These terms are borrowed from Gérard Genette's formulations of *"historire, récit, et narration"* (usually translated from the French as story, narrative, and narrating) on which subsequent narratologists rely. See Gérard Genette, *Narrative Discourse*; Shlomith Rimmon-Kenan, *Narrative Fiction: Contemporary Poetics*; and Mieke Bal, *Narratology: Introduction to the Theory of Narrative*.

23. Gérard Genette, *Narrative Discourse*, 22.

24. Tvetzan Todorov, *Littérature et Signification*, 20, cited by Shlomith Rimmon-Kenan, *Narrative Fiction: Contemporary Poetics*, 8.

25. Arthur Danto, *Narration and Knowledge*, xi.

26. Roland Barthes, *S/Z*, 3–6.

27. Roland Barthes, *S/Z*, 4, 5.

28. John Updike, "At War with My Skin," in *Self-Consciousness: Memoirs*, 66. See Mary Ann O'Farrell's discussion of psoriasis as an emblem and curse of identity in "Self-Consciousness and the Psoriatic Personality."

29. G. Thomas Couser, *Recovering Bodies: Illness, Disability, and Life Writing*, 11.

30. E. M. Forster, *Aspects of the Novel*, 86.

31. Seymour Chatman, *Story and Discourse*, 45–47.

32. Peter Brooks, *Reading for the Plot*, 4–5.

33. Tod Chambers and Kathryn Montgomery, "Plot: Framing Contingency and Choice in Bioethics," 81.

34. Richard Zaner, *Conversations on the Edge*, 101.

35. Frank Kermode, *The Sense of an Ending*, 179.

36. Slavoj Žižek, "The Ongoing 'Soft Revolution,'" 18.

37. Paul Smith, *Discerning the Subject*, xxvii.

38. Charles Taylor, *Sources of the Self*, 36.

39. Edward Husserl, *Cartesian Meditations: An Introduction to Phenomenology*, 91.

40. Barbara Herrnstein Smith, "Narrative Versions, Narrative Theories," 228.

41. Groundbreaking work by the early Russian formalists and French structuralists, the predecessors to today's narratologists, formed taxonomies of different sorts of narrators, narratees, and narrative situations. The difference between a first-person narrator and a third-person narrator has profound influence on the meaning and the consequences of a text. So-called homodiegetic narrators who take part in the action differ in trustwor-

thiness and impact from heterodiegetic narrators, who speak to the reader from "off the page" and outside the scene. By conceptualizing the narrative levels that can occur when someone tells someone else that something happened—first-hand, second-hand, and the like—narratologists have mapped out quite specifically the consequences of the actual *sites* of telling and listening. See Dorrit Cohn, *The Distinction of Fiction;* Jonathan Culler, "Omniscience"; and Nicholas Royle, *The Uncanny* for recent studies of narratorial knowledge.

42. Georges Poulet, "Phenomenology of Reading"; Wolfgang Iser, *The Implied Reader;* Norman Holland, 5 *Readers Reading;* Richard Gerrig, *Experiencing Narrative Worlds.*

43. See Roland Barthes's *Pleasures of the Text* for a remarkable examination of the state of bliss engendered through textual acts.

44. See an early essay of mine called "Medical Interpretation: Implications of Literary Theory of Narrative for Clinical Work" that develops this notion of the patient as author and the doctor as reader.

45. See Wayne Booth, *The Company We Keep;* J. Hillis Miller, *The Ethics of Reading;* and Tobin Siebers, *The Ethics of Criticism* for three quite divergent approaches to the questions of reading's ethical consequences for reader, writer, and text.

46. Adam Zachary Newton, *Narrative Ethics,* 48, 24.

47. J. Hillis Miller, *The Ethics of Reading,* 2, 3. Subsequent page references to this work appear in parentheses in the text.

48. Martha Nussbaum, *Love's Knowledge,* 143.

49. Marshall Gregory, "Ethical Engagements over Time," 284–85.

50. Geoffrey Hartman, "Shakespeare and the Ethical Question," in *A Critic's Journey,* 89.

51. Henry James, *Art of the Novel,* 347. See Hillis Miller's wonderful discussion of James's prefaces in *Ethics of Reading,* chapter 6, "Re-Reading Re-Vision: James and Benjamin."

52. Geoffrey Hartman, *Scars of the Spirit,* 12.

53. Dori Laub, "Bearing Witness, or the Vicissitudes of Listening."

54. Cathy Caruth, *Unclaimed Experience: Trauma, Narrative, and History* (italics in original), 92.

55. Louise Rosenblatt, *Literature as Exploration,* 38.

56. See Pamela Gilbert, *Disease, Desire, and the Body in Victorian Women's Popular Novels* for an examination of one time's concerns that reading can be dangerous for the reader. More generally, such reader-response critics as Jane Tompkins and Wolfgang Iser have struggled with the inherent power and potential exploitations of the reading transaction. Harold Bloom's *Anxiety of Influence* typifies the complementary caution that the writer exercises demonic possession over his or her reader.

57. See G. Thomas Couser's *Vulnerable Subjects* for a wide-ranging examination of the ethics of representing others in personal and professional writing.

58. Emmanuel Lévinas, *Time and the Other,* 90.

59. Gilles Deleuze sees psychoanalysis as "a fantastic project to lead desire up blind alleys and stop people saying what they wanted to say. A project directed against life, a song of death, law, and castration, a thirsting after transcendence, a priesthood," *Negotiations,* 144.

PART II

Narratives of Illness

4 ▣ Telling One's Life

I have had in my practice for many years a now 89-year-old African American woman with hypertension, breast cancer, spinal stenosis, insomnia, and uncontrollable anxiety. She lost her husband to congestive heart failure, her son to lung cancer, and a granddaughter to a hit-and-run accident near Jones Beach. For years, she took Librium for her nerves, unwilling to enter psychotherapy and unable to really talk about the source of her anxiety. She has considered herself sickly ever since she fell off a horse as a girl on a farm in South Carolina. I realized that her great-grandfather must have been born into slavery.

For years, I was baffled by her illness. Recently, she told me the core of her sickness. She did not fall off a horse as a 12-year-old girl. She had been raped by a white boy from the neighboring farm. She knew at the time, young as she was, that she could not tell anyone about this. Her mother would not be able to keep the secret from her father, and if her father knew, he would have acted on his rage and would, in the Southern justice of the time, have died as a result. So for almost 80 years, she kept this secret, disfiguring her heart with wrath and fear. It took more than 20 years for me to become trustworthy enough to hear her tell it. And, once she told her secret—in tears, in anguish, in fury—her health improved. She slept. Her back pain got better. She stopped the Librium. Her heart had room to expand, not being in the grip of the untold.

▣ Listening for Stories

The healing process begins when patients tell of symptoms or even fears of illness—first to themselves, then to loved ones, and finally to health professionals. That illness and suffering must be told is becoming clear, not only in treating trauma survivors but in ordinary general medicine. The powerful narratives of illness that have recently been published by patients reveal how illness comes to one's body, one's loved ones, and one's self. These narratives, or pathographies as they are sometimes called, demonstrate how critical is the telling of pain and suffering, enabling patients to give voice to what they endure and to frame the illness so as to escape dominion by it.[1] Without the narrative acts of telling and being heard, the patient cannot convey to anyone else—or to self—what he or she is going through. More radically and perhaps equally true, without these narrative acts, the patient cannot himself or herself grasp what the events of illness mean.

The patient might not know what needs to be told. Often times, the signs and causes of illness are very unclear to everyone, the patient included. All the patient might know is that she is not feeling herself. To tell her doctor or nurse or therapist about feeling unwell enables her to put her out-of-the-ordinary feelings into words and then to hear, right along with the doctor or nurse, what is said. Familiar to psychoanalysts, this unrehearsed spontaneous telling of sensations and feelings begins all the time in doctors' offices, but ordinarily it is permitted to proceed for less than a minute. (A study published in 1984 found that the average amount of time between the opening of a medical interview and the doctor's first interruption was 18 seconds.[2]) Sadly, health care professionals are not equipped to listen to such telling of the self with a diagnostic and interpretive ear, so that too soon, the narrative is derailed by such questions as, "Is the pain sharp or dull?" or "How long did it last?"

The telling need not even be in words. Once, a young woman came to see me with severe and relentless abdominal pain. She was fidgety, spoke in fragmented speech, seemed clearly to be suffering. She had already seen a gastroenterologist, a gynecologist, and an expert in colitis, all of whom had found no abnormality to account for her symptoms. Since this was my first meeting with her, I asked as a matter of routine about the health of her family members. Her father, I learned, had died of liver failure. As she spoke of his horrible suffering—his abdomen swollen with fluid, his muscles spent, his mind clouded—she put both her hands, fingertips interlocked, almost protectively, over her own upper abdomen. I told her that she used the same gesture to discuss her own symptoms as she had to describe her father's illness. For the first time in the interview, she became still. She looked down at her hands, now in her lap. We were both silent. And then she said, "I didn't know this was about my father."

The novelist and short-story writer Eudora Welty describes herself as always having been a listener of other people's stories. "Long before I wrote stories, I listened for stories. Listening for them is something more acute than listening to them. I suppose it's an early form of participation in what goes on."[3] Listening for stories is what we in health care must learn to do. To listen for stories, we have to know, first of all, that there are stories being told. We have to notice metaphors, images, allusions to other stories, genre, mood—the kinds of things that literary critics recognize in novels or poems. When doctors or nurses listen to patients in this way, related to what psychiatrists call "listening with the third ear," they will ask themselves readerly questions: "Why is she telling me this now? How come I'm feeling irritated or distracted or sad as I listen to her? How come she started with the end of the story and told it backward? Why did she leave out the chest pain until the very end? Why has she included her sister's accident in the story of her bellyache?" What I am trying to convey is the kind of listening that will not only register facts and information but will, between the lines of listening, recognize what the teller is revealing about the self.

Conventional medical care has not considered this kind of listening to be its responsibility. Except for some psychiatrists and psychoanalysts, health care professionals cannot give the time or get the training needed to listen for stories. Without knowing what is salient to an illness and what is not, many doctors and nurses fear that such listening will trap them for hours hearing information that is unrelated to disease. Listening to it, they think, will only distract them from the task at hand—to deal with the insomnia or to treat the abdominal pain. Unfortunately, sickness does not travel in straight lines, and we who care for sick people have to be equipped for circuitous journeys if we want to be of help. Although many health care professionals worry that they do not have the time to listen for stories, many of us who have incorporated listening into practice find that time invested early is recouped quickly. Indeed, the first few visits with a patient may take more time than in conventional practice, but time is saved shortly down the road by having developed a more robust clinical alliance from the start. The serious consequences of not being able to do this kind of narratively sophisticated listening is that patients' symptoms get dismissed, their nonmedical concerns get ignored, and treatable disease gets missed. More compellingly, only this kind of narrative listening will hear the connections among body, mind, and self, and disease recognition and treatment cannot proceed, we are beginning to believe, without simultaneous attention to all three.

Health professionals have begun to do research and to write about how doctors and nurses can more effectively listen to their patients.[4] Patient-centered care and relationship-centered care require respectful authentic relationships with patients that come about through attentive and creative listening. How to talk with and listen to patients is being taught in medical schools and nursing schools. In some cases, mechanical communication skills—establish eye contact within the first minute of the interview, repeat the last words the patient said to show you are listening—are taught to unwary students who might then appear to be listening, whether they know how or not. More genuine efforts to teach health professionals to listen to patients include sophisticated training in self-awareness and mindfulness.[5]

The more we learn about how human beings tell of themselves in general, the more we can respect the diagnostic importance of what our patients tell us and, perhaps, the more effectively we can really listen. Patients are by no means the only ones to be telling of themselves. They join with the culture at large in doing so, thereby enacting the continuity between being sick and being alive. A great deal is known by those who study autobiography and life-writing about what happens when one person tells another person about his or her life, and medicine stands to benefit enormously by learning the basics of how such life-writing or life-telling works.

There are many ways outside of the medical setting in which we tell of ourselves—in formal autobiographies, in memoirs, in letters to friends, on television talk shows, in Internet chat rooms, and in private conversations and journals. "Who am I? How did I get to be this way? How can I be true to myself? May I choose to be another self?" are asked with increasing frequency and pressure, not just in confessionals or psychoanalytic sessions but in the routines of life. Contemporary fiction has been transformed into memoir, or at least those who read and write fiction have tacitly agreed that the boundaries between fiction and so-called truth no longer hold. Such phenomena as the *Oprah Winfrey Show* and reality television shows demonstrate the craving of ordinary people to tell their life stories, however humiliating or private, to as wide an audience as can be found and to eavesdrop as others tell of theirs.

We answer questions about our identity in many ways. Religious rituals prompt examination of one's goodness and sinfulness. Citizens grapple with questions of identity whenever they file their tax returns or decide to stop at a red light, demonstrating who they are in terms of lawfulness, generosity, and civic duty. American responses to the terrorist attacks of September 11, 2001—the horror, the loss, the sorrowful outrage—exposed an underlying sense of being identified by their culture and a new vulnerability, by virtue of belonging to it, to harm. All the means of identity—party politics, racial/cultural self-awareness, sexual preference, class-action suits, gang membership, language of origin—have taken on particular forcefulness in a situation of globalized and commodified sameness of McDonald's, Home Depot, and Wal-Mart.

Everybody gets to ask questions about the self. My neighbor asks these questions when he wonders whether or not to hire undocumented noncitizens off the books in his landscaping business, weighing the savings for himself against the illegality of the act. My hairdresser asks these questions when she laments the loss of a regular client who, she thought, valued her services but went with a cheaper salon. The doorman of my apartment building asks these questions when he struggles to provide services to homebound elderly residents, even after his shift is over. All these people are probing questions of identity, self-worth, and genuine action. Simultaneously they ask questions about ethics and selfhood, the "What should I do?" and "What do we owe one another?" merging into and powering the "Who am I now?"

Although in a different register, academics ask such questions too. Philosophers, psychologists, sociologists, literary scholars, and even biologists focus on the vexed and proliferating questions about subjectivity and the sources and manifestations of a sense of identity.[6] Beliefs about the self have, of course, been the central preoccupation of philosophers, phenomenologists, psychologists, literary scholars, linguists, and semioticians.[7] Over the centuries, our most influential scholars and writers from Plato and Homer to Freud and Marx have grappled with the nature of being—whether it is constant, preformed at birth, given by God, present before language, unitary or various, provable, transcendent, or ever-developing through actions. Philosophical, religious, scientific, and humanistic traditions contribute to and culminate in our complex and evolving notions of the received and created self.

The philosopher Charles Taylor draws a fittingly vast frame in pondering the question of what constitutes the self:

> Perhaps the best way to see this is to focus on the issue that we usually describe today as the question of identity. We speak of it in these terms because the question is so often spontaneously phrased by people in the form: Who am I? But

this can't necessarily be answered by giving name and genealogy. What does answer this question for us is an understanding of what is of crucial importance to us. To know who I am is a species of knowing where I stand. My identity is defined by the commitments and identifications which provide the frame or horizon within which I can try to determine from case to case what is good, or valuable, or what ought to be done, or what I endorse or oppose. In other words, it is the horizon within which I am capable of taking a stand.[8]

We search the horizon—astronomers, oceanographers, artists, musicians, doctors, novelists, geneticists—seeking ways to recognize ourselves and those who surround us, yearning to place ourselves within space and time (and infinity), dramatizing our stubborn beliefs that life means something and that we ourselves matter.

Scholars who pose questions about identity answer them within their discipline's own language and patterns of thought, thereby reenacting their disciplinary forms of knowing about the self. The philosopher asks questions about the self in terms of autonomy and morality, the psychologist in terms of interpersonal behavior, the sociologist in terms of individuals' social roles, the literary scholar in terms of the texts that result from the search for identity or the processes entailed in reading them, and the biologist in terms of the body and brain that support and display whatever the self might turn out to be.[9]

What all these scholars are doing, if considered from a metaposition high enough up to blur the specifics, is to examine who they are, how they got to be that way, and how many selves are available to them to become. Their examination is simultaneously a demonstration: it is in the very acts of discoursing about identity that they identify themselves. No one is born a philosopher or psychologist or sociologist or literary scholar or neurobiologist but, instead, one becomes that way by virtue of preferred ways of looking at the universe and the self in it. Those preferences, in turn, probably have something to do with life experience and heredity, that is to say, with autobiography. Sociologists are not merely being true to their field in conceptualizing social roles as sources of identity; they are also being true to self!

THEORIES OF LIFE-WRITING

We see, then, that both in popular culture and in academia, individuals do what they can to probe the self and to declare what is found. Judging from the explosion in the publication of autobiographies and memoirs, writing one's life story is a choice made with increasing urgency today.[10] Psychologist Jerome Bruner writes that "it is through narrative that we create and re-create selfhood. . . . [I]f we lacked the capacity to make stories about ourselves, there would be no such thing as selfhood."[11] Telling our story does not merely document who we are; it helps to make us who we are.

The writing of autobiography has been extensively studied by literary scholars and psychologists, and so considering autobiographies is a useful way to come to grips with the processes of telling of the self. [12] Whether one's narrative of self is published or not, the same yearnings propel its telling, and the same outcomes result from it. As we tell of ourselves—in psychoanalysis, in private journals, in e-mails to friends, or in formal autobiographies—we seek out the clarity available only from putting into language that which we sense about ourselves. The gesture of telling of ourselves is a plea for affirmation while it puts into action an honest, sometimes brutal, but always creative, knowledge of one's self.

Writing an autobiography is usually a pivotal event in the life of its writer. Any time a person writes about himself or herself, a space is created between the person doing the writing and the person doing the living, even though, of course, these two people are identical. Called the "autobiographical gap," this space between the narrator-who-writes and the protagonist-who-acts confers the very powerful distance of reflection, without which no one can consider his or her own actions, thoughts, or life. Within this reflective space, one beholds and considers the self in a heightened way, revealing fresh knowledge about its coherent existence.

Defying ordinary time, writing the story of one's life allows past and present to coexist not only in the mind of the author but in the resultant text, past and present transforming one another and leading to a future impossible without the act of having written the autobiography.[13] The literary scholar Roy Pascal wrote, in 1960, that autobiography entails living in the present: "Autobiography is then an interplay, a collusion, between past and present; its significance is indeed more the revelation of the present situation than the uncovering of the past."[14] More recent students of autobiography go even further, suggesting that the gesture is always toward the future: "Remembrance, reflection, and reconstruction all are indispensable elements of the enterprise, but (contrary to the usual preconceptions) they are all aimed mainly at the life that lies ahead, not at the one already lived."[15]

Autobiography cannot be considered apart from fundamental beliefs about the self, which in turn are influenced by beliefs regarding the nature of language, thought, consciousness, time, memory, and relation. To write or tell one's autobiography makes one ask intimate questions about the truthfulness of one's memory, the authenticity of one's self-regard or self-condemnation, the foundations of one's taste, and the continuity or discontinuity achieved throughout one's life. Where is the self recoverable—if, indeed, there is a recoverable self—in memory, in external reality, in others, or in language? Is there a factual and objectively retrievable past, or is the past a construct of recollection and desire? How is memory related to experience, and how are they both related to imagination? What, finally, is the relation between writing of the self and being that self, that is to say, does the identity exist outside of its textual representation by the hand of that self?

Looking at autobiographies and autobiographical theory through time helps us to understand how the self has sequentially been constituted and understood. St. Augustine's fourth-century *Confessions*, usually considered to be the first published autobiography, remains the touchstone for contemporary ideas of temporality and personal reflection, not only in autobiographical writings but also in life experience. Augustine's realization that the past and the future can only exist in the present—the past as memory and the future as anticipation—grounds reflective life-writing today.[16] Life-writers since Augustine—Jean-Jacques Rousseau, Anne Bradstreet, William Wordsworth, Benjamin Franklin, Henry James, Marcel Proust, Gertrude Stein, Virginia Woolf, Malcolm X, and Roland Barthes, to name some of the highlights—have adopted the genres of po-etry, fiction, history, biography, manifesto, and the writer's notebook in which to represent their lives or to declare who they think they are. How we have read life-writing over time traces, in microcosm, the evolving—and often dramati-cally contradictory—stages of our comprehension of what might constitute a self and what, indeed, might constitute a life.[17]

Until the mid-1950s autobiography was treated by scholars, if at all, as a mar-ginal source of information for historians, literary critics, or biographers. When Rousseau or Benjamin Franklin or Henry Adams reported their lives, they were setting forth master narratives of the evident truth, stamping one version of their lives as the authoritative and unquestionable one. These life-writers repre-sented fully formed, autonomous selves who exerted power in the world and who remained whole and the same throughout their lives. These selves, their readers realized, were there for the describing, larger than life, confident of their integrity and their permanence. If the existence of a self worth reporting was not in doubt, the enterprise of so reporting was therefore not a remarkable act. Early students of autobiography, inspired by anthropologist Georges Gusdorf, read autobiographies as straightforward and authoritative reports of a cohesive self.[18]

Beginning in the 1960s intellectual life in general was rocked by so-called French critical theory, asserting, among other things, that the subject, or the self, is not contained within the person but instead is socially constructed, a figment of language or culture, stripped of supremacy outside of the words it might produce. Once Roland Barthes, Michel Foucault, and Jean Paul Sartre redefined the "author" as figural, functional, ventriloquistic, place-keeping, or dead, the author's report of self underwent ironic critique.[19] Psychoanalytic concepts of the unconscious had been an essential component of the belief in the autonomous self by providing a model of a self-contained, however layered, in-dividual self. When French psychoanalyst Jacques Lacan reinterpreted Freud to suggest a textual unconscious and a self born through its relation with other, the belief in the reportable and indivisible individual self was further eroded.

By the late 1960s French critical thought—including the work of Jacques Derrida and Paul de Man as well as Foucault and Barthes—challenged the until-then widely accepted belief in the autonomous individual who, within limits, could both direct his or her course in life and then tell about it.[20] In the place of an intact and permanent self, we inherited a self conceptualized as a fragmented, ambiguous, and ever-changing cultural construct. Who you are, that is to say, is not an established consequence of your birth, biology, social station, historical period, individual experience, and free will but instead is forever being created by subjective sensations, by power relationships over which you have no control and by evanescent changes in how you envision and make temporary sense, through language, of your world. According to this thinking, we have lost the closure conferred by classical notions of the self; in return we endure the contingency of never, exactly, knowing who we are but enjoy the freedom to create that identity anew and every day.

Meanwhile, scholars continued to find novel ways in which to contemplate life-writing, perhaps in part as a means to retain the comfort of the solid old "self." By declaring that autobiography is a "retrospective prose narrative written by a real person concerning his own existence, where the focus is his individual life, in particular the story of his personality," literary critic Philippe Lejeune tried to salvage autobiography as a distinct genre with a tradition and a future, and at the same time to assert that the author of that work was, indeed, a "real person."[21] Other readers, including linguist Elizabeth Bruss, argued that autobiography is a genre because one has to "do" different things to write and read them than one does when faced with fiction or expository prose.[22] Meanwhile, others took the opposite strategy, suggesting that autobiography was not restricted to a particular sort of self-report but could be widened, conceptually, to include just about all artistic writings.[23] This last gesture was a splendid effort to maintain, over the objections of critical theory, the existence of a self who has, after all, the last word. Whatever one writes, they suggested, one cannot help but write about oneself, therefore proving that self's existence.

By the late 1970s literary critics admitted that autobiography offered not so much factual and temporal coherence as poetic and expressive unity.[24] One did not set out, in writing one's autobiography, to report on the self but rather to eavesdrop on oneself, writing about it so as to learn what it might have become.[25] Deconstructing the gesture altogether, Paul de Man suggested that "[a]utobiography, then, is not a genre or a mode, but a figure of reading or of understanding that occurs, to some degree, in all texts."[26] Other scholars, agreeing with de Man, contested traditional notions that autobiography reported on the self and replaced these with the notion that autobiography is a field in which conflicts among self, identity, and discourse could be observed—productively—to play themselves out.[27]

But if autobiography was no longer to be considered the referential record of an individual's reportable life, it certainly was evidence of the vortex of cultural, political, economic, artistic, and intellectual forces that influenced the situation of any one person. And so, life-writing was seized by scholars in women's studies, ethnic studies, and African American studies as primary texts that recorded not so much individual lives as situations that influenced all lives lived out under their sway. Life-writing became a means to track the power of gender, race, culture, and class in forming personal lives, enabling scholars and activists to critique the impact of these societal forces.[28] Furthermore, identity scholars defined members of groups—women, slaves, historically oppressed groups—by the conventions they adopted in writing of their lives. For example, feminist scholars argued that women write autobiographies that reflect relationships and context, while men write linear reports of autonomous accomplishments.[29] The process of autobiographies was as telling of the lives and times of their authors as was their content.

We can see, in looking at life-writing over time, how dramatically and continuously transforming is our notion of what it means to be an individual and how and why one might want to tell about being this individual. These changes have practical implications for all of us: an autonomous "classical" or "essentialist" self will expect more control and less interference from the outside than will a fragmented "postmodern" self who realizes that he or she reflects all the discontinuities and ambiguities in the culture. Certainly sick people and those who care for them will behave very differently depending on their beliefs about the boundaries of and control over the self.[30] An illness interpreted as God's punishment for one's own sins will be experienced differently from an illness interpreted as a consequence of a corrupt culture in which the self is blameless. By reading and understanding life-writing, we are schooled in these changes, better able to understand how we ourselves inhabit our own lives and how patients might respond to challenges to their health.

POSTMODERN AUTOBIOGRAPHY: NARRATIVITY, RELATION, AND THE BODY

Three features of contemporary understanding of the self are of great practical significance in the effort to understand the events of illness and medicine. Recognizing—or even being—one's self unfolds in narrative language, includes attention to others, and takes account of the body.

Narrativity is a hallmark of postmodern theorizing about autobiography, that is, that identity is both declared and created with narrative. As Eakin writes, "When it comes to autobiography, narrative and identity are so intimately linked that each constantly and properly gravitates into the conceptual field of the other. Thus, narrative is not merely a literary form but a mode of phenomenological and cognitive self-experience, while self—the self of autobiographical discourse—does not necessarily precede its constitution in narrative."[31] Scholars in social science and psychology join their literary colleagues in the shift toward narrativity as the source of identity. Theodore Sarbin, architect of the field known as narrative psychology, writes that "[p]eople conceptualize the first order self, the I, by treating self, metaphorically and literally, as a storyteller."[32] No longer demeaning, to be called a storyteller means not that the teller is telling lies but that the teller is creating self.

Much of human knowledge, suggests philosopher Paul Ricoeur, exists in prenarrative or quasi-narrative form. In order for one to capture what one knows—about the self or, more globally, about anyone or anything—this knowledge has to achieve the status of narrative language.[33] Ricoeur's descriptions of "untold stories" bring home forcefully the realization that our experience has a protonarrative, or "prefigured," quality that becomes visible or "readable" upon framing it in words: "[A]re we not inclined to see in a given sequence of the episodes of our lives '(as yet) untold' stories, stories that demand to be told, stories that offer anchorage points for narrative?" (1:75). By seeing narrative "shadows" of events, Ricoeur can explain the relation between existing and knowing, for the story ultimately told is "in 'continuity' with the passive entanglement of subjects in stories that disappear into a foggy horizon." (1:75). In adopting the image of the horizon, both Taylor and Ricoeur emphasize the effort to place ourselves as we learn about ourselves, to be oriented cosmically, physically, and intersubjectively and, they submit, it is through narrative acts that such placing occurs. "Experience," summarizes Anthony Paul Kerby in his study of narrativity, "naturally goes over into narration," helping us to grasp the elusive connections between being and telling.[34]

Psychologists and neural scientists have studied the development of memory and knowledge of the self through childhood.[35] What emerges from these landmark studies is a picture of a highly dynamic and ever-changing self-knowledge, not laid down permanently in the brain but always reengineered by new experiences that alter old memories. The research findings of psychologists and neurologists support the abstractions of postmodernism: careful empirical studies of children's evolving sense of self document the fluid, dialectical relationships between a child's actual experience and the narrative frames into which these experiences are filed. What happens to you, what you remember, and how you tell about it are mutual forces that contribute to your sense of your self over time.

Very young children narrate their experiences to themselves, almost as if trying to relive or recapture or reflect on what has happened. My grandson Julian used to practice his newly mastered words as he fell asleep, and he would also narrate the events of the day. After an evening during which he and his grandfather had played with letters of the alphabet and then seen a group of deer in the forest, he said, as he fell off to sleep, "Ice, star, O, M, N, deer, pa." Autobiographers do the same thing as they write of the self. A continuum of telling of the self starts in infancy, develops through adolescent diaries, and sometimes results in written and published life-writing. The drive in all these activities is the same: to tell and simultaneously listen to a story that reflects and constitutes the self. Such acts of telling are ultimately ethical acts determined by collective responsibilities toward ourselves and others. As Ricoeur notes, " We tell stories because in the last analysis human lives need and merit being narrated." (1:75)

Relation with others has become far more prominent within recent theories of life-writing than it used to be, replacing the monolithic loyalty to the Western concept of the individually construed self with a realization of the relationally created self. "Selfhood," writes Bruner, "involves a commitment to others as well as being 'true to oneself.' . . . [S]elf-making and self-telling are about as public activities as any private acts can be."[36] Autobiography is still recognized as the effort by a writer or a narrator to reflect on, recapture, reinterpret, and represent to readers the events in his or her life that, taken together and in the particular sequence and frame in which they are provided, make sense (in one of many possible ways) of it. But instead of stolidly and reliably recounting the events of one's life, the autobiographer is understood, now, to be seeking and not merely repeating the grounds of meaning in a life, and to search not only among his or her memories but also among his or her intimates for that meaning.[37]

The most urgent change in autobiographical theory, perhaps voiced most influentially by feminist scholars describing how women's autobiographies differ from men's, is to acknowledge that the autobiographer tells the story of his or her self within his or her significant relationships with others. Human beings do not become—or create—themselves in autonomous and deracinated acts of will but instead develop over time in concert with others. Postmodernism's fragmentation here gives way to a quilt-unity of virtual wholeness made up of disparate but interweavable pieces.

Many autobiographies begin their lives as biographies of other people. Henry James writes *A Small Boy and Others*, the first book of his masterful autobiography, as a memorial to his brother William. Simone de Beauvoir's *A Very Easy Death* refers, directly anyway, to the illness and death of the author's mother while metaphorically to the deaths of us all. Mary Gordon writes *Shadow Man* about her father, thereby telling of herself as both a girl and a grown woman. Annie Ermaux writes of her mother's deepening dementia in *I Remain in Darkness*, articulating and exposing the deepest parts of her own interiority by way of telling of her aging mother. Many memoirs of illness are written by children about parents or by parents about children, recounting not only an illness but a family.

When health care professionals write reflectively about their practice, they learn how interwoven are stories of patients and story of self. Abraham Verghese writes of his young gay AIDS patients in rural Tennessee at the start of the HIV epidemic, describing their alienation from the Southern Christian culture that judges them with great harshness. What powers Verghese's description of his patients is his own otherness—as a physician of color, from India by way of Africa. His own experience of cultural marginalization informs and deepens his ability to care for his patients who, too, are on the edge.[38] The family physician Peter Selwyn writes about his care of HIV-infected patients in the South Bronx at a time when there was no effective treatment and many, many deaths. It was the deaths of his patients that enabled the doctor to relive his own early loss of his father to suicide. Only in the face of his patients' losses and deaths could Selwyn mourn fully his horrible loss, begin to survive it, and as a result become more available to his patients in their illnesses.[39] The pediatrician and psycho-oncologist Rachel Remen writes movingly and earnestly about her patients facing terminal cancers, telling of her own experiences living with Crohn's disease in the process of probing their suffering and celebrating their resilience.[40]

As these authors wrote the biographies of their patients, they came to understand how urgent it is for them as health care professionals to reflect on and tell of their own lives. As Selwyn writes, "[T]he process of becoming aware of my past was ultimately beneficial not only in my life but also to my work. . . . I have learned that the greatest gift that I can give to patients is to allow the awareness of my own pain and loss to deepen my solidarity with them, as they stand facing their illness and death."[41]

If identity emerges from one's relations with others, making the boundaries between biography and autobiography hard to place, identity also declares itself in one's differences from others. Jacques Derrida's famous concept of différance combines the two meanings of the French word, difference and deferral. A thing or subject or word or text is "itself" to the extent that it differs, in both space and time, from not-self. In Derrida's words, "Some interval or gap must separate it from what is not itself in order for it to be itself."[42] This important idea helps us to incorporate awareness of identity with awareness of otherness and suggests that the individual is constituted in reference to the other, either in similarity or in contradistinction.

The body has taken on great importance in understanding the self. The self has—and is—a body. It is because corporeality has become such an urgent touchstone of much recent work in autobiography that autobiography is featured prominently in this book about medicine. Despite the extraordinary disagreements surrounding autobiographical truth, all roads in contemporary autobiographical theory lead to the body. Almost all the papers presented at a 1994 symposium on autobiography dwell on the body—trauma survivors, sexual abuse, suicide, sexuality, cross-gender identification, and AIDS.[43] Philosophers and literary scholars have resoundingly dismissed Descartes's cogito that separated body from mind—and then treated the body as unimportant—to embrace a far more complex understanding of the self's relation to the body.[44] Not only is the body the exterior of the self—the shell for the kernel of the self—but the body is also the interior of the self, the dark and noisy beating of the heart, borborygmi of the intestines, wheezing and rheuming of the lungs, visited by surgeons in the OR, heard by internists through the stethoscope, signifying beyond interpretation. The feminist literary scholar Judith Butler could just as easily be commenting on the body as on sex: "'Sex' is thus, not simply what one has, or a static description of what one is: it will be one of the norms by which the 'one' becomes viable at all."[45]

The body has become our most legible signature. In autographs ever more demonstrable as the self's own—the face, the voice, the fingerprint, the DNA sequence—corporeal evidence proclaims the individuality, the authenticity, the singularity of the self. I am me, the body attests, I and only I am me. The body is regaining respectability in philosophy and letters, because we have outgrown the binary opposition between body and mind (or the physical and the spiritual) that relegates the body to effacement or contempt.[46] At the same time that individuals are able to transcend their definition by their bodies—such, after all, is the basis for racism, sexism, and discrimination against the other-abled—they are also able to incorporate their experience of being embodied into their concept of self and their movement through the world and through life.

Autobiography with the body in view becomes an enterprise different from the humanist/Rousseauean tradition of the grand narrative of self or the Augustinian confession of moral weakness and boast of moral strength. With the body in view, autobiography cannot claim immortality but must succumb to temporality. It refuses allegory for singularity, for there can be but one body that is mine. It insists on intersubjective relation, because bodies have surface, needing contact—suckling, grooming, copulating—not "disembodied" and hence able to float, unconnected, alone. It has to concern itself with the actuality of its build, the how and the why of its organic construction while it gives heed to its unknowable and ungovernable parts. (Lewis Thomas once wrote something like, "If you were put in charge of your liver, you'd be dead in a day.") And autobiography with the body in view opens fields of ethical duties unspoken by classical life-writing, if only the duties to be responsible curators for the bodies we have been given for our lifetimes.

LISTENING FOR STORIES THAT PATIENTS TELL

This short review of autobiographical theory lends some terms and concepts to our project of listening for the stories of self that patients tell us. Considering life-writing as narrative self-creations bent toward poetic unity that are experienced by the writer as personal discovery and cultural declaration alters how readers might receive such texts. These concepts suggest where, ideally, readers might position themselves vis-à-vis the teller. The writer of a life story needs a reader of a specific sort who will donate his or her presence to that which the teller tries to convey. Because of autobiography's risky self-disclosure, its reader has to be peculiarly attuned to the project in order to qualify as its witness. Like those who listen to the testimonies of trauma victims or survivors of the Holocaust, the reader of autobiography implicitly signs a pact to read, at least initially, from the perspective of the teller. Anyone can become critical of an autobiography's writer, of course, yet taking up the book to become its reader demands, perhaps, a different readerly loyalty from that demanded by fiction or other nonfiction prose.

The reader says, by virtue of the act of opening the autobiography, "I am your listener; I willingly agree to join with you in the project of manifesting and finding your self." A readerly act positioned otherwise—I open this book to collect information about you that will be used against you—is an act of narrative bad faith. (That some autobiographies may be written toward self-aggrandizement, or narcissistic self-indulgence, or willful deception and cannot be read genuinely will be bracketed for now). What Patrocinio Schweickart asserts about the feminist reader—that she acts as "witness and intimate confidante of the textual subject, engaged in a dialogic process"—can be generalized, I submit, to all readers who read autobiography with authenticity.[47]

Although listening to a patient in an office differs from reading Augustine's *Confessions* and is, I think, much harder, learning how life-writing works opens fresh ways of contemplating the tasks of listening for stories that patients tell. The triad of narrativity, relation, and the body seems particularly salient to the clinician's task, the clinician who may indeed be responsive to the body and, perhaps, to the relations within a patient's life but may not yet be equipped to be dutiful toward the narrativity of both their patients' telling of and living of their lives.

Although some health care professionals may feel that they listen to a very restricted version of self-telling (what does the rotator cuff really have to do with the whole person?), illness, no matter how minor, reminds one of one's mortality and frailty and ultimate end. When patients talk about themselves to their doctors or nurses, they are revealing aspects of the self closest to the skin, having pared away the optional layers, if you will—occupation, habits, even history and culture—to get down to the core of who they are. Hence, the listening that goes on in the clinical setting qualifies as a consequential reception of autobiography. Health care professionals might be among the few trained confidantes available to individuals in ordinary life, replacing the confessors or spiritual advisors of former times as the vessels, sworn to secrecy, of others' fears and sorrows. Doctors and nurses are the ones who hear what others tell of themselves in the destabilizing times of illness when questions of self and worth naturally emerge. Even though doctors or nurses or social workers focus, in training, mainly on health-related matters, they incur obligations toward patients' total well-being by virtue of what their patients tell them. Bearing witness to such telling becomes the responsibility of these listeners.[48]

Medicine, in turn, has important contributions to make to the field of life-writing and, indeed, to the study of the self. All who want to learn of the self may be deeply interested in the unique, genuine strain of life-telling that goes on in medicine. The self-who-tells in the medical context begins in the relation with the body or, if anything, is eclipsed by bodily concerns. Clinical telling ordinarily at least touches on important life relationships in the course of the telling. Now, the listening ear in medicine is often deaf to story, and so the narrativity of the patient's account may not be appreciated. However, when told freely and heard expertly, the self-telling that occurs in medical settings can reflect a rich and earthy unity of body, mind, and life and can give voice to body, relation, and narratively achieved identity. Unlike the more intellectual or aesthetic or casual presentations of self that might be encountered in art or academy or popular culture, the self-who-tells to a trusted doctor who knows how to listen can afford to sound all channels, including the soma, the psyche, and the anima. Honored to hear evidence from this unusual perspective on selfhood, we health professionals are obligated to contribute what we learn to the ongoing discourse about the postmodern self, not only about disease and treatment but about who the self has become and how to be true to it.

A short essay/story entitled "Communion" appeared in the *Annals of Internal Medicine* in 1995. Written by the gastroenterologist Richard Weinberg about his care of a young patient, the text lays bare the perilous telling that patients must accomplish and the potential dividends of careful clinical listening. This text seems to me to display the unity possible in the postmodern autobiographies and biographies created in the clinic. "I am not an intimidating person but I found my last patient of the day huddled in the corner of the examining room, as if awaiting an executioner. She was in her mid-twenties, and she clutched a sheaf of medical records against her chest like a shield. She had made the appointment to our clinic herself. The face sheet on her chart said 'chronic abdominal pain.'"

The doctor introduces himself, takes an unrevealing gastrointestinal history, and studies the patient's medical chart to learn that she has already had the routine diagnostic procedures, which were unremarkable, and she been on all the medications that usually help her symptoms, with no relief. She appears anxious and desperate, and yet she strikes him as courageous and defiant.

> What, I asked myself, kept her trudging from doctor to doctor on this medical odyssey? And what could I possibly do for her?
> She seemed so uncomfortable talking about herself that I moved on to inquire about her family history. Her parents had emigrated from Italy. Her mother had died when she was a young girl, and although she was not the oldest child, it had fallen to her to play the role of mother to her five siblings. She was a devout Catholic who, like her mother, attended Mass every morning. "But I don't take communion," she added. Her father was a baker, and through years of hard work now owned his own bakery, which she managed.

The gastroenterologist himself is a good cook, but baking is one thing he has yet to master. He engages the patient in spirited conversation about the relative merits of French and Italian Napoleons, but as soon as he shifts the conversation back to medical matters, the patient again becomes withdrawn and monosyllabic. Despite his inability to do much for the patient, she returns to his clinic week after week. He talks mostly about baking, having learned that this was the only point of contact that kept her from withdrawing.

Eventually, she tells him of her insomnia from recurrent nightmares, lurid nightmares decisively signifying a history of abuse.

> "Were you ever sexually assaulted?' I asked gently.
> "Yes."
> "When?"
> "When I was fourteen." . . .
> "What happened?" With great effort she told me. She had been raped by her oldest sister's boyfriend. . . . "There's nothing dirty he didn't do to me," she sobbed, and now unstoppable, she poured out the grim details of her ordeal.

The patient tells her doctor about her sense of defilement and her inability, from shame and fear, to tell anyone. "You're the only person I've ever told."

> I felt completely out of my depth. I consoled her as best I could, and when her sobbing had subsided, I gently suggested a referral to a psychiatrist or a rape counselor. I'm a gastroenterologist, I told her, this is not my area of expertise. I had neither the knowledge nor the experience to help her, I explained. But she adamantly refused to consider a referral to anyone else. She didn't trust them. I then understood that having unearthed her dark secret, I had become responsible for her care.

The gastroenterologist reads about sexual trauma and consults with a psychiatrist colleague, who helps him decide that he is doing as much as anyone could do for the patient. He sees her weekly, mostly to listen, as she tells of her efforts to purge herself of the stain of the rape through bulimia, a self-inflicted punishment that felt so deserved. Gradually, she recovers, renews her college studies, comes to his clinic less and less frequently, until she appears on a last visit, bestowing on him a gift of six perfect Napoleons she had baked for him.

> "Thank you for believing in me," she said.
> "I should say the same," I replied. . . .
> I had been chosen to receive a gift of trust, and of all the gifts I had ever received, none seemed as precious. That afternoon, I left the clinic feeling exhilarated and full of love for my profession. That evening after dinner, I opened my present and partook of the communion from the baker's daughter.

I don't mean, by beginning and ending this chapter with stories about rape, to suggest that all medical illnesses stem from sexual assault. And yet these twin stories of abuse—the first heard from an elderly woman whose telling came too late for the sake of her health and the second heard from a communicant whose telling may have salvaged her life—suggest the therapeutic urgency of listening to narratives of body/self and what might be required to hear them. Dr. Weinberg becomes an effective witness for his patient by virtue of his curiosity, his patience, his willingness to devote time to most likely unbillable visits, his ability to tolerate his own inexperience and lack of knowledge, and his humble acceptance of the role his patient has assigned to him. He adopts a stance not of passive hearing but of active attending, enabling the patient to articulate that which has been latent and corrosive for years. While he attends to the emotional and sexual dimensions of what the patient tells, he is also, simultaneously, listening diagnostically for any evidence of gastrointestinal disease that might be causing his patient's symptoms. The resultant text braids biography of patient—body and life—with autobiography of doctor—diagnostician and witness—exposing to the reader interior elements of both conversants. What we have here indeed is the story of "someone telling someone else that something happened," and both "someones" contribute meaning to the transaction.

Their clinical work enacts the many aspects of the postmodern self. The injuries to self home in to one part of the body, typically. What is being told in this case, again typically, is not an injury in isolation but an injury familialized—the patient is running her father's bakery, assaulted by her sister's boyfriend, trying her best to fulfill her mother's role. The treatment is performed intersubjectively, this doctor having been chosen as the one who must hear her out—him and him alone. What chooses him as the obligatory listener is that he unearthed her secret, suggesting the hidden power entailed in the very process of beginning to tell another of what the body conceals. Most powerfully, this story displays the redemptive force of narrative itself to heal, and to heal not only the shame and humiliation but also, almost as a dividend, the eating disorder and the abdominal pain.

Not all conversations that take place in the medical setting are earthshaking personal disclosures. Indeed, the kind of disclosure described in "Communion" takes place side by side with the most banal and trivial conversations, making it all the harder for health professionals to understand the importance of the talk they hear. Not all patients will look back on their conversations about their hypertension or osteoarthritis as particularly meaningful, and yet the clinical listener has to be alert all the time for the gleam of self-telling, to pick up the thread offered—sometimes so very casually or tentatively—by a patient who is prepared to begin a story of a life.

Whether or not they choose to be, health care professionals are the listeners as relative strangers tell of themselves. Because the contemporary "self" is constituted in the way it is—ever evolving, becoming through narrating, constituted through relation, and inflected by the body—and because of social practices that have selected health care as the locus for much that concerns personal meaning, it falls to doctors and nurses and social workers to be the ones to listen to the lives of others. Whether we like it or not, it falls to us to record what patients tell us of themselves, to respect the value of their telling it, and to trust that what is said means something. It becomes our great challenge and privilege to absorb, over time, that which patients choose to tell us about their health, their past, their lives, their hopes. It becomes our duty to reflect back to the teller whatever unity or coherence or meaning emerges from their brave telling and our courageous listening.

NOTES

1. Anne Hunsaker Hawkins, in *Reconstructing Illness,* and Arthur Frank, in *The Wounded Storyteller,* have provided masterful summaries and analyses of pathographies, or illness narratives, giving evidence of the massive cultural forces bending toward the telling of illness.

2. Howard Beckman and Richard Frankel, "The Effect of Physician Behavior on the Collection of Data."

3. Eudora Welty, *One Writer's Beginnings,* 14.

4. A robust educational and research enterprise has evolved from origins in the Society for General Internal Medicine, now centered in the American Academy on Physician and Patient. See Mack Lipkin Jr., Samuel Putnam, Aaron Lazare, eds., *The Medical Interview;* Moira Stewart and Debra Roter, eds., *Communicating with Medical Patients;* Robert Smith, *The Patient's Story;* John Coulehan and Marian Block, *The Medical Interview.*

5. See the review essay by Dennis Novack et al. on developing self-awareness in physicians, "Calibrating the Physician: Personal Awareness and Effective Patient Care" and Julie Connelly's work on mindfulness in clinical practice, "Being in the Present Moment: Developing the Capacity for Mindfulness in Medicine."

6. Theodore Sarbin, in Sarbin and Scheibe, eds., *Studies in Social Identity,* gives a powerful overview of recent theories of identity-formation emerging from psychology and social sciences. Paul John Eakin summarizes literary theories of autobiography in *How Our Lives Become Stories,* and James Olney capitulates particular theories of telling of memories in *Memory and Narrative.* Sidonie Smith and Julia Watson offer a comprehensive and commonsense summary of autobiographical theory and practice in *Reading Autobiography.* Charles Taylor's *Sources of the Self* represents philosophy's efforts to understand the making of modern identity.

7. Anthony Paul Kerby, *Narrative and the Self.*

8. Charles Taylor, *Sources of the Self,* 27.

9. Eakin, in *How Our Lives Become Stories,* summarizes contemporary discourse and debate about the subject and sources of identity. See also Roy Schafer's chapter "Narratives of the Self" in *Retelling a Life,* 21–35, for a survey of concepts of the self in analytic thought.

10. Sidonie Smith and Julia Watson, *Reading Autobiography.*

11. Jerome Bruner, *Making Stories: Law, Literature, Life,* 85–86.

12. We owe particular thanks to two scholars—James Olney and Paul John Eakin—who committed themselves to autobiographical theory and practice in the 1960s and 1970s, functioning as conveners of conferences, editors of collected papers, and intellectual curators and nourishers of this emerging theoretical field. See James Olney, *Metaphors of Self: The Meaning of Autobiography; Autobiography: Essays Theoretical and Critica;* and *Studies in Autobiography.* See Paul John Eakin, *Fictions in Autobiography: Studies in the Art of Self-Invention* and *Touching the World: Reference in Autobiography.*

13. Elizabeth Bruss, *Autobiographical Acts: The Changing Situation of a Literary Genre* and John Paul Eakin, *Fictions in Autobiography: Studies in the Art of Self-Invention* championed the notion of the autobiographical act as a central biographical event in the life of its writer, deflecting attention away from the factual content of autobiography toward its performance content in the writing present.

14. Roy Pascal, *Design and Truth in Autobiography,* 11.

15. Larry Sisson, "The Art and Illusion of Spiritual Autobiography," 99.

16. Paul Ricoeur discusses Augustinian temporality at length in *Time and Narrative,* vol. 1, "The Aporias of the Experience of Time: Book II of Augustine's *Confessions.*" See also James Olney in *Memory and Narrative.*

17. For summaries of theoretical studies of autobiography, see James Olney, "Autobiography and the Cultural Moment: A Thematic, Historical, and Bibliographical Introduction," in *Autobiography: Essays Theoretical and Critical,* 3–27; William Spengemann, "The Study of Autobiography: A Bibliographical Essay," in *The Forms of Autobiography: Episodes in the History of a Literary Genre;* and Suzanne Nalbantian, "Theories of Autobiography," in *Aesthetic Autobiography: From Life to Art in Marcel Proust, James Joyce, Virginia Woolf, and Anaïs Nin,* 26–42.

18. Georges Gusdorf, "Conditions and Limits of Autobiography."

19. Roland Barthes "The Death of the Author," in *Image-Music-Text,* 142–48; Michel Foucault, "What Is an Author?"; Jean Paul Sartre, "What is Literature?" in *What Is Literature? and Other Essays,* 21–245.

20. Jacques Derrida, *On Grammatology* and *Writing and Difference;* Paul de Man, *Allegories of Reading.*

21. Philippe Lejeune, *Le pacte autobiographique.* Collected works appeared in English as Philippe Lejeune, *On Autobiography,* 4.

22. In an effort to bring speech act theory to bear on the generic study of autobiography, Elizabeth Bruss refocused critical attention onto the autobiographical act itself, the *performance* of telling of self the source of its truth. See *Autobiographical Acts.*

23. William Spengemann, *The Forms of Autobiography.*

24. See John Sturrock, "The New Model Autobiographer," and Christine Downing, "Re-Visioning Autobiography: The Bequest of Freud and Jung."

25. Avrom Fleischman, *Figures of Autobiography: The Language of Self-Writing in Victorian and Modern England* and Paul Jay, *Being in the Text: Self-Representation from Wordsworth to Roland Barthes.*

26. See Paul de Man, "Autobiography as De-Facement" for a seminal challenge to

all notions of referentiality and the possible excision of the self from the task of writing about it, with the side effect of declaring autobiography not a genre but a figural mode.

27. See Jeffrey Mehlman, *A Structural Study of Autobiography: Proust, Leiris, Sartre, Lévi-Strauss;* Louis Renza, "The Veto of the Imagination: A Theory of Autobiography"; and Michael Sprinker, "Fictions of the Self: The End of Autobiography" for deconstruction-inspired challenges to classical autobiographical theory.

28. Patricia Meyer Spacks, "Women's Stories, Women's Selves" and "Reflecting Women"; Sidonie Smith, *Subjectivity, Identity, and the Body: Women's Autobiographical Practices in the Twentieth Century;* Stephen Butterfield, *Black Autobiography in America;* Joseph Brooches, "Black Autobiography in Africa and America."

29. Although a comparison of women's pathographies with men's pathographies along these lines has not been undertaken, one wonders how these gendered differences in telling of the self would maintain when the self is ill.

30. See David Morris, *Illness and Culture in the Postmodern Age* and Arthur Frank, *The Wounded Storyteller* for accounts of the postmodern self within the context of health and illness.

31. Eakin, *How Our Lives Become Stories,* 100.

32. James C. Mancuso and Theodore Sarbin, "The Self-Narrative in the Enactment of Roles," 236.

33. Paul Ricoeur, *Time and Narrative* vol. 1. See also Anthony Paul Kerby, *Narrative and the Self,* chapter 2, for an introduction to the notions of prenarrative knowledge and the narrative and temporal requirements for self-knowledge.

34. Anthony Paul Kerby, *Narrative and the Self,* 43.

35. See Katherine Nelson, *Narratives from the Crib,* on crib narratives; Jerome Bruner, *Making Stories: Law, Literature, Lives.*

36. Jerome Bruner, *Making Stories: Law, Literature, Life,* 69–70.

37. See G. Thomas Couser and Joseph Fichtelberg, eds., *True Relations: Essays on Autobiography and the Postmodern* for proceedings of a 1994 conference on autobiography. The collection includes essays on photographic life-writing essays, multiauthored autobiographies, and life-writing of gays, Native Americans, and tribal Africans.

38. Abraham Verghese, *My Own Country.*

39. Peter Selwyn, *Surviving the Fall: The Personal Journey of an AIDS Doctor.*

40. Rachel Remen, *Kitchen Table Wisdom.*

41. Peter Selwyn, *Surviving the Fall,* 125–26.

42. Jacques Derrida, "La différance," 51–52, cited by Barbara Johnson in *The Critical Difference,* xi, translation Johnson's.

43. G. Thomas Couser and Joseph Fichtelberg, eds., *True Relations.*

44. See, for example, Eduardo Cadava, Peter Connor, and Jean-Luc Nancy, eds., *Who Comes after the Subject?;* Anthony Paul Kerby, *Narrative and the Self;* Judith Butler, *Bodies That Matter;* and Elizabeth Grosz, *Volatile Bodies: Toward a Corporeal Feminism* for recent repudiations of the Cartesian dualism.

45. Judith Butler, *Bodies That Matter,* 2.

46. Shirley Neuman, "'An appearance walking in a forest the sexes burn,'" 293.

47. Patrocinio Schweickart, "Reading Ourselves: Toward a Feminist Theory of Reading," 17–44. Marie Lovrod adopts Schweickart's concept of the feminist reader in an essay on survivor narratives written by survivors of sexual abuse. See Marie Lovrod, "'Art/i/fact' Rereading Culture and Subjectivity through Sexual Abuse Survivor Narratives," 23–32.

48. See chapter 9 for an extended treatment of bearing witness to suffering.

5 🔲 THE PATIENT, THE BODY, AND THE SELF

A 51-year-old man came to see me with diarrhea and abdominal pain. A successful writer of nonfiction, he had been physically healthy except for a completely resolved sports injury of some years ago. He had suffered through a major depression about 20 years ago, had undergone intensive long-term psychotherapy, and was now not clinically depressed. When he experienced persistent left upper quadrant abdominal pain and developed a dramatic change in his bowel habits, he came to the quick and irrevocable decision that he had pancreatic cancer. A rapid loss of around eight pounds confirmed this medical suspicion in his own mind.

His diagnostic certainty, however, was not the central aspect of his presentation.

What most impressed me upon learning of his symptoms and what he made of them was that he discovered—to his great astonishment and sadness—that he felt ready and even eager to die. His uncle had died of pancreatic cancer (this autobiographical fact contributed to his self-diagnosis), and so he knew of the clinical nihilism surrounding the disease. He made up his mind not only that he *had* pancreatic cancer but also that he would choose to die of it as quickly as possible. Having an incurable disease felt like a release, an escape from life. His only regrets were that his wife would become a young widow and that his mother, now in her late 70s, would have to suffer the death of her son. For their sakes, perhaps, he lamented his early death, but not for his own.

A GI workup revealed a simple, benign, and treatable cause for his abdominal pain and diarrhea. And yet, by virtue of this episode, he was a changed man. He now had to grapple with the relative ease with which he found himself able and eager to call an end to life. Recognizing his feelings as passive suicidality, he had to confront his heretofore submerged feelings that he had had enough of his life.

As he talked to me about these feelings, I could recognize the depth to which he had traveled within himself upon the onset of symptoms. Not an unreflective man, he had always appeared to me to embrace his life, to be passionate about his work, and to be fully committed to and engaged in his marriage. With my encouragement, he reentered analytic treatment, and he is at the time of this writing doing physically well and no longer suicidal.

▣ Our Bodies, Our Selves

This brief clinical vignette highlights the intimate relationships between our bodies and our selves. From neurobiology to phenomenology, much of the sciences and the humanities probe these relationships—the connections between brain and mind, perception and understanding, speech and language, and consciousness and imagination. The disagreement between Descartes and Spinoza in the seventeenth century—is there division or unity between mind and body?—is repeated today in cultural studies, anthropology, and literature as we human beings try to imagine or come to grips with our mysterious existence as simultaneously material and metaphorical beings. Religious doctrines confront the spiritual consequences of carnal existence while schools of psychology and psychiatry argue about both the body's transparency to emotion and emotion's source in the body's neural mechanisms. Beliefs about death and the hereafter—beliefs, of course, that drive faith, culture, philosophy, even law—pivot on attitudes about our ability to transcend materiality and live beyond our corporeal limits. With the explosion of new knowledge about the brain's contributions to pain, emotion, and consciousness, these questions multiply, as do their conflicting answers.[1]

It is in the shadow of all these discourses about body and self that medicine grapples with the relation between body and self in health and illness. Accepting the power and privilege of touching another's body, interfering with it, hurting it, perhaps healing it incurs in health care professionals profound duties to acknowledge the inviolability of the patient's body as a locus of the person's self. While doctors and nurses might breach the body's unity, we do our best to maintain the "wholeness" of the patient. Even if we do not always act as if we remember, we remember that the body is the proxy for the self, and that demeaning or disrespecting the patient's body demeans and disrespects the patient's self. Many of the concerns of bioethics and health law have to do precisely with these questions of the body's owner, guardian, curator, and protector.

Personal writings by sick people and health care professionals can contribute to this ongoing discourse. By presenting autobiographical writings of patients and doctors from many settings and venues—published pathographies, students' writing in Parallel Charts, health professionals' reflective writing, and transcribed medical interviews—I hope to bring perspectives of sick people and those who care for them to bear on these questions. Answers to some of these questions are available, I am convinced, by looking carefully at the subgenre of life-writing called illness narratives, for it is here that the body speaks and can be observed to constitute the self.

Neither prison nor temple of the soul, the body has always been an important refuge of the self. The body cannot be expropriated by another, except in a dark science fiction vision of whole-body transplantation. It cannot be plagiarized, no matter how good the cosmetic surgeons get, until human cloning becomes commonplace.[2] Its ownership cannot be collectivized, except perhaps during pregnancy. He or she who "has" any one body gets to keep it, enjoy its pleasures, and suffer its breakdown, whatever miracles are at his or her disposal to fix it as it breaks. The body is the passport, the warrant, the seal of one's identity.[3] "This," said as one firmly pounds one's chest with the flat of one's hands, "is me."

What appears to be a common destination on the pilgrimage for identity is the shrine of flesh and blood. Teenagers and punks tattoo, embellish, and scarify their bodies. The heights of personal redesign attained by Michael Jackson or Oprah Winfrey through surgery, pigmentary alteration, or weight change are imitated not only by supermodels and anorexics but also by ordinary lipstick appliers and dieters. So-called enhancement treatments—growth hormones for height, estrogenic hormones for breasts, androgenic steroids for muscles, even selective serotonin reuptake inhibitors for mood stabilization—fuel the efforts to "fix" the self by fixing the body or the brain.[4] Transsexual surgery perhaps gives the most extraordinary evidence of the carnal roots of identity and the biological means to fix a failed one. By these aberrations as well as by the commonplace efforts to be healthy by eating well, exercising, and refraining from smoking and using drugs, members of the culture assert more and more loudly and unambiguously that their identities are clearly, directly, and irrevocably tied to their bodies.

Illness intensifies the routine drives to recognize the self. It is when one is ill that one has to decide how valuable life is, which relationships are most meaningful, and what terrors or comforts the end of life holds. When people become sick or disabled, they question their existence in new ways. They ask particular versions of universally asked questions about the self. Instead of "How can I be true to myself," they ask "What did I do to deserve this disease? What will become of me? Now that I am blind, or without legs, or can't hear, or can't talk, am I still 'me'?" When the religious scholar John Hull lost his vision in middle age from retinal disease, he felt unmoored from the easy and natural connection with who he was, unable to "glance down and see the reassuring continuity of my own consciousness in the outlines of my own body, moving a distant foot which, so to speak, waves back, saying, 'Yes, I hear you. I am here.'"[5] He lost the integrity of his body, and without it, he realized how one's corporeal integrity anchors one's sense of self.

The body, as my story about the patient convinced he had pancreatic cancer demonstrates, coauthors the story of the life being lived in it. Illness occasions the telling of two tales of self at once, one told by the "person" of the self and the other told by the body of the self. How the body communicates its tale is very mysterious. Sometimes its signals are very clear—my left knee hurts since I ran 13 miles or my period is coming and giving me cramps. Sometimes its signals are obscure, like the paralysis suffered by Freud's hysterical patients. Even though the body is material, its communications are always representations, mediated by sensations and the meanings ascribed to them. It is sometimes as if the body speaks a foreign language, relying on bilingual others to translate, interpret, or in some way make transparent what it means to say.

The self depends on the body for its presence, its location. Without the body, the self cannot be uttered. Without the body, the self cannot enter relation with others. Without the body, the self is an abstraction. John Hull says that without vision, "I often feel I am a mere spirit, a ghost, a memory. . . . This is such a profound lostness."[6] And yet the body itself can become invisible in this transaction. It is a commonplace that we disregard our bodies until they cause us trouble. The anthropologist Robert Murphy experienced fleeting neurological symptoms of muscle spasms and numbness of his feet. Eventually, he learned that a tumor had grown around his spinal cord from the level of his neck to midchest, compressing the cord and eventually causing quadriplegia. Murphy bent all his skills and conceptual powers as an anthropologist to write a "participant-observer" report on himself, called *The Body Silent*. He understands this dual nature of the body: "People in good health take their lot, and their bodies, for granted; they can see, hear, eat, make love, and breathe because they have working organs that can do all those things. These organs, and the body itself, are among the foundations upon which we build our sense of who and what we are, and they are the instruments through which we grapple with and create reality."[7]

Healthy people, who enjoy the "silence of health," have little reason to dwell on their bodies or their bodies' relationship with the world.[8] If they did, they might notice that their body enables them to collect experience through vision, hearing, smell, taste, and touch. Hull laments that his blindness prevents him from storing memories because, without visual images, he has no trace of the people he had been with or the places he had visited. Although extreme, this claim—that memories depend on the bodily machinery for collecting them—must be heard as a report from the frontier of the body/self relationship, a frontier accessible only through Hull's illness.

The observations of Murphy and Hull compel us to ask what our bodies do for us. My body is the medium through which I obtain sensory sensations and information. It is through the instrument of my body that I become aware of hunger, thirst, cold, heat, pain, passion, and pleasure. My body is what I use to get where I want to go, and it is what I use to know where I am in space. I cannot separate the bodily components from the mental components of such phenomena as dreams, fantasies, thoughts, and emotions. Nor can I dismiss the bodily contributions to such states as religious fervor, creative force, intellectual transport, or aesthetic glee.

The identity of a person is not determined by the state of his or her body. Otherwise, we would have to endorse sexism, racism, ageism, and discrimination against the disabled. And yet, the way a person experiences the world and accumulates and metabolizes experience depends directly on that person's body and its senses. The body is not a trivial or meaningless aspect of self at the same time that it mustn't be allowed to determine and unduly limit self. How can we transcend an essentialist bodily definition of self while acknowledging the body's shaping of experience?

The body defines the self from the inside, but the body does not define the self to the outside. There are two bodies: the one lived in and the one lived through. One body absorbs the world, and one body emits the self. Poised between world and self, the body simultaneously undergoes the world while emanating to that world its self. Or again, the body is simultaneously a receiver with which the self collects all sensate and cognate information about what lies exterior to it and a projector with which the body declares the self who lives in it. The body is in the copulative position between world and self.

An account from someone whose body can absorb the world but cannot emit the self demonstrates how these two bodies differ. Jean-Dominique Bauby was the editor of the French fashion magazine *Elle*. He suffered a massive stroke, injuring his brain stem and leaving him what is eloquently if brutally called "locked-in": he was unable to move or to speak but was fully alert to his surroundings and his predicament. His left eyelid alone was in his voluntary control, and so he "dictated" a book, called *The Diving Bell and the Butterfly*, to an amanuensis who could transduce eyelid blinks into letters that formed text. This remarkable report from another extreme bodily frontier details the suffering Bauby undergoes in being able to absorb but not transmit: he is cut off from those he loves, unable to reach them, unable to do anything more than exist in front of them.

On Father's Day, his son and daughter come to visit him at his nursing home. His son, Théophile, perhaps eight years old at the time, invites him to play:

> "Want to play hangman?" asks Théophile, and I ache to tell him that I have enough on my plate playing quadriplegic. . . . I guess a letter, then another, then stumble on the third. My heart is not in the game. Grief surges over me. His face not two feet from mine, my son Théophile sits patiently waiting—and I, his father, have lost the simple right to ruffle his bristly hair, clasp his downy neck, hug his small, lithe, warm body tight against me. There are no words to express it. My condition is monstrous, iniquitous, revolting, horrible. Suddenly I can take no more. Tears well and my throat emits a hoarse rattle that startles Théophile. Don't be scared, little man. I love you. Still engrossed in the game, he moves in for the kill. Two more letters: he has won and I have lost. On a corner of the page he completes his drawing of the gallows, the rope, and the condemned man.[9]

In brilliant counterpoint, Bauby describes his boundless longing for what his body can no longer do for him. He is denied the "right" to collect the sensory details of being with his little boy while, even more tragically, he cannot transmit the fullness of his love to his son except through a hoarse rattle whose meaning is not grasped.

The matter is not simple. Bauby is not "merely" quadriplegic. He is denied the automatic, usually unconscious transparency of the triple relationship of self/body/world. Without the body in position, Bauby can neither absorb world nor enact self in it. That he writes this book despite his extreme disability is an achievement of magnificent scale, rescued from the ruins of his body.

Simone de Beauvoir writes that "the body is not a thing, it is a situation. . . . [I]t is the instrument of our grasp upon the world, a limiting factor for our projects."[10] The evidence provided by Bauby, Hull, and Murphy contests de Beauvoir: the body indeed is an object, a space-occupying thing, a very complex organism. This object that is my body I control to some extent by my will, my behavior, and my reflexes (many of which remain unknown to and unwilled by me). This object is at the same time controlled by its genetic inheritance, its environmental surround, its random hits and accidents, and by the passage of time. Not only do I use this object to move through space and to absorb information about what else is in it but I also use this object to transmit to other such objects my thoughts, feelings, and desires. Through the avenues of speech, gesture, expression, appearance, movement, artistic production, and textual production, I emit or transmit what goes on inside my body into the milieu outside the body.

⬚ TELLING OF THE BODY

The body is and is not the self. No wonder the telling of the self that occurs in the doctor's office becomes complicated. Such telling follows the rules for autobiographical telling or writing in general: the teller splits into a narrator and a protagonist, generating the autobiographical gap. The narrator tells what the protagonist has done in the past, even if the past is but milliseconds away.[11] When one tells of one's body, though, one doubles the autobiographical charge: "I first noticed the pain in my chest after I brought the groceries home from D'Agostino's. It went away when I sat down in the kitchen, but then it came back when I picked up the baby, and so I started worrying that it might be my heart." The autobiographical gap here is accompanied by another gap that we might call the corporeal gap. The teller of the self tells of the body of the self. The act of telling separates, momentarily, the teller-who-reports from the body-that-feels. The teller is called upon to become the voice of the body or the medium through which the body can convey its message to the listener.

Telling of the body uses the corporeal gap in a simultaneous gesture of avowal and disavowal. The poet Lucy Grealy writes in *Autobiography of a Face* of her ordeal with Ewing's sarcoma of the right lower jaw, diagnosed when she was nine years old, whose treatment required years of chemotherapy and radiation and more than 15 operations. She reports that her life has revolved around her face from grade school to her adulthood. After a long graft operation for reconstruction, she reports, "When I awoke I was in a lot of pain, but the pain was in my hip, where the graft came from, far away from my face, my 'self,' so it was easier to deal with."[12] Here, one part of the body is self while the other is nonself. Earlier, Grealy describes a disembodied experience of disavowal in preparation for transport to the operating room, "I felt as if I were watching someone else shyly try to hold the short gown down over her legs as she awkwardly wiggled along the rough sheets" (144). And again, "I remember having a surreal vision of myself as if I were a bystander in the room" (170). This corporeal gap places distance between the person of the self and the self's body, especially when it must undergo humiliating or painful manipulations.

Such experiences of fragmentation or dissociation, although not restricted to illness, recur in illness narratives as frightening but also self-protective devices.

In her candid and sorrowful account of living with Stage 4 breast cancer, Christina Middlebrook describes similar episodes of disembodiment, here during her bone marrow transplant:

> I had not stayed inside my body to suffer the death of every fast-growing cell. My body was a poisoned wreck: all mucous membranes shed, the inside of my mouth and gastrointestinal tract filled with ulcers, eyelids glued shut with blepharitis. In the mornings, I would open my eyes with my fingers. . . . To save myself, *I*, the me of me, retreated to a far corner above the room. From there, I think, I turned my soul away to contemplate the firmament, to stare at the heavens, the stars and the moon. I found a large psychic cloak and gathered my endangered identity within. Who *I* am could not endure the torture of that room.[13]

These brave authors donate to us readers a truth of illness, the record of living with a body that has, temporarily anyway, abandoned its inhabitant, turning against the person to make impossible the simple things—like opening one's eyes without using one's hands—that in health are mindless background.

If illness allows the body to separate from the person who lives in it, it may prompt conflict or struggle between them. The body can, for example, keep secrets from the person who lives in it and from the person who takes care of it, not only in aspects that might be shameful to talk about—like bowel habits or sexual problems—but in its ordinary constitution. The corollary of keeping secrets is, of course, telling secrets—in my clinical vignette above, the writer's *body* harbored and then exposed his passive suicidality.

Two scenes from modern fiction illustrate the body's secrecy and how its secrets might be pierced. In Joseph Heller's *Catch 22*, bombardier-narrator Captain Yossarian, lying sick in a field hospital bed, feeling very cold, recalls when his buddy Snowden was hit by shrapnel in a bomber. Snowden, too, felt very cold: "Yossarian's stomach turned over when his eyes first beheld the macabre scene. . . . The wound Yossarian saw was in the outside of Snowden's thigh, as large and deep as a football, it seemed. It was impossible to tell where the shreds of his saturated coveralls ended and the ragged flesh began." Yossarian calms his nausea and assuages his anxiety by expertly exposing and then bandaging the large leg wound. He is proud of his corpsmanlike accomplishment.

But Snowden keeps complaining that he is cold, and suddenly the fatal wound comes into sight: "[Yossarian] saw a strangely colored stain seeping through the coveralls just above the armhole of Snowden's flak suit. Yossarian felt his heart stop, then pound so violently he found it difficult to breathe. Snowden was wounded inside his flak suit. . . . Yossarian ripped open the snaps of Snowden's flak suit and heard himself scream wildly as Snowden's insides slithered down to the floor in a soggy pile. . . . Here was God's plenty, all right, he thought bitterly as he stared—liver, lungs, kidneys, ribs, stomach and bits of the stewed tomatoes Snowden had eaten that day for lunch."

What had seemed fixable was completely out of control. "Yossarian was cold, too . . . as he gazed down despondently at the grim secret Snowden had spilled all over the messy floor. It was easy to read the message in his entrails. Man was matter, that was Snowden's secret. Drop him out a window and he'll fall. Set fire to him and he'll burn. Bury him and he'll rot like other kinds of garbage. The spirit gone, man is garbage. That was Snowden's secret. Ripeness was all."[14]

The wounded body bargains, offering up a trivial bid as if in hopes that, if accepted, it will get to keep its fatal secret. Borrowing King Lear's summative realization that "ripeness is all," Yossarian and maybe even Heller behind him acknowledge the time-bound, embodied, material, and mortal place that is all we have to call home, spicing up with savage irony (the stewed tomatoes in among the organs) the mournful doom of death.

The opposite bid is tendered in the poet and physician William Carlos Williams's short story "Old Doc Rivers" in which the wounded body surrenders itself into the hands of others. Doc Rivers is called to an East Hazelton, N.J., apartment because the elderly harness maker, Mr. Frankel, has abdominal pain. The anesthesiologist-narrator explains that the kitchen table was set up as a makeshift operating table.

> As soon as I had entered, Rivers called into the hall for the old fellow to come on along, we were ready for him. He had been in bed in the front of the house and I shall never forget my surprise and the shock to my sense of propriety when I saw Frankel, whom I knew, coming down the narrow, dark corridor of the apartment in his bare feet and an old-fashioned nightgown that reached just to his knees. He was holding his painful belly with both hands while his scared wife accompanied him solicitously on one side.
>
> The old fellow was too sick for that sort of thing. . . . Rivers made the incision. He took one look and shrugged his shoulders. It was a ruptured appendix with advanced general peritonitis. He shoved in a drain and let it go at that, the right thing to do. But the patient died next day.[15]

See how these examples bring the body center stage? Yes, Yossarian, man is matter, and ripeness is all. It is the very *matter* of the body that compels our interest. It is the time-boundedness of its ripening, whether in the youthfulness of the soldier killed in warfare or in the advanced age of Mr. Frankel succumbing to infection, that we pay heed to the body's power. In both fictional scenes, the sick body defamiliarizes ordinary sights and events. The bombardier is driven to physical symptoms himself by the sight of his buddy's wound—and, in fact, it is his remote experience of being cold that brings the event to mind at all. Doc Rivers's anesthesiologist is disoriented by the view of the harness-maker moving down the hallway with painful belly in hand, his sense of propriety shocked. Both viewings of the injured body involve the viewers in complex actions—blame, guilt, efforts to respond to the violence done to the other's body—that reflect fundamentally on their own sense of self.

Keeping secrets from one another is only one of the ways that the body and the person who lives in it can work at cross-purposes. Sometimes, especially in the clinical setting, the body and the person who lives in the body actively disagree. They can tell contradictory stories that either baffle the auditor or make him choose sides. The following transcript is a tape-recorded interview between a patient and an internist, chosen almost at random from a research database of audiotaped medical interviews. This doctor and this patient are meeting for the first time in a general medical clinic in a teaching hospital. (Permission has been granted to publish the interview, anonymously, for educational purposes.[16]) In the earlier part of the interview, the patient, a 65-year-old retired truck driver, has explained that he has had chest pain, back pain, and shortness of breath.

D: Now tell me about the shortness of breath. You had that, obviously, back in 1982, when you were in the hospital.
    P: I been having that.
    D: And . . .
    P: It start getting worse
D: When?
P: Well, like I was when I, just a little I say a little before I quit work.
    D: Un-hunh . . .
P: It started, you know, I started working, I be working and I be flipping that heavy stuff, and all of a sudden you know I mean it would hit me and I would have to stop.
D: When did you actually stop working?
P: I stopped working in 87, I think it was.
D: 87. So between 82 and 87, you worked heavy labor, uh, working that truck, fruit produce.
P: All my life.
D: Un-hunh . . .
P: For 50 years I been doing it.
D: Long time.
P: Yessir.
D: Yeah. Uh, so in 87 you started getting more short of breath.
P: Well, since I stopped work, see, I haven't been getting that exercise.
D: Well, did you stop work because you were getting more short of breath or did you get more short of breath after you stopped working?
P: Well, I got to tell you, this leg went on me.
D: Un-hunh [laughter].
P: I mean, it got so I couldn't hop up in the truck no more.
D: So it was really your leg that made you stop work.
    P: My leg is what knocked me out of work.
    D. I see.
P: This leg here went on me, I think I had a slight stroke, I'm not sure, but I think I did.
D: Well, did you see a doctor to ask him if you.
    P: No, I didn't bother, [shared laughter] but you know it got so I couldn't, couldn't walk, see, I figured it was my back, I didn't know what it was, you know. But as it was I couldn't climb into the truck. And what good was I, you understand me, to the man?
    D: Right.

P: And I had recently, and I'm now 65, at the time I was 62. So they let me [retire] on the job.

D: Okay, let me go back to your shortness of breath for a minute and then we'll talk about this leg pain. . . .

The patient and the doctor struggle to identify the plot, or the causality, of what led the patient to retire from his job as a truck driver. Was his shortness of breath a consequence of hard work or a consequence of stopping hard work? Was the patient's retirement dictated by leg pain and not the shortness of breath at all? We hear overtones of class—"what good was I to the man?"—along with the patient's evident pride in his history of physical strength. The doctor and patient also struggle to establish the temporal structure of this plot. Notice how temporally complex is this short segment of conversation, starting with the doctor's "Now," going back and forth between 1982 and 1987, and the patient's renegotiating to begin the story 50 years earlier when he started work.

Later in the same interview, the doctor learns more about the patient's heart:

D: You wake up at night short of breath?

P: Right.

D: You do. How long has that been going on?

P: I think about a year. I be sleeping.

   D. Uh-hunh . . .

P. where for { } pretty much out of nowhere, and all of a sudden I wake up and I can't get my breath back and I sit up.

D: And how often has that happened in the last year, is it, you know, once a month, every week, every night?

P: Not every night, not every night. I figure maybe once a week, sometime every two weeks, it all depends, you know it varies.

D: Un-hunh, so and then you, and then what happens?

P: I set up. I'm in pretty good shape.

   D. Un-hunh . . .

P: I be alright, you know.

D: How long does it take before you, your, your breathing calms down?

P: Maybe about five minutes.

D: Five minutes. Anything else when that happens, do you sweat a lot, or?

P: Once in a while I might break into a sweat, if it be real warm, but that don't happen too often.

D: Most of the time, what about chest pain when that happens, do you have chest pain or not?

P: No, no, no.

D: You're not.

P: Not.

D: Okay. And, um, uh, uh, do you sleep with one pillow, more than one pillow?

P: Three pillows I sleep on.

D: Three pillows. How long you been doing that?

P: Past two or three years.

D: Past two or three years

       P: Since I quit work

D: Is that because your breathing is easier on two or three pillows?

P: In a way, yes. It helps.

D: It does.

P: Un-hunh.

The patient seems to be trying to tell a story of himself as a strong working man who drove a produce truck until retirement age, leaving his job only when his leg gave way, but who continues to be "in pretty good shape." The doctor interferes with this story, eliciting instead a shadow story of severe congestive heart failure told unwittingly by the patient. Although the patient does not know the significance of his nighttime breathlessness and his reliance on three pillows for comfortable sleep, the doctor does. In effect, the patient's body tells the doctor—over the patient's shoulder, as it were, whispering out of his hearing—about his heart disease. The patient's statement of health—"I be alright, you know"—is overpowered by the voice of his own body. In effect, the body colludes with the doctor to negate what the patient says.

However, this doctor seems to have heard the body at the expense of hearing the patient. He does not acknowledge the patient's story of being in pretty good shape, except by the parenthetical "un-hunh" now and then, because the conflicting story of heart failure told inadvertently by the patient's symptoms drowns it out. The body has material warrant, and if the patient says otherwise, his word is dismissed as untrue. The patient would be better off, most would agree, were he to have a realistic view of his compromised cardiac condition. And yet, in order to educate him about his heart disease and motivate him to accept treatment for it, this doctor needs to hear, recognize, confirm, and work with the patient's vision of himself as a strong lifetime worker who slowed down because of leg trouble and not heart trouble.

But, however distinct, the body and the person who inhabits it need not be at odds with one another. As often as they might be in conflict, the body and its inhabitant can be intimately related, the body echoing the inhabitant's interests, metonymically standing for its totality. A third-year medical student wrote in her Parallel Chart about taking care of a woman with AIDS who had a dangerously low platelet count, leaving her at risk for serious bleeding. How the student relates to the patient's platelets conveys the extent to which she has merged, in imaginative identity, with this dying woman:

> The day you started to bleed out I ran to the lab with a tube of your blood to find out how many platelets you had left. I told the lab lady that it had to be STAT, STAT, STAT because you were bleeding. She STAT, STAT, STAT-ed her way to the automated blood count machine and promptly put your tube in line behind eight others. I said No!—My blood—I meant your blood—goes in first— and I managed to get us six tubes ahead on the conveyor belt. As the row of purple tops advanced, I watched the tubes ahead of ours be picked up and stirred

by the science-fictiony robotic arm. Then it disappeared into the machine and the computer screen told us that someone named Milly Brand had 110 thousand platelets. I never thought there was such a thing as "platelet envy"—but when your count came back as two thousand, I found that I was very resentful of Milly Brand.[17]

The student leaned toward this patient in her care through the intermediary of this peripheral blood component. Treating her platelets with tender regard tinged with envy demonstrates the power of her advocacy, the congruence of the student's interest with the patient's interest. This nearness is demonstrated in several of the pathographies I've introduced in this chapter. Even at the same time that a body may be in revolt against its inhabitant, and even when the body and person have to split off in radical dissociation, we also see how the body enacts the concerns of the person, how the illness distills the essence of the person's identity.

As I read the accounts of John Hull, Robert Murphy, Lucy Grealy, and Christina Middlebrook, I find myself thinking that their ordeals are overdetermined, although the authors treat them as if they are underdetermined. Here is what I mean. Lucy Grealy suffers from bone cancer of the face, and she has to undergo horrible pain, loss, and disfigurement. And yet, much of her suffering might have happened without the illness. The dysfunctionality of her family, the irresponsibility of her father, the remoteness of her mother, the psychotic illness of her brother conspire with her illness and perhaps would, even without her cancer, have bracketed the joy of her childhood and adolescence. She didn't *need* the cancer to have undergone her ordeal. John Hull may not have needed his blindness to experience his limits as a father and husband, his caution as a scholar, his reserve from sociality. Blindness, of course, concentrated all these aspects of self but did not create them.

We see these ill people digging deep down into their strengths as they navigate illness, declaring *who they are* by virtue of how they face their disease. "Blindness is, for me, a kind of religious crisis," writes Hull, and yet for a person built with his elegant and earthy connection to faith, so would have any reversal of health or happiness.[18] Robert Murphy's professional training as an anthropologist endows him with powerful frames within which to behold his own losses. His account is peopled not by family members or friends as much as it is buoyed up by favorite scholars—Merleau-Ponty, Victor Turner, Lévi-Strauss—and their ideas. *He lives through his illness the way he lives through his life.* "Paralysis is an allegory of life," he writes. "[T]he battle of life's wounded against isolation, dependency, denigration, and entropy . . . is the highest expression of the human rage for life, the ultimate purpose of our species—paralytics, and all the disabled, are actors in a Passion Play, mummers in search of Resurrection."[19] And Christina Middlebrook finds within her practice as a Jungian analyst the concepts, the beliefs, and the cosmic unity that illuminate her best path through the pain and loss of early death toward meaning. It is who she is that shines through her illness. *Who she is and not what she has* is what marks her illness.

Audre Lorde makes this point irrevocably clear. In her *Cancer Journals,* this feminist lesbian African American poet writes, "Each woman responds to the crisis that breast cancer brings to her life out of a whole pattern, which is the design of who she is and how her life has been lived."[20] Although an illness might trigger dissociation from life, it can also distill the life, concentrate all its deepest meanings, heighten its organizing principles, expose its underlying unity. This is not to say that illness is a gift (even though several authors of illness narratives indeed describe gifts—the heightened sense of hearing for the blind person, the realization of the worth of the mind for the paralyzed person) but rather that, as it takes away, illness also gives searing clarity about the life being lived around it.

NARRATIVE TRUTH, CORPOREAL TRUTH

How, then, can the tales of illness be heard? If illness prompts secrets, conflicts, and contradiction along with brave sincerity and distilled identity, how must those professionally committed to caring for the sick adequately hear them speak? What is asked of those who sit by the bed of the patient, those who sit across the desk from the patient, those who hear demands for information and guidance? What is required is the skill of stereophonic listening, the ability to hear the body and the person who inhabits it. What is required is the capacity to recognize the many voices of sickness—in their contradiction, their secrecy, and their exposure of the self.

When Christina Middlebrook underwent her bone marrow transplant and the radical dissociation it occasioned, she relied on her witnesses to keep her alive. "Without the periodic witness . . . who knew who I was, *I* could not know myself. . . . I was blessed with sympathetic witnesses . . . who came regularly to my bedside and, unwittingly, held my identity for me when I dared not."[21]

This insight, remarkably clear, tells health professionals what to do at the bedside or in the office. "The staff was diligent in involving me, the me that acted as though *I* was present, in each procedure. . . . They were witnesses too" (65). How little we know about the country of pain and the nearness of death—and yet, we have these treasured communiqués from there to guide us, to teach us what we, the healthy, can do. If we listen to Middlebrook, to Hull, to Murphy, to the unnamed truck driver with heart disease, to my student talking to her dying patient, we can know with ever greater truthfulness what sickness means and what it ought to call forth in us. Middleton continues: "Like the lucky soldier in war, like some physically abused children, some concentration-camp survivors, *I* am still here. We lucky ones who have not gone mad have had witnesses who bore the truth when we could not. I think that's the only way the soul survives (72)."

These lessons about the tales of illness have immediate and practical implications for routine medical care. Once we know how both the body and the person who lives in it speak, we must seek the means to hear them both accurately with professional skill.

The body has various avenues through which to convey its messages. Visible lesions of all kinds—from Snowden's wound to Frankel's painful abdomen—signify the existence of underlying disease processes. Findings on the physical examination—an enlarged liver, blood in the stool, narrowing of the retinal arteries—suggest pathological states. Measurements of substances in the blood—sugar, cholesterol, Lyme disease antibodies, platelets—can signal disease. Looking at biopsy samples or images with enhancements of various kinds can let one *see* evidence of sickness.

As the body tells through these various ways what might be wrong with it, the person whose body it is tells what *feels* out of the ordinary. Sometimes these two sources of information are congruent, as when the patient describes pain in the leg and the X-ray documents a fracture of the tibia. At other times, these sources of information conflict, as when the patient describes abdominal pain but the abdominal CT and the liver function tests are, as we say, unremarkable.

Sadly, we know that it is not always easy to tell doctors what the matter is. Medical training enforces a particular method of listening to patients' narratives of illness. Most North American medical schools teach doctors to report a patient's history using a standard outline: chief complaint, history of present illness, past medical history, social history, family history, review of systems (questions about all organ systems of the body), physical examination, laboratory test results, formulation, assessment, and plan. Doctors, especially inexperienced doctors, *elicit* information from patients in this sequence too. You will hear a doctor saying to a patient who has just disclosed the death of a parent, "We'll get to that in Family History." Because many health professionals are uncomfortable around emotion and uneasy when the medical interview is not crisply and evidently focused on the physical problem at hand, they structure the conversation as it unfolds by interrupting the patient and redirecting him or her to furnish only medically relevant information in the order dictated by the doctor's outline.

Students of literature know that the news given by a story is imparted both by its content and by its form. I understand Joseph Heller's message about the madness of war not only by taking in what happened to Yossarian and Snowden. In addition to the plot itself, I get Heller's news by virtue of the black-comedic genre of the novel, the mood of intense irony, the images of desecration and profiteering that course through the whole text, the surreality of much of what happens, and his allusions—here to Shakespeare—that signal to me what else I should be thinking about as I read. I also gradually gather the meaning of the novel by paying attention to my own response to it—what is it that I, as reader, undergo in the course of living through the reading experience? All these formal aspects of the text *convey* very important information about the narrative world, information that is just not available in the content of what is represented.

When patients try to tell their doctors about their illnesses, they are attempting to represent something personal, frightening, meaningful, death-related and therefore far more complex than the plot of a novel. How wasteful that doctors can revoke from patients the *form* of their telling, restricting them to bare content. Instead of listening silently while a patient makes the countless narrative

decisions that must be made in conveying anything, the doctor spoils the patient's narrating by forcing it into medicine's preferred outline and sequence.
Doctors think that they are streamlining the process of telling of symptoms by
asking for the history of present illness first and then, when they are ready for
it, moving to family history. In all but the most mechanical and straightforward
problems, this streamlining sacrifices information of the most valuable sort.
Were medical listeners able to listen *for* stories with narrative sophistication,
they would mine far, far more knowledge about their patients from an equal
amount of time spent with them. If the professional listens stereophonically for
what the person says and also what the body says, he or she has the rare opportunity not only to hear the body out but also to translate the body's news to the
person who lives in it.

A NARRATIVE-CLINICAL IDEAL

We are realizing more and more how complex is the effort to *hear* both the body
and the person speak. It is folly to expect that a sick person can tell a professional what the matter is. If some oral narratives of illness sound chronological,
well organized, and coherent, it is probably because the patient wrote an outline
and rehearsed its performance. Usually, the story of sickness comes out chaoti-
cally, achronologically, and interwoven with bits of life and the past.

Like narrative truth, corporeal truth may not be immediately available
through its telling but is recoverable through its authentic hearing. There is
truth to be heard in however the patient chooses to tell of illness, body, or self.
Sometimes, though, this truth is obscured by uncertainty or emotion and must
be actively taken up from the diction, the metaphors, the genre, the mood, and
the allusions of what a patient might tell over time. The nature of the body is
such that patients cannot ordinarily just *tell* in words what needs to be heard
about it. Instead, patients convey through all sorts of ways what a good clinical
listener should be able to cohere into corporeal truth. The headache of the
healthy but anxious woman or the nausea of the child who does not want to go
to school need not be seen as lies or fabrications. Instead, these reports may
fruitfully be received as messages—about fear, about rebellion, about unac-
knowledged desires—that require more than the usual expertise to decode but
that are nonetheless replete with news, and even replete with truth.

Two clinical examples may illustrate what I mean. The general internist Julia
Connelly writes of seeing a new patient, Andrew, in the office, an elderly man
with dementia.[22] Her impulse was to turn to the patient's sister Emma, who accompanied the patient to the visit and whom the doctor knew, for the clinical
history. However, Dr. Connelly had just heard a presentation by Cary Henderson, an author himself mildly demented, who made a plea that people with
Alzheimer's disease be "talked to and respected as if we were honest to God real
people."[23] "I wanted to be a 'good' doctor, and I did not want to embarrass Andrew or hurt him by asking simple questions impossible for him to answer. . . .

Also, I was pressed for time. A discussion with him, I feared, would take forever.
. . . My own denial, too, pushed me away from him. I didn't really want to experience the depths of his dysfunction and feel the dreadful impact of these
changes on him. . . ."

However, being a "good doctor" meant that she had to surmount these disin-
centives against engaging fully with this profoundly ill man: "[H]e needed to
know through my actions that I saw him as a person and respected him as such,
normal or not. I knew I must listen to his halting and confused speech, no matter how difficult it was for me and how long it took. I must try to understand
whatever he wanted or needed to tell me (141–42)."

The doctor lets her patient tell of his problems, and in the process, he demonstrates through his language difficulties and disorientation how impaired by dementia he has become. Through circuitous channels of associative conversation
and old photographs the patient displays, the doctor learns of the patient's
childhood, his military history, and his current symptoms. She is able to join
Andrew, despite his memory deficit, in a wide range of feelings—his laughter
on looking at childhood photos of himself, his terror at recent wind storms, and
his gratitude toward her for her kindness.

> We sat quietly for a while. What should I say or do? I told him he had a disease
> that results in progressive memory loss. "This is the reason you have problems
> recalling names." I told him he would get worse and that he should move to a
> place where he could have assistance during the day. He listened and nodded his
> head. Finally he agreed to visit the nursing home. . . . I promised to visit him
> there if he needed me to. . . .
>
> As I became fully aware that Andrew's mind was severely limited, several
> things happened to me. I slowly *became* his physician, and I became aware of my
> wish to protect him from even the harm that I might cause him in exposing the
> secret of his confusion. . . . Slowly, I began to realize that I was the one who
> might be embarrassed and that I was hiding behind my personal concerns. An-
> drew's loss is a horrible one, and it will continue until his total disconnection
> from the human race occurs. I did not have the capacity to be empathic with
> him. (143–44)

Dr. Connelly demonstrates the consequences of listening for stories, even if to
do so she has to push against the gradients of habit, time pressure, and her own
reluctance to accept the reality of the patient's profound losses. Her actions ex-
emplify several of the features I have described of narrative medicine. She speci-
fies that this orientation toward her patient unfolded slowly over the time of
several office visits, that it had to encompass the singular about her patient and
not just the general knowledge she had about Alzheimer's disease, and that the
therapeutic work was accomplished within the intersubjective medium of her
fulfilling her ethical duties toward a compromised and vulnerable patient. In a
further turn of the spiral toward skilled narrative medicine, Julie both acknowledges her narrative debt to Cary Henderson for giving her the insight and
courage to *be with* her patient and offers her narrative of Andrew in a like spirit

of clinical benevolence, showing how effective medicine both begins and ends in narrative: "[K]nowing at least some of Cary Henderson's narrative encouraged me to write Andrew's narrative as a way to help me face his losses. I asked Emma to read what I had written about her brother and for permission to publish it here. Emma as well as her daughter were grateful to have read what I wrote and granted me permission to publish the essay. At the time of writing, Andrew has agreed to move into the adult-care facility (145)."

The second clinical example is written by a literary scholar about the death of her child.[24] At two months of age, Lisa Schnell's daughter is diagnosed with lissencephaly, a fatal congenital neurological disease that prevents seemingly all cognitive, motor, and sensory functions. As the mother comes to grips with this horrible diagnosis and the realization that her baby will not live beyond a year or two, she herself develops neurological symptoms of muscle twitching, difficulty swallowing, and eye spasms. She decides she must have multiple sclerosis or amyotrophic lateral sclerosis.

Her internist sees her regularly in the office. He steadfastly postpones doing invasive neurological procedures, instead treating her with gentle mood stabilizers and plenty of opportunity to talk about what she is going through:

> My doctor is a very smart, very engaging man whom I've known for about four years and who is properly sympathetic about my situation, even truly compassionate. He takes a lot of time in this first visit just to listen. He then does a bunch of rudimentary neurological tests . . . , asks me how much I'm sleeping, how much I'm eating, and reassures me that I almost certainly don't have a degenerative neurological disease. . . . "What you have," he tells me without a trace of condescension or dismissal, "is stress." . . . He tells me I am doing amazingly well given the circumstances, that I am brave and kind of inspiring. He tells me how much he admires me. (267)

When her symptoms persist for months over many visits, the doctor seems to lose his patience:

> "Lisa," he says sharply, "is there something really bad happening to you?" I look at him in confusion. "That's why I'm here," I say. "*You're* the one who's supposed to tell me that." "Lisa," he repeats, . . . "is there something really bad happening to you?" . . . I can only stutter, "I don't know, I just don't know." Then the sharpness is gone and he says to me, as though he's resigned to the futility of this exchange and maybe even a little sad about it, "Lisa, something really bad *is* happening to you . . . but it isn't this." And I sit there in paralyzed silence as he gets out a pen and writes me a referral to a neurologist. Handing me the referral, he tells me to schedule my regular follow-up for four weeks out, and he walks out of the room, shutting the door quietly behind him. (268–69)

Only after this strange interchange does it fully dawn on the mother that her symptoms are related to her daughter's illness. "The body has an amazing way of 'thinking' for itself. And my body was doing the only thing it could do to connect me with my child—it was imitating her." She realizes that she had almost surrendered to the master narrative of disease, assuming her own abnormal sensations connoted biological disease, when in truth they were telling her of her emotional loss. Once she can leave off worrying about her biological health, she recognizes clearly if mournfully her body's efforts to answer the dreadful loss dealt to her though her baby's illness. "It was my doctor's very refusal to tell his own story about my illness that allowed me to regain my health. . . . I did, gradually but certainly, get better after my narrative revelation. . . . There was no trip to the neurologist, there were no CAT scans, no MRIs, no muscle biopsies. Just a slow climb back to health. And an enduring sense of gratitude for, and the irony of, a medical doctor who was wise enough to give me a dose of my own medicine (278)."

Professor Schnell's internist was able, in effect, to listen to his patient's body when it told a nonbiological story. When he asks sharply, "Lisa, is there something really bad happening to you?" it is almost as if he addresses her body directly, knowing that the body and the self are, at that moment, telling contradictory things. His realization, in turn, enables the patient to widen the register within which she hears her symptoms and lets her hypothesize an emotional source for her distress. The physician takes the lead in guiding the self away from the body. Without his guidance (which took a measure of courage), the patient might not have found her way toward the most helpful interpretation of her body's communications.

If autobiographies tell truths about their writers of which their writers are unaware, then patients' narratives tell truths about themselves of which they are unaware. And if patients' narratives bear any resemblance to life-narrating in general—and how could they not?—then the *hearing* of these narratives is, like reading autobiographies, a demanding and daring intersubjective act, positioned between individual teller and individual listener. The autobiographical scholars Sidonie Smith and Julia Watson suggest that "autobiographical narration . . . cannot be read solely as either factual truth or simple facts. As an intersubjective mode, it lies outside a logical or juridical model of truth and falsehood."[25] When a doctor listens to a patient, he or she is not only verifying knowledge and collecting facts but also creatively reaching for a mutual interpretation of all that the patient might disclose about the self. And how terribly tragic a state of affairs that, when the contemporary Mr. Frankel walks down the hallway ready to hand over his ailing belly, the receiving doctor will not recognize him. The receiving doctor will recognize neither body nor self, much less the self-in-body. The reason that doctors' impersonality has achieved the status of crisis is not that it is any worse than it used to be but that, today, to fail to recognize the body is to fail to recognize the self.

Reflecting on their sessions with their physicians, some patients realize a particular comfort and satisfaction in telling a serious auditor about their physical symptoms. What in other settings might be draped with humiliation and reported with shame is here matter for full disclosure. The telling of private bodily sensations not only seems permitted here but also is oddly (and not perversely) pleasurable, for the auditor is equipped not only to bear witness to the telling but also to interpret what is heard, based on professional knowledge of the body. The doctor will be able to pierce through the patient's symptoms to reveal meanings that the patient himself or herself cannot find, and so the telling is not only done in order to unburden oneself of information but to obtain a specialized reading of it unavailable except through the medium of a health professional.

While a patient speaks, the doctor writes down what she says, giving evidence of its importance and worth. The tone of the doctor's voice is grave; the gaze at the patient is direct and sad. The patient feels during this exchange that what has happened to her matters to the doctor and that what she tells is important information. During the time that she tells and he listens, it is as if nothing else matters for the doctor but the patient. The pact between them is sealed not by virtue of his displaying his professional licenses or her exercising her patient's rights but by the directness of his gaze, the deliberate movement of his hand writing in her chart, and the informed drift of his questions that reveal that he has heard her answers.

Narrative medicine proposes that health professionals, as a matter of routine, be equipped with the skills that allow them to competently and naturally absorb, recognize, interpret, and comprehend the value of all that patients tell. Through training in reading, in writing, in reflecting, in decoding these many gestures of life-writing, health professionals can readily become dutiful and powerful readers of their patients' illness narrative. They can do more. Through their own powers of reflection and clinical imagination, they can recognize the plights of patients sometimes more clearly than can the patients. They can then, with deep empathy, name the suffering they see, offer themselves humbly as one who recognizes, who listens, and who cares.

NOTES

1. See, for example, Antonio Damasio, *Descartes' Error* and *Looking for Spinoza;* John Searles, *Strange but True;* Daniel Dennett, *Kinds of Minds;* Gerald Edelman, *Bright Air, Brilliant Fire* for recent contributions to this ongoing conversation.

2. This realization, I believe, explains the extraordinary popular worry surrounding genetic testing, genetic treatment, and cloning. Such medical advances raise the possibility that one can fundamentally alter the body one lives in. These advances threaten the unity of the body, even as transplants do not. If, as Richard McCann wonders after his liver transplant or as one with a titanium hip or cyborg-prosthetic limb realizes, one can no longer tell the limits between self and nonself, what would be the effect of an ability to change the very basic genetic "instructions" for the body?

3. See Fernando Vidal, "Brains, Bodies, Selves, and Science: Anthropologies of Identity and the Resurrection of the Body" for a meditation on the life-after-death of the body.

4. See Carl Elliott, *Better than Well;* Jonathan Metzl, *Prozac on the Couch;* Sheila Rothman and David Rothman, *The Pursuit of Perfection.*

5. John Hull, *Touching the Rock*, 64.

6. John Hull, *Touching the Rock*, 25, 145.

7. Robert Murphy, *The Body Silent*, 12.

8. That moving phrase, "the silence of health," is the subtitle of a book by Felix

Guyot, *Yoga: The Silence of Health.* I thank Norman Holland for finding the source of this phrase we both admired. See Drew Leder, *The Absent Body,* for a meticulous and inspired investigation of the phenomenological understanding of embodiment and its frequent absence from consciousness.

9. Jean-Dominique Bauby, *The Diving Bell and the Butterfly,* 71–72.

10. Simone de Beauvoir, *The Second Sex,* 34.

11. See a report written by an eminent narratologist on her experience in trying to narrate her own life through a serious illness. Shlomith Rimmon-Kenan, "The Story of 'I': Illness and Narrative Identity."

12. Lucy Grealy, *Autobiography of a Face,* 170. Subsequent page references to this work appear in parentheses in the text.

13. Christina Middlebrook, *Seeing the Crab: A Memoir of Dying,* 62.

14. Joseph Heller, *Catch-22,* 446–50.

15. William Carlos Williams, "Old Doc Rivers," 85–86.

16. This research project was completed in the Department of Medicine of Columbia University with support from the Andrus Foundation and the American Association of Retired Persons. With Columbia University Institutional Review Board approval, patients and physicians gave their consent for the anonymous publication of audiotaped and transcribed interviews. Interview transcribed by author following sociolinguistic conventions outlined by Elliot Mishler in *Research Interviewing* in which overlaps in speech are noted (here by tabulated turns), uninterpretable utterances are marked by curly brackets, and nonlexical utterances are preserved.

17. Permission has been granted by the author to publish this excerpt of the Parallel Chart. The name Milly Brand is an alias.

18. John Hull, *Touching the Rock,* 51.

19. Robert Murphy, *The Body Silent,* 222, 230.

20. Audre Lorde, *The Cancer Journals,* 7.

21. Christina Middlebrook, *Seeing the Crab,* 62. Subsequent page references to this work appear in parentheses in the text.

22. Julia Connelly, "In the Absence of Narrative."

23. Cary Smith Henderson, Ruth D. Henderson, Jackie Henderson Main, and Nancy Andrews, *Partial View: An Alzheimer's Journal,* 7. Subsequent age references to this work appear in parentheses in the text.

24. Lisa J. Schnell, "Learning How to Tell." Page references to this work appear in parentheses in the text.

25. Sidonie Smith and Julia Watson, *Reading Autobiography,* 13.

PART III

Developing Narrative Competence

6 ▣ CLOSE READING

Narrative medicine makes the case that narrative training in reading and writing contributes to clinical effectiveness. By developing narrative competence, we have argued, health care professionals can become more attentive to patients, more attuned to patients' experiences, more reflective in their own practice, and more accurate in interpreting the stories patients tell of illness.[1] The last chapter gave us some specific terms and concepts with which to sharpen these arguments: health professionals have to learn to hear the body and the self telling of illness, in whatever forms, dictions, and discourses they find themselves giving utterance to their reality. If patients' reports do not limit themselves to answers in our reviews of systems, then we must be prepared to comprehend *all* that is contained in the patient's words, silences, metaphors, genres, and allusions. Listening and watchful clinicians must become fluent in the tongues of the body and the tongues of the self, aware that the body and the self keep secrets from one another, can misread one another, and can be incomprehensible to one another without a skilled and deft translator.

We are beginning to conceptualize what intermediates and mechanisms might power the process from narrative competence to clinical effectiveness.[2] Scholars have postulated several candidates: development of the clinical imagination, deepening of empathy for patients, awareness of the ethical dimensions of clinical situations, and the development of the capacity for attention have all been suggested as the clinical dividends of narrative training.[3] Ongoing outcomes research—with medical students, nurses, social workers, and physicians at Columbia University, University of North Carolina, University of Massachusetts, and elsewhere—are now under way to collect information and generate data that will help us understand the nature, direction, and magnitude of the changes attributable to our teaching.[4] The more clearly we understand *why* and *how* narrative training benefits clinicians, the more fully we will achieve its benefits.

Early work in literature-and-medicine focused on teaching literary texts to health professionals and students, and much of the inaugural theoretical work in the field examines the teaching of reading in clinical settings.[5] To begin with, reading in the clinical setting will exert the same influences reading exerts everywhere. Since antiquity, readers have known that their readerly actions influence them deeply. Aristotle described the transformative powers of the pity and the fear that follow the reading or witnessing of drama, both from the spectacle and from the plot itself. In 50 B.C. Horace reminded poets that their task is "to teach and to delight" their readers. The Renaissance poet Sir Philip Sidney sharpened Horace's point, making virtue the ultimate outcome of reading and writing. Two hundred years after Sidney, Percy Bysshe Shelley proposed the imagination as the muscular mechanism for this move toward virtue.[6] Contemporary scholars continue to examine the consequences of reading, not only as technical concerns but also as matters that concern both beauty and goodness.[7]

Many of us have been struck by the parallels between acts of reading and acts of healing. One person tells a story, either writing it down or articulating it in person, while another receives that story with the obligation to make sense of it. What the reader or listener does with the writer's or teller's story will depend on the receiver's absorptive powers, interpretive accuracy, characterological tendencies, and the bank of stories in the receiver's possession with which to compare or align this one. The fate of the received story will also depend on the receiver's stance. Is the reader/listener positioned as a critic, a helper, or one seeking entertainment or distraction? What, in effect, does the receiver want to derive from the story, and for whose benefit? Unlike communication theory or interpersonal relations theory, a reading theory of the clinic encompasses the dynamics of the relationship between two people, the teller and the listener, but also conceptualizes the narrative itself as a dynamic partner in their intercourse, able of its own to alter what happens between them.

All the ground covered by the reader-response theorists over the latter half of the twentieth century is being recapitulated from a fresh start within clinical disciplines.[8] Whether in a textual relationship with a book or a clinical relationship with a patient, the reader/listener/receiver uses the self to share in the creation of discourse, neither passively containing nor rigidly dominating the production of the other. Georges Poulet claimed in 1972 that "the extraordinary fact in the case of a book is the falling away of the barriers between you and it. You are inside it; it is inside you; there is no longer either outside or inside." Such claims are repeated and updated in contemporary examinations of the ethical duties incurred in the reader by texts. In the words of James Phelan, "the very act of reading has an ethical dimension: reading involves doing things such as judging, desiring, emoting, actions that are linked to our values."[9] The reader becomes actively engaged in the matter of the book, agreeing to become in some way an agent for its use—whether to endorse it, condemn it, or join with it in finding meaning.

Posing a clinical theory of reading lets us probe claims that can be made almost frivolously when referring to fiction but that have practical and demonstrable consequences for clinicians and patients. The literary scholar Sander Gilman asserts, in assessing the field of critical theory, that in the medical humanities one can "find a model for the importance of theory as an inherent component of pedagogy. The very acts of reading and seeing in their most abstract and critical modes become one of the means by which young physicians are trained."[10] The same could be said not only about clinical training but also about clinical work itself. If so, then inspecting reading in the clinical setting may enable us to demonstrate what reader-response theorists suggest about how the reading self is used to attain meaning for the text. The clinic becomes the literary scholars' laboratory, while their theories contribute to clinicians' daily work.

As we amplify the theories and practices of narrative medicine, we lean on traditional understandings of narrative acts while being nourished by the most contemporary movements in critical theory. We see the reading practices of the New Critics from the 1950s and the analytic thinking of the structuralists of the 1960s become useful again to new readers, while their work is, of course, "corrected" or "refreshed" by the knowledge posteriorly available from scholars who have followed them. In the process of transposing literary theories to clinical work, we find ourselves making fresh use of work sometimes today overlooked, while we allow postmodern rethinking to lead us in new directions. The following account of reading borrows across the recent past within critical theory toward an emerging practice, committed to meaning, and designed to be of help as we bear witness to our storytellers.

⌷ HOW SHOULD ONE READ A BOOK?

In her essay "How Should One Read a Book?" Virginia Woolf answers her own question, provisionally, with a number of observations: "Open your mind as widely as possible, then signs and hints of almost imperceptible fineness . . . will bring you into the presence of a human being unlike any other" (235).[11] One enduring effort of literary criticism throughout the evolution of schools and stages—from the early formalisms, through New Criticism, to linguistically oriented structuralism, and through the deconstructive turn to postmodernism and now on to the new formalisms—has been to understand the reader's act. Jonathan Culler suggests in *Structuralist Poetics* that "[t]o read is to participate in the play of the text, to locate zones of resistance and transparency, to isolate forms and determine their content and then to treat that content in turn as a form with its own content, to follow, in short, the interplay of surface and envelope."[12]

To translate this sentence into ordinary English, what Culler suggests is that a text's meaning is carried in the dynamic relationship between what it is about and how it is built, and that the good reader can both understand the text's content and identify aspects of its structure that lend to its meaning. When we read Culler's sentence in the context of clinical work, its charge is doubled, for we realize that our "reading" of disease takes place at the level of the body's surface and its pathophysiological structure underneath the skin, while our reading of what a patient says takes place at the level of the evident meaning of the words and their implications buried in the clinical and/or personal state of affairs represented. It is this that we want to teach our students. We are not committed to the project of teaching medical students and health care professionals the complexities of literary theory or even the criticism of particular works. We want to make them transparent to themselves as readers, and we want to equip them with the skills to open up the stories of their patients to nuanced understanding and appreciation.

Virginia Woolf and her colleagues over time have provided some answers to her question—and not normative answers but radically descriptive ones—by looking at readers themselves, the narrator, and the process that obtains between them.[13] The reader entering a text has many tasks to perform. One task is to seek out the most fruitful "implied reader" for each text, selecting among countless possible readers the most promising one for this story or novel or poem. In his seminal work, *The Rhetoric of Fiction*, Wayne Booth explains that a "distinction must be made between myself as reader and the often very different self who goes about paying bills, repairing leaky faucets, and failing in generosity and wisdom. It is only as I read that I become the self whose beliefs must coincide with the author's."[14] A reader can deploy any number of interpretive approaches to a text, much as a clinician can mobilize any number of therapeutic approaches to a patient. The skilled reader or clinician learns to select an interpreter who "fits" the particular text or patient—for example, some texts need a forgiving reader instead of a skeptical one, and some patients need an authoritarian doctor instead of a collegial one. Developing skill as a reader or a clinician entails knowing which of one's countless registers to bring to bear on each interpretive situation. The reader adopts his or her readerly stance toward the work—based in part on the makeup and behavior of the narrator but also based on the reader's own makeup and behavior—which will *alter* the work. A sentimental person will not get the savagery of Thomas Pynchon. An obsessive person might be unable to surrender to the metaphoric travels of W. G. Sebald. It follows, then, that each reading is singular, based on the coupling of this narrator and this reader.

Readers are not static or single entities. Lionel Trilling reminded us how our assessment of stories changes as we mature: "A real book reads us. I have been read by Eliot's poems and by *Ulysses* and by *Remembrance of Things Past* and by *The Castle* for a good many years now, since early youth. Some of these books at first rejected me; I bored them. But as I grew older and they knew me better, they came to have more sympathy with me and to understand my hidden meanings."[15] In this lighthearted way, Trilling voices the power of books to read us, to alter us, to become real forces in our lives. Inexperienced readers—and the medical students and health care professionals who come to our seminars are often reading seriously for the first time—are impressed to see their store of stories accrue. They realize that stories influence one another, almost as if, within the individual reader, the works of Flannery O'Connor talk to those of Richard Wright or Toni Morrison's to Faulkner's. What literary scholars call "intertextuality" is simply this power of stories to add to the meanings of their neighbors. Students discover that stories, when read seriously and skillfully, get into their bones and have a say in what they think and what they do and who, ultimately, they are. Arthur Frank's model of "thinking *with* stories" is enacted at the start of this process, and we teachers in the clinic are the happy midwives of this life change.[16]

One of the preliminary tasks of the reader is to identify a story's teller. Although the teller or narrator is a virtual creation of the flesh-and-blood author and must not be confused with him or her, the reader forms a palpable relationship with this being in the course of reading the work. Because the reader has access to the text's characters or situations only through the one who tells the story, the narrator's position—ironic, forgiving, skeptical, naively accepting, hostile—will inflect all aspects of reading.

The good reader learns to distinguish among many kinds of narrators with differing levels of reliability and authority. Much of narratology has been consumed with the examination of the narrator. Some stories are told by a first-person narrator and others by a third-person narrator or, more uncommonly, a second-person narrator. A narrator can be situated outside the action of the plot or can be situated as a character within the plot, either as an active agent or passive observer.[17] Narrators can, by virtue of age or cognitive equipment or motivation, be reliable or unreliable. Benjy in William Faulkner's *The Sound and the Fury* is, by virtue of his mental retardation, unreliable in some aspects of telling. Maisie in Henry James's *What Maisie Knew* grows up in the course of the novel from a 6-year-old girl, accruing reliability as she grows. The governess in James's "Turn of the Screw," on the other hand, accrues *unreliability* in the course of the story as she displays herself more and more to be governed by something other than logic and careful observation.[18]

The narrator can change or multiply over the course of a work. Some stories—Henry James's "Turn of the Screw" and Mary Shelley's *Frankenstein* are prominent examples—are told by a series of nested narrators, one of whom tells the story to the next, and eventually the story, passing through many tellers, reaches the reader. Astute readers of such tales have to adopt many reading tasks at once. They must attend to each of the nested "tellings" and tolerate the confusion and contradiction inherent in reading multiple versions of one story. Ultimately, they are able to interpret each level of the story within its proper set of intentions and perspectives. Each stage of this narrative activity has its own limitations in perspective and warring motivation, although of course the potential dividend of multiply told stories is to provide a picture close to "booming, buzzing life," faithful to the dazzling complexity of ordinary reality. To make the clinical parallel, such confusing and contradictory sets of tellings obtain regularly in the hospital—the patient tells the history of present illness to the medical student, who tells the intern, who presents it to the attending physician, who writes the note in the chart!

Once the reader has entered the text and made the acquaintance of the narrator, he or she has to be ready for the reading act's transformations. Some psychologists and literary scholars conceptualize the act of reading as composed of three stages: departure, performance, and change.[19] The reader is transported to alien worlds and times, able imaginatively to partake of landscapes and events in the past and the future, given access to conversations and interior musings of actual people and fictional ones, and, in an oddly *real* way, entering personal relation with both the writer who creates characters and those characters thereby invented. For the duration of reading, disbelief is suspended so that fictional events can be experienced *as if* believable and actual. Good readers develop the cognitive and imaginative skills to conjure up for themselves in earthy and seemingly real ways that which the author and the narrator represent in the text. The town of Middlemarch is *seen* by the good reader of George Eliot's masterpiece, and the reader of Thomas Mann's *Magic Mountain* feels like an inhabitant of the tuberculosis sanatorium in the Alps. When the good reader enters a text, he or she notes and lives by its rules. Gabriel Garcia Marquez's world of magical realism sets different rules from Honoré de Balzac's world of clinical realism. A reader might be considered a guest in the home of the text, eager to see it all and take in its aspects while extending to those who live there gratitude for the welcome, agreeing to live according to the place's rhythms and demands, and taking care not to disturb its routines. Of course, when a reader finds the narrative world inhospitable or revolting, he or she can either just leave—by closing the book—or can register the distress in the critical literature or in the classroom.

What is particularly salient to clinical practice is that the reader is an active instrument for the creation of the text. The world of the text does not exist until it is taken up, imagined, configured, and undergone by the individual reader. In the words of the literary scholar Wolfgang Iser, "The literary text activates our own faculties, enabling us to recreate the world it presents. . . . The way in which this experience comes about through a process of continual modification is closely akin to the way in which we gather experience in life."[20] The reader must "climb aboard," as Iser says, a journey of not insignificant consequences (277).

While away, the reader is not a passive viewer but rather a most active participant in the events, and upon return from the reading journey, the reader realizes that he or she has been altered by the voyage.[21] This is not to suggest that critical faculties are abandoned by the reader who surrenders to the text. Not unlike the clinician's efforts to think diagnostically about a patient and at the same time to develop a therapeutic alliance with him or her, the reader categorizes, analyzes, measures up successes and failures, and deploys critical judgments of the work at hand while at the same time submitting to the world of the text. One's susceptibility to imaginative transport does not cause one's critical feet to leave the ground.

Through the cognitive and imaginative processes of transport, transformation, and merging with the teller and the told, intersubjectivity is achieved. The subject-position of the reader can be temporarily abandoned in favor of—or enriched by—the subject-position of the character or, indeed, the patient. We can choose, that is, to see the world from another's position in it. As Virginia Woolf writes, in "How Should One Read a Book?" "To read a novel is a difficult and complex art. You must be capable not only of great fineness of perception, but of great boldness of imagination" (236). This boldness of imagination is the courage to relinquish one's own coherent experience of the world for another's unexplored, unplumbed, potentially volatile viewpoint. *This* is the process we in health care must understand. One need not have experienced the patient's ordeal or even have felt sorry for him or her in order to achieve a clinical stance from which one can help: one needs to *see* the world from the vantage point of the patient and to *experience*, vicariously, events from that stance.[22]

Anne Hudson Jones has called the literature-and-medicine pedagogical approach that is aimed at such shifts in the subject-position the "aesthetic" approach, and I applaud her for doing so, for the name suggests that clinical work asks us to behold, value, and become humble in front of patients while we perform purposeful and active work for them.[23] To recognize that one goal in teaching literary texts to clinicians is to build their capacity for aesthetic appreciation sharpens the task at hand: I am not trying to train literary scholars, and I am not trying to train doctors or nurses or medical students to provide psychological care to troubled patients. Instead, I am trying to strengthen those cognitive and imaginative abilities that are required for one person to take in and appreciate the representation—and therefore the reality—of another. Whether that representation is in visual art, a fictional text, or the spoken words of a patient in the office, the one who absorbs and *confirms* the representation must have the capacities to witness and give meaning to the situation as depicted. Only then can its receiver be moved to act on behalf of its creator.

When I say that good readers make good doctors, I am thinking about very particular kinds of readers. "Close reading" is the kind of reading taught in graduate programs in literature in which the reader, as a matter of habit, pays attention not only to the words and the plot but to all aspects of the literary apparatus of a text. A phrase introduced by the New Critics in the 1940s, close reading began its career as a brash response to earlier forms of literary scholarship dominated by bibliographic or biographical interests.[24] The New Critics (including, for example, I. A. Richards, William Empson, T. S. Eliot, Cleanth Brooks, and Kenneth Burke) espoused close attention to the text itself and all the ambiguity, irony, paradox, and "tone" contained within the words themselves. Criticism since then has taken many turns away from the strong commitment to the text itself to frame those texts historically, politically, semiotically, economically, in terms of gender or sexuality or colonial status, and yet subsequent critics cannot but ground their critique in their own close readings of texts. What texts "do," we all ultimately realize, they do in the resonance achieved between the words themselves and the worlds that surround them, elicit them, and are reflected and transformed by them.

By the time a student has been coached in close reading for a period of time, he or she develops the reflexes to notice many, many aspects of a text. Training for close reading of literary texts is not unlike training for more clinical kinds of reading that health professionals assimilate. If I were to put a normal chest X-ray up on a view box (or, as we often used to do in the old Presbyterian Hospital, whose conference rooms were not equipped with such fancy equipment, up against a Hudson River–facing window), any doctor would say something like the following: "This is a well-penetrated, nonrotated film. The inspiration is adequate. The bony structures are unremarkable. The mediastinum is normal. The cardiac silhouette is normal. The lung parenchyma is without consolidation. There are no effusions." The reader has learned to pay attention to various features of the visual text, moving sequentially through a drill of specific aspects so as to capture all the news that the chest X-ray has to offer. Without the drill, the eager medical student might go straight for the signs of pneumonia without having noticed the metastatic lesion in the sixth right rib.

I have developed a drill of sorts for reading texts in which the reader examines five aspects of the narrative text—frame, form, time, plot, and desire—which I would like to share with other teachers of literature to health care professionals. It is not, of course, a coincidence that some of these aspects of the narrative text echo what I called the narrative features of medicine—temporality, singularity, causality/contingency, intersubjectivity, and ethicality. The reading drill mobilizes consideration of these features during the examination of an individual narrative text, crystallizing the abstract ideas discussed in earlier chapters through the reader's experience of each particular text. In the same way in which a medical student is trained to look at film quality, bones, mediastinum, heart, and lungs, readers can be reminded to consider explicitly each of these five textual aspects. When this drill becomes reflexive, the reader will not overlook important elements of the narrative. I have learned that my drill helps to open texts up even to inexperienced readers and that the same drill is effective whether the text is a short story, a novel, a scientific paper, a hospital chart progress note, or an entry written by a medical student in a Parallel Chart. At the risk of appearing to routinize the highly singular, creative, individual feat of reading, let me define each of these elements and show how they might be used.

🔲 FRAME

First, the reader frames the text, locating it in the world by considering many questions—where does this text come from? How did it appear? What does it answer? How was it answered? How does it change the meaning of other texts?[25] Historians refer to this kind of textual locating as "historicizing." A paper published in the *New England Journal of Medicine* has a different sort of authority than does a paper published in a clinical throwaway journal. The signature short story of a seasoned author's tenth collection of stories will be read differently from an unknown author's first story posted on the web. A progress note dated July 3 written by a medical intern should be read differently from a note written by the same author the next May, for July's intern is saturated with uncertainty and excitement over new authority and has little practical experience in treating disease. In all these cases, the particular frames of the texts ask for specific assumptions about its goals and herald particular consequences to be brought about from its reading.

We can follow Gérard Genette's tripartite description of narrative discourse as consisting of the *story*, or the actual events being represented; the *narrative*, or the text with which these events are represented; and the *narrating*, or the act of telling of what happened. In this case, our framing efforts attend to the *narrating* being accomplished. What is the narrative situation of this particular reading or listening? Who is gathered to hear this tale being told? The differences between the *New England Journal of Medicine* and *Resident Physician* include, most fundamentally, who the readers are—their status, their professional citizenry, what they had to pay to gain access to the text, how long they might keep the pages in their files for future rereadings, and so on. Some narrative situations confer either oddness or reverence on their texts. In search of the results of a patient's chest CT, my internal medicine ward team enters the radiology reading room, a dimly lit cavernous space about 40-by-60 feet subdivided by shoulder-high room dividers into sections for reading images of the chest, bones, abdomen, and head. Groups of white-coated people wander its maze, quiet as if in response to the darkness. We find the chest board, a triptych of screens in front of which sits a young woman radiologist, face illuminated by the soft blue glare. When she calls up our patient's chest CT on her monitors, she talks to the images and not to us. She stares at the pictures and, as if a medium of an absent other, she intones that which she receives from the source while we do our best to eavesdrop on her monologue. Never does she turn to talk to us; rather she gives voice to the pictures that she beholds. My intern said that if all the lights suddenly went on, everyone would blink in distress, the radiologists now evidently pale from their cave, the spell having been broken.

As a reader frames a text, he or she pays attention by necessity to its source and its destination, that is, its writer and its reader. A seemingly exasperated former reader of my first edition of Henry James's *The American Scene* wrote in the margin of a particularly mandarin stretch of prose, "What is he *after?*" In framing this text, the reader had to query the author's intention (no matter how out of fashion in literary studies such an interest might have fallen); by the act of querying the author's intention, of course, the reader exposes his or her own affective experience undergone in the act of reading. Indeed, framing the text always reveals something about the forces holding this particular writer and reader together. Each reading has its own frame, depending on the text, of course, but also on the situation of the reader and the writer—personally, temporally, and culturally.

The spatial meaning of the word "to frame" is also salient for the reader. What, in effect, is left in and what is left out of this text? How did the author draw borders around events, people, time periods, or emotions in determining the purview of the work? The power of some works depends on the narrowness of its frame. Hemingway's story "Hills Like White Elephants" achieves its force by leaving out any explicit mention of the abortion the couple is contemplating. Jane Austen's *Sense and Sensibility* and *Emma* have all the more savage an effect on the contemporary reader by limiting their overt interest to the domestic lives of their protagonists, leaving readers to fill in the enraging blanks of gender and class injustices. What needs to be contested in medicine is seldom the accuracy of observations but the restriction of interest—the frame drawn so tightly—to the biological.

Feminist critics have become acutely attuned to the gaps within texts or to what goes on beyond their endings.[26] The close reader can give voice to that which is present by inference or effect or silence alone. Like Sherlock Holmes's awareness of the dog that did not bark, the reader who adequately inspects the frame of the text will actively wonder about what's left out and will supply—if only in hypotheses—that which leaves, at best, a shadow or a trace. Deconstructionist critics spoke of the *aporia,* or gaps in meaning inherent in language itself.

Never, indeed, does one speaker of a language fully "get" what another speaker does with it. I can assume that my blue is akin to your blue, or that my use of the word "unfortunate" is not unlike yours, but I had better understand—and make room for—the limits of this assumption. Readers who develop the habit of wondering what has been left out of a text are all the more capable of decoding its meaning, and clinicians who develop this habit will, through their resultant curiosities, learn medically salient facts about the lives and health of their patients.

▣ FORM

The *form* of the text may be invisible except to those with training and skill. As Percy Lubbock writes in *The Craft of Fiction*, "The form of a novel . . . is something that none of us, perhaps, has ever really contemplated. It is revealed little by little, page by page, and it is withdrawn as fast as it is revealed; as a whole, complete and perfect, it could only exist in a more tenacious memory than most of us have to rely on."[27] We inherit from the structuralists a keen appreciation of how a text is built and how the formal elements of the text—its genre, its divisions into parts, its diction, its metaphors, the characteristics of its narrator—endow it with meaning beyond the denotation of the individual words or particular plot events. In the following sections, I pay attention sequentially to genre, visible structure, narrator, metaphor, allusion, and diction, among the more important elements of literary form. When we teach close reading, we encourage readers to pay explicit attention to each of these elements of form, the better to take the measure of not only what a text is about but how it exerts its influence on the reader. I have developed the habit of asking students to grapple with each of these categories in inspecting any text, especially when they seem inapt. Identifying the metaphors in an intern progress note or realizing that the genre of a discharge summary dictated upon a patient's death is an obituary are fresh ways to open texts—and authors and readers—to consciousness of what work the text accomplishes.

Genre: Is this text a short story, an obituary, an epistolary novel, a gothic tale, a black comedy, or a lyric poem?[28] Each type of literary text, or genre, has its own rules and conventions, requiring particular skills from the writer and calling forth particular forms of attention from the reader. A reader can be altogether misled if he or she applies the rules of reading memoir to the reading of science fiction or the rules of reading Elizabethan drama to the reading of a Beckett play.

Because a literary genre is an active, living organism that evolves in relation to its time and culture, it refreshes itself and strikes out on new ground while it recapitulates itself and gives homage to what preceded it. Much like diseases, genres are not static entities. New genres arise from old ones, old ones are revitalized, combinations of several genres appear and take the reading world by storm.[29] What is Michael Ondaatje's *The English Patient?* It is a novel, of course, but inserted within the novel are climatological disquisitions about desert sands and African winds, the physics of bomb neutralization, and ancient history as told by Herodotus. What is W. G. Sebald's *Austerlitz* but a seamless combination of dream, national memory, psychoanalytic monologue, and artist's notebook? When we realize that the hospital chart is a genre with its own strict rules of composition, we unlock a powerful method of studying the text itself as well as the actions it tries to represent.[30]

I am impressed with the impact that the identification of genre can have for inexperienced readers. The suggestion that Tillie Olsen's story "Tell Me a Riddle" is, generically, a riddle helps my students tolerate their own uncertainties through reading about Eva. A student taught me last year that Richard McCann's meditative essay "The Resurrectionist" is itself the letter of gratitude to the liver donor that is alluded to in the text. Flannery O'Connor's "The Lame Shall Enter First" might be all the more productively read in the realization that it is, indeed, like its title, a parable.

One of the implications of addressing genre directly is to make sure to include many genres in our teaching. Hugh Crawford cautioned us years ago that the conventional restriction of literature-and-medicine teachers to the genre of the short story limits the work we are able to do with students.[31] Students need the experience of living with a narrator through a long work of fiction as well as the short form. Poetry, drama, life-writing, film, and biography each bring their own generic lessons to readers and, ideally, all will be offered over time as clinicians gain competence as readers.

Visible Structure: Some works are divided into books and chapters. Some chapters have subdivisions within them. Even short stories can be built with either named or numbered sections, or at least with sections set off from one another by a double return. Observing the structural subdivisions of a text often raises productive questions. That the sections in Charlotte Perkins Gilman's story "The Yellow Wallpaper" get progressively shorter provides important information about the narrator's state of mind. Book 1 of Henry James's *The Wings of the Dove* is shorter than Book 2, leading to what James calls the "foreshortening" of his fictional development. The break between sections 1 and 2 in Lawrence's "The Odour of Chrysanthemums" occurs at the point of Walter's death, signifying what makes for meaning in these lives. Jamaica Kincaid's "The Girl" is not only one breakless paragraph—it is one breathless sentence. The chapters in "The Death of Ivan Ilych" address shorter and shorter periods of time, demonstrating, if plotted on a graph with chapter on the x axis and year on the y, an asymptotic curve toward death.

Explicitly examining the visible structure of the text allows the reader to query the meaning of the breaks, the impact of the tempo, and the message of the rhythm of the work. Even the relative length of sections can give a clue to their importance or weight. As a matter of course, I ask students to write out lists of chapters or sections, with page numbers and a few words of plot summaries, so as to alert themselves to the potential meanings of these formal elements of the text.

Narrator: Although clinical readers do not have to master all of Genette or Rimmon-Kenan, they can develop the habit of identifying in some detail aspects of the narrator. I insist that students comment on the narrator's engagement in the story, his or her access to events and character's knowledge, and position of view or focalization. I encourage them to characterize their own relation to the narrator and whether this changes over the course of the text or over the course of multiple readings.

Besides making the overarching distinctions raised above regarding the narrator's reliability and his or her positioning vis-à-vis the plane of the story and the action of the plot, students should examine experiential aspects of the story's teller. A narrator can be intimate, like Chekhov's narrator of "Ward Number Six," who invites the reader into a perilous story environment with a virtual arm over the shoulder and comforting inviting presence. Other narrators are experienced as remote, skeptical, unforgiving, or judging. The narrator of Flannery O'Connor's "The Lame Shall Enter First" judges the protagonist Shepherd so caustically and relentlessly from the beginning of the story that the reader might feel the need to defend the character against the narrator's assault. Toni Morrison in *Beloved* allows the telling of the story to gradually be taken over by the murdered baby's ghost. There are special cases in which one text has multiple narrators, either nested within one another, like *Frankenstein*, or turn-taking, like *The Sound and the Fury*.

The narrator's position toward the story or the characters may change over the course of it. James Joyce represents profound human and universal communion in "The Dead" by letting his narrator slowly move from a distant and judging stance toward the character Gabriel to an intimate, forgiving presence right by Gabriel's side. The angle of vision of the narrator in Chekhov's short story "Gusev" widens over the course of the story to include, by the story's end, the whole cosmos. The key that opens meaning in "The Death of Ivan Ilych" is the movement of the narrator over the course of the story. The early scornful, distanced, judging teller of Ivan's life slowly moves in toward Ivan, closer, more forgiving, until, by chapter 4, he or she has attained Ivan's interior and can speak *for* him as well as of him. By chapter 9, the speaker is Ivan's soul. This is the extraordinary accomplishment of Tolstoy, to have shown us how to cross that boundary into the subjectivity of the other.

The practice one accumulates in identifying narrators and focalizers in narrative fiction is of enormous benefit when one then reads such clinical texts as progress notes or admission write-ups. Who speaks? is often the pivotal question when trying, for example, to understand a patient's decision about end-of-life care or, less dramatically, about whether or not the time has come to stop smoking.

Metaphor: Metaphors can be local and fleeting images that crystallize meaning through a fresh juxtaposition or an enduring governing image that runs through or coheres a work. The nightingale is Keats's governing image in his "Ode to the Nightingale" to represent the creative spirit. The snow, general over Ireland, is Joyce's governing image in "The Dead," to suggest the forgiving universality of the condition of being human. The stuffed parrot in Flaubert's "A Simple Heart" reproduces, within its own ridiculous sentiment, Felicité's creatureliness, earnestness, and godliness. Without the parrot, Flaubert would not have been able to convey to his reader the peasant woman's contradictory stance as at once doomed and transcendent. When a British medical student reminded me that "Mum" was the word used in England both for chrysanthemums and mothers, Lawrence's "The Odour of Chrysanthemums" revealed itself to me whole.

To identify such a governing image in a work often helps to orient the reader toward its figural or even figurative meaning, a meaning in excess of the work's plot. The silver sounds of the creek in Sandra Cisnero's "Woman Hollering Creek" give voice to the entire writing project, including both the protagonist's laughter and the narrator's verbal production of the story itself. Grappling with the metaphors of the light and the sack at the end of "The Death of Ivan Ilych" enables the reader to come to terms with dying. The work of such linguists and anthropologists as Cynthia Ozick, George Lakoff and Mark Johnson, and James Boyd White help us to understand the primacy of metaphorical thinking in not just literary acts but also all our acts of thinking and living. All thinking, they claim, including scientific and mathematical as well as poetic, is metaphorical, because metaphor is how the human brain travels.[32]

Allusion: All texts speak to other texts—they cannot help it—and the close reader is alert to the echoes of these intertextual conversations. For example, the monster in *Frankenstein* learns English by reading a found copy of *Paradise Lost;* only once the reader has identified *Frankenstein* as a retelling of Milton's dramatic poem can he or she fully understand the meaning of Shelley's masterpiece. Henry James's story "The Beast in the Jungle" includes a deathbed scene—in which the dying heroine, May Bartram, forgives the thick-skulled protagonist, John Marcher—that seems to many readers to be the scene missing from James's *Wings of the Dove.* By reading "The Beast," readers finally know what *Wings* heroine Milly Theale might have said to her less-than-courageous suitor Merton Densher. Readers get anxious at their paltry store of stories early in their reading careers, and their teachers have to help them through this affective state while they accumulate—patiently, over time—the great expanse within the narrative intertext.

Diction: Diction is the linguistic register in which a work is written. Some texts are written conversationally or casually, like Raymond Carver's "Cathedral" that opens with "This blind man, an old friend of my wife's, he was on his way to spend the night." Others have biblical dictions, like "Odour of Chrysanthemums": "She was afraid with a bottomless fear, so she ministered to him" and "And now she saw, and turned silent, in seeing." By characterizing the manner of language as casual or formal, breezy or bureaucratic, contemporary or timeless, the reader can identify the mood, level of gravity, kind of authority being sought, and kind of intimacy with the reader being desired by the work. Some works have inserted dictions or texts within them—of dialect, stream of consciousness, dream sequences, letters, or quoted works—that might contrast productively with the diction of the narrator.

Hospital charts have a most exhaustively controlled diction, prescribing the grammatical tense and voice in which one may write and prohibiting terms of emotion. Young students learn lessons of medicine *by virtue of the diction* in which they find themselves writing—if, they muse to themselves, I have to write "40 mg of Lasix was pushed" rather than "I pushed 40 mg of Lasix," then there must be something funny about the "I" in this world.

TIME

In teaching close reading in clinical settings, it is helpful to ask students to identify the text's temporal scaffolding in as much detail as possible. Readers who pay disciplined attention to order, duration, story-time, discourse-time, and velocity can *enter* that narrative world with new ease. Once oriented to the text's temporal structure, even inexperienced readers seem able to comprehend otherwise baffling plot dislocations or multiply narrated storylines. A simple look at the verb tenses of the story can tell the reader something about the immediacy or reflectivity of the story. That Chekhov's short story "Gusev" is told in the present tense draws the reader into that ship's infirmary and does not let up on the suspense of wondering which of us will be next to die. Iterative or progressive forms, like the sentence, "In good weather, they would go early to the farm at Gefosses" from "A Simple Heart," confer a sense of chronicity or endlessness. Time becomes cyclic instead of pointed toward a goal, suggesting either timeless, mythic universality or that the reader is simply trapped in the text.

The story-time, or the time traveled in the course of the narrative's plot, lends to a text its scope and lends to the reading act its tempo. Generations elapse in Tolstoy's *War and Peace;* a day in June elapses in Virginia Woolf's *Mrs. Dalloway;* the time it takes to iron a blouse elapses in Tillie Olsen's "I Stand Here Ironing." In Susan Mates's "Laundry," the phone that starts ringing at the beginning of the story is still ringing at the end of the story, signaling a story-time of seconds. Even though the reader learns of events beyond these time periods through memories and flashbacks, the story-time is a *lived* experience for the reader, conferring acuteness or chronicity on the reading act itself.

Temporal dislocations and synchronicities are, of course, the signature of modernism. Woolf and Joyce and Proust, among others, revolutionized the act of reading and shocked readers into experiencing time anew. Mrs. Dalloway undergoes the day of her party *at the same time* that she undergoes former times bidden sensually or associatively on that day. The door hinges' squeak brings back early days at Bournton; anticipation of seeing Peter arouses the sensation of having loved him; the intoning of Big Ben asserts and contrasts conventional timefulness with each experienced achronological moment. This protagonist experiences herself at all moments of being, as it were, at once! The reader, dizzy with the suggestion that the 4-year-old and the 24-year-old of the past are indeed *within* the self as parts of the present, cannot help but open to his or her conventionally considered "former" selves. Authors will often mark their own time within texts, making specific reference to the time it has taken them to narrate a particular action or reflecting on the duration of their own attention to the story they are telling. By attending to temporal shifts within the fictional world and metanarrative statements about time outside the text, the reader can come to some provisional grasp of what this particular teller is able to do in uncloaking truth of its masquerade of time.

In his novel *So Long, See You Tomorrow,* William Maxwell adopts the governing image of the open frame of a house under construction (which he enforces by also invoking Giacometti's sculpture *Saturday 4 A.M.*) to convey the shape of life. Under Maxwell's hand, the unnamed boy protagonist plays in his future house while it is being built—no floors, no walls, no roof, but only two-by-fours framing sky, passage possible as will soon be impossible between the kitchen and the living room or between adjoining bedrooms. The openness and the blankness and the space for the sky utter, as words cannot, the yearning to be simultaneously in all rooms of one's life at once, the past, the present, and the future permeable to one another, their order random and therefore indeterminate and free from the force of fate.[33]

Alas, for the protagonist in the novel as well as the reader reading it, the walls of time come up, the past recedes—done, irretrievable—and the future waits, while the present oscillates between inevitable and unbearable. Maxwell embodies, in this work of fiction, the connection Ricoeur asserts between temporality and narrativity. The boy and the old man that the boy becomes together tell the story, not necessarily in chronological order but in an order that exposes meaning. The very structure of this or any novel—like any prose, any sentence—makes one unit follow another, in sequence, one sound and idea and step at a time, unabsorbable whole, but needing to be experienced in time.

Like many stories and novels, Maxwell's novel is *about* time. Time is its plot. Repetition, recapitulation, and working through are not only the temporal structures adopted in the telling; they are the plot elements as well (the protagonist, after all, is telling this story to his analyst in treatment long after the events occurred). What this novel, and arguably all postmodern fictions, *tries* for is a space within time, for both writer and reader, during which regret is stilled, anxiety is muted, memory is transparent, and the repetition can cease. What it achieves, more modestly, is a mournful awareness of our embeddedness in our past and a humble acceptance of the inevitability of our fate.

The reason to insist that medical readers be attuned to narrative time is to train them to be attuned to illness time. Clinical work unfolds in a highly regulated temporal frame—clinicians are anxious to nail down the chronology and duration of symptoms. Most interruptions in patients' accounts of themselves, I would think, are to ask such questions as For how long? or When did it start? Because temporality is a signature for disease, diagnosticians cannot dwell in a Woolfian or Joycean simultaneity. Nonetheless, the doctor's regimented diachrony may be at odds with the patient's expressive synchrony. Because the experience of time might be one of the most telling aspects of the divide between the sick and the well, health professionals have an urgent need to examine and make at least imaginative sense of how patients might experience time.

Patients exist within temporal caesurae, the experience of pain or suffering indivisible into "then" and "now." States of suffering erase all distinctions in time except for "before it started" and "since." Jean Stafford's short story "Interior Castle" depicts the state of pain of a young woman who has been in a car accident: "All she had been before and all the memories she might have brought out to disturb the monotony of, say, the morning bath, and all that the past meant to the future when she would leave the hospital, were of no present consequence to her."[34] These states are neither willed nor controllable, but are merely to be endured.

Our bodies age, but they also exist simultaneously in all times. We don't lose the organs we had when we were children. They merely see us through or fail us. A woman in renal failure receives her son's kidney in transplant, accepting back within her pelvis the kidney she had grown there decades ago for him. Richard McCann in "The Resurrectionist" wonders about the body he had as a child, as a teenager, now that his liver has failed him in adulthood: "I could still recall the body I'd had when I was ten, the body in which I carried what I called 'myself,' walking along the C&O Railroad tracks. . . . I could recall the body I'd had, nervous and tentative, when I first made love at seventeen. But these bodies were gone, as was the body into which I'd been born, these bodies I'd called 'mine' without hesitation, intact and separate and entire."[35]

Everything that has happened to our bodies is with us still—scars, infarcts, stenoses, adhesions. Kathryn Montgomery once told me that you could accomplish an entire medical interview by asking a patient, "Tell me about your scars." Our bodies are texts, then, clerking the records of what we have been through, hoarding evidence of past hurts, remembering as only bodies can the corporeal stabilities that keep us alive.

Teaching medical readers to attend to temporality in fictional or poetic texts can equip them with hardy tools for empathy.[36] Our own temporality can act as a silo, effectively stripping us from the existential experience of others. If we do not know what looks blue or red to someone else, how much less might we understand what an hour or a day feels like to another. This most fundamental creaturely dimension of time can separate us from others unless we take measures to imagine the times of others and to envision the inner experience of its passage. If schooled in this attention to other people's temporality, the doctor or nurse or social worker has gained access to a powerful and often unsaid aspect of patienthood and is better able to imagine the day or the hour of the life of the sick person for whom she cares.

PLOT

Readers turn with some relief from the exacting intellectual tasks of parsing a text's formal elements of frame, diction, metaphor, and time to pay attention to what happens in it. "Reading for the plot," of course, has been derided as the thing learned readers do not do. However, as Peter Brooks insists in his influential *Reading for the Plot,* the most accomplished readers never outgrow their hunger to find out "what happened" or their thirst to read to the end of the story. Indeed, any true textual desire has to be built on the youthful, spontaneous desire to travel, with one's author, toward wherever the plot might lead. "Plot . . . thus comes to appear one central way in which we as readers make sense, first of the text, and then, using the text as an interpretive model, of life."[37] Getting to know and living with a story's characters, entering imaginatively into its setting, and undergoing its events seem to many to be the fundamental things one *does* with a story.

The plot of a story is like a protein, a string of amino acids. The bare sequence of amino acids does not suffice for the protein to do things. In addition to an *order,* the protein needs a *shape* to work. It needs to be curled upon itself to form contact points or sites for other molecules. The hemoglobin molecule, for example, is a long string of amino acids that is looped in a way to accommodate, in its interior, an atom of iron. Only when configured so that there is a nest for the iron atom can the protein fulfill its duty of carrying oxygen. In like manner, the plot begins as a string of chronologically related events. Usually, such events can be spoken in a few sentences: "John Marcher and May Bartram meet in Naples and are caught in a thunderstorm in a small boat in the bay. Many years later, they meet again at a mutual friend's country home and fall into a casual intimacy. They never marry, in part because of Marcher's fatalistic belief that something terrible will happen to him. May offers her love to Marcher, but Marcher does not hear her. Only upon May's death of a disorder of the blood does Marcher realize his terrible mistake in not having accepted and returned May's love." Built on this slim scaffolding of plot, James's "The Beast in the Jungle," deploys tremendous intensity and meaning by virtue not of "what happened" but by virtue of how what happened unfolds, curls upon itself in reflective flashbacks and frightened efforts to see into the future. What is "held" within the nests of this curled up string of events is May's silent love, Marcher's odious solipsism, the place of marriage in ordinary lives, the sources of the anguish of grief, and the sense of how one's worth depends on other's mournfulness on one's death.

One cannot, of course, separate the plot from the form in which it is given. In describing the relation of the plot (James calls it the "idea") to its form in the essay "The Art of Fiction," James writes that "in proportion as the work is successful the idea permeates and penetrates it, informs and animates it, so that every word and every punctuation-point contribute directly to the expression, in that proportion do we lose our sense of the story being a blade which may be drawn more or less out of its sheath. The story and the novel, the idea and the form, are the needle and thread, and I never heard of a guild of tailors who recommended the use of the thread without the needle, or the needle without the thread."[38] In the same way that a biologist today would never distinguish between anatomy and physiology, the reader knows not to assert that plot is ever separable from form.

Nonetheless, something *happens* in stories—quite beyond the language used or the style adopted. And "that which happens" is not always evident— ambiguities proliferate in such modernist works as Woolf's *To the Lighthouse* or

Joyce's *Finnegan's Wake* and in such postmodern novels as Martin Amis's *Time's Arrow* or Paul Auster's *New York Trilogy*. Inexperienced readers worry that the plot is not visible to them whole. They look for *Cliffs Notes* or other kinds of assurances that they are "getting" what is meant to be gotten from a reading. Over lives of reading, they accrue confidence that their own probing into the meaning of a work will measure up to anyone else's. When Frank Kermode writes that "fictions are for finding things out, and they change as the needs of sense-making change," he hints at fiction's pluripotency, its flexibility in different hands.[39] "For the world is our beloved codex. We . . . do, living and reading, like to think of it as a place where we can travel back and forth at will, divining congruences, conjunctions, opposites; extracting secrets from its secrecy, making understood relations, an appropriate algebra."[40] He convinces us that our task as readers may be as consequential as the task of the writer, although in different ways, because we configure the events of plot into meaning.

Without doubt, the teller and the listener in the clinical setting work together to discover or to create the plot of their concerns. The better equipped clinicians are to listen for or read for a plot, the more accurately will they entertain likely diagnoses and be alert for unlikely but possible ones. To have developed methods of searching for plot or even imagining what the plot might be equips clinicians to wait, patiently, for a diagnosis to declare itself, confident that eventually the fog will rise and the contours of meaning will become clear. I do not mean to suggest that there is a straight line connecting Mrs. Ramsay of *To the Lighthouse* with the diagnostic criteria for rheumatoid arthritis or Alzheimer's disease, but that a similar combination of cognitive, affective, imaginative, and characterological abilities are called into play in finding plot in narrative and making a diagnosis in unwellness.

▥ DESIRE

In teaching inexperienced students close reading, the category of desire is both the most obscure and the most accessible. What appetite is satisfied by virtue of the reading act? What hunger seems to have been fulfilled in the teller by virtue of his or her writing act? These questions do not pertain to the desires of the characters in the work or of the flesh-and-blood author behind the work as much as to the desires of the narrator and the reader themselves. Desire powers the production and the consumption of a text, and recognizing the satisfactions of reading—Roland Barthes calls them the "pleasures of the text"—enhances not only the reward but also the accuracy of our appreciation of the text.[41]

Almost the last questions I have learned to pose to a reading class are questions about desire: What was satisfied in you by virtue of reading this text? What seems to be satisfied by the writing of it? Akin to although not identical with intention, which usually pertains to the author and not the narrator, the desire in the text connotes an almost physical experience of need fulfilled, drive attained, and state of bliss achieved. In an odd way, close reading can often be experienced as physical exertion, in which readers feel spent by a demanding activity that uses many parts of themselves and that leaves them in a state of satisfied exhaustion. Perhaps this state of exhaustion distinguishes close reading from casual reading. The casual reader reads for relaxation or distraction, fulfilling only a desire for entertainment or rest. The close reader deploys full powers of intellect, concentration, imagination, metaphorical thinking, and moral confrontation, fulfilling desires for identity, self-examination, facing up to challenge, and attaining new clarity about the world and self and other. As James describes in the preface to *The Wings of the Dove*, "The enjoyment of a work of art, the acceptance of an irresistible illusion, constituting, to my sense, our highest experience of 'luxury,' the luxury is not greatest, by my consequent measure, when the work asks for as little attention as possible. It is greatest, it is delightfully, divinely great, when we feel the surface, like the thick ice of the skater's pond, bear without cracking the strongest pressure we throw on it."[42]

Asking readers to articulate the desires awakened by a text has been, in my teaching, a reliable method of guiding them to the heart of their encounter with the text. The reader experiencing his or her desires in response to a text is *living* the penetration and transformation that takes place when incorporating a story into self. We nourish ourselves with the stories we hear and read; we metabolize them and incorporate them into our tissues, derive energy from them, become more of who we are by virtue of their fuel. To call attention to these appetites and desires acknowledges the fundamentality of reading as a human act, realizing that we do what we do as readers not only for our own good but also because our lives depend on it.

To talk about appetites and desires puts a physical slant on the actions of reading. I mean to do so, for these desires are experienced with the full body and mind of the reader. Literary scholars have become very interested in such phenomena as memory, immunity, genetics, and reproduction, not as scientific puzzles but as means by which to make sense of human experience. I believe that the root *interest* in these topics is in their corporeal reality. How we live our lives within our bodies—including, of course, our brains and synapses and memory traces and sexual passions and the like—is more and more being recognized as a critical element in our efforts to find or make meaning out of one another's creative productions.

Many contemporary critical approaches to texts are highly inflected with notions of the body. Such influential critics as Julia Kristeva, Judith Butler, Michel Foucault, and Eve Kosofsky Sedgwick base their textual concepts on aspects of the body. Butler asks, in *Bodies That Matter:* "Are certain constructions of the body constitutive in this sense: that we could not operate without them, that without them there would be no 'I,' no 'we'?"[43] One's experience of oneself, that is to say, devolves in part from one's status as embodied, and so narrative acts by definition engage reader and writer in processes of discovery and transformation that include dimensions of the actual physical processes of memory, perception, sensation, creativity, and response.

The desire arising from a text usually combines some aspect of actual physical sensation or response with intellectual or emotional desires. Perhaps "The

Lame Shall Enter First" satisfies an urge to challenge oneself with the morally revolting in order to better distinguish the saintly from the satanic. Perhaps "The
Death of Ivan Ilych" satisfies a desire to look death full in the face while recognizing and absolving all who muddle through ordinary days, ordinary lives,
with pettiness and selfishness and dread. Perhaps "The Beast in the Jungle" satisfies an unexamined desire to save oneself from the perils of intimacy and love.
The close reader will come to the end of a text having undergone something,
having experienced an event, having been altered by his or her reading. The
better one can identify the needs or longings that are satisfied in one's readings,
the more accurately can one name what the text has accomplished.

This final aspect of my reading drill differs from the preceding four—frame,
form, time, and plot—in being peculiarly well suited to literary study in the
medical setting. Facing one's desires vis-à-vis one's texts may be something more
aptly and expertly done in the department of medicine than the department of
English. It may be an area in which narrative medicine can make original contributions to literary studies, if only by virtue of our familiarity and ease with aspects of the body. By concluding with an examination of desire, my readers can
come back to earth, back to materiality, grounded again after the abstractions of
temporality and metaphor, home once again in lives of bodies and health.

🔲 Coda

As we teach health professionals and students how to read, we realize that these
habits of readerly reflection are highly valuable for the clinician who listens to
the patient, reads a note in a medical chart, or rereads what he or she has written
about practice. The simple drill to train readers to identify frame, form, time,
plot, and desire can mobilize their consideration of the enduring narrative features of medicine and of illness—temporality, singularity, causality/contin-
gency, intersubjectivity, and ethicality. The drill reconstitutes, that is to say, at a
local and textual level the more abstract features of narrative medicine and
brings them to bear on a single act of reading. It is hoped, of course, that the clinician will do the same kind of *bringing to bear* not only when reading a short
story but also when listening to a patient tell of illness.

When these reading skills are brought to bear on a clinical encounter with
an individual patient, they do their work, in part, by bridging some of the relentless divides—arising from the conflicting understandings of mortality, contextualization, causality, and emotional suffering—that separate clinicians from
patients. The clinician equipped with the skills of close reading will, we hope,
be better able to reach across these divides once equipped with the wherewithal to absorb form, understand plot, hail narrator, follow metaphor, track
time, and live in the face of desire. These clinicians will then have the capacities to attend to what patients tell them and to represent that which is heard
in a form that honors the narrative acts performed by the patient. These two
moments in the clinical encounter—attention by one as another tells and rep-

resentation by one of what another has told—are the powerful and reciprocal engines that permit the bearing of witness and development of healing affiliation in a clinical encounter. The next chapter explains how, once equipped with the formal and textual skills of close reading, the doctor or nurse or social worker can develop and sustain tremendous power to listen, to recognize, and to *matter* for the patient.

NOTES

1. A few examples of recent narrative medicine conferences and workshops give a sense of the increasingly widespread reach of the field, both geographically and conceptually: "Narrative, Pain, and Suffering" at Rockefeller Study Center, Bellagio, Italy, October 2003; "Psychoanalysis and Narrative Medicine," Gainesville, Fla., February 2004; "Narrative Medicine," panel at Modern Language Association Annual Meeting sponsored by the Society for the Study of Narrative Literature, Washington D.C., December 2005.

2. The National Endowment for the Humanities funded a two-year project specifically to address this question of the mechanisms and intermediates of narrative training in health care. I have convened an intensive study group of Columbia faculty and graduate students—Sayantani DasGupta (pediatrics), Rebecca Garden (English), Craig Irvine (family medicine and philosophy), Eric Marcus (psychiatry and the Psychoanalytic Institute), Tara McGann (English), David Plante (creative writing), Maura Spiegel (English), and Patricia Stanley (health advocacy at Sarah Lawrence College)—to think through, articulate, and test potential conceptual means by which narrative training exerts its beneficial effects for health professionals and trainees. The following chapters owe much to our deliberations over the years 2003 to 2005.

3. See Kathryn Montgomery Hunter, Rita Charon, and John Coulehan, "The Study of Literature in Medical Education"; Anne Hudson Jones, "Literary Value: The Lesson of Medical Ethics"; Jack Coulehan, "Empathy"; Rita Charon et al., "Literature and Medicine: Contributions to Clinical Practice" for some recent statements of hypotheses. Anne Hunsaker Hawkins and Marilyn Chandler McEntyre summarize these theories in their "Introduction: Teaching Literature and Medicine: A Retrospective and a Rationale" in *Teaching Literature and Medicine,* 1–25. Robert Coles had visionary ideas about these mechanisms in his *Call of Stories: Teaching and the Moral Imagination* and "Medical Ethics and Living a Life."

4. See Sayantani DasGupta and Rita Charon, "Personal Illness Narratives: Using Reflective Writing to Teach Empathy" and David Hatem and Emily Ferrara, "Becoming a Doctor" for examples of empirical studies starting to be published that systematically examine what happens in the course of narrative training in health care.

5. Anne Hunsaker Hawkins and Marilyn Chandler McEntyre, eds., *Teaching Literature and Medicine.*

6. Aristotle, *Poetics;* Horace, *Ars Poetica;* Philip Sidney, "An Apology for Poetry"; Percy Bysshe Shelley, "A Defense of Poetry."

7. See Walter Benn Michaels, *The Shape of the Signifier* for a major review of concepts of the reader's experience since midcentury.

8. See Jane Tompkins, *Reader-Response Criticism* and Wallace Martin, *Recent Theories of Narrative* for useful introductions to the school of literary criticism.

9. Georges Poulet, "Criticism and the Experience of Interiority," 42, and James Phelan, "Dual Focalization, Retrospective Fictional Autobiography, and the Ethics of *Lolita*," 132.

10. See Sander Gilman's contribution to the thirtieth anniversary issue of *Critical Inquiry*, "Collaboration, the Economy, and the Future of the Humanities."

11. Virginia Woolf's essay, published in *The Second Common Reader*, presciently visits many of the tenets of twentieth- and twenty-first-century reader-response criticism and reception theory, 235.

12. Jonathan Culler, *Structuralist Poetics*, 259.

13. See James Phelan, *Living to Tell about It* for a masterful treatment of many of the elements I have chosen to display in this brief visit to narrative theory, including the implied author, the unreliable narrator, the ethics of reading, and the desire inherent in the reading act.

14. Wayne Booth, *The Rhetoric of Fiction*, 137–38.

15. Lionel Trilling, "On the Teaching of Modern Literature," 7. Marshall Gregory makes much the same case in a recent essay, "Ethical Engagements over Time: Reading and Rereading *David Copperfield* and *Wuthering Heights*."

16. Arthur Frank, "Asking the Right Question about Pain: Narrative and Phronesis."

17. This area of narratology is plagued or blessed with a highly technical and discriminative language, distinguishing between extradiegetic narrators (outside the action of the plot) and intradiegetic narrators (within the plot's action) who are further differentiated into homodiegetic narrators (participants in the plot's action) and heterodiegetic narrators (absent from the plot's actions). I have chosen not to include this terminology in my text, but point to it here for readers who may want to consult Rimmon-Kenan or Chatman for further details.

18. See Shlomith Rimmon-Kenan, "Narration: Levels and Voices" in *Narrative Fiction*, 87–106; Seymour Chatman, "Discourse: Covert versus Overt Narrators" in *Story and Discourse*, 196–262; and Wayne Booth, "Types of Narration" in *The Rhetoric of Fiction*, 49–165 for useful summaries of these concepts.

19. See Martha Montello's marvelous discussion of the reader as traveler, relying on the work of psychologist Richard Gerrig, in "Narrative Competence." See also Charles Anderson and Martha Montello, "The Contributions of the Reader" in *Stories Matter*, edited by Rita Charon and Martha Montello.

20. Wolfgang Iser, *The Implied Reader*, 279–81.

21. A major theme of reader-response theory and of psychoanalytic approaches to literature, the personal transformation undergone by the reader extends not only to knowledge gained or emotions fleetingly experienced but deep characterological restructuring of the self. In addition to previously cited works by Norman Holland and Richard Gerrig, see the psychoanalytic literary criticism as practiced by Shlomith Rimmon-Kenan in *Discourse in Psychoanalysis and Literature*, Meredith Skura in *The Literary Use of the Psychoanalytic Process*, Norman Holland in *The Dynamics of Literary Response*, Peter Brooks in *Psychoanalysis and Storytelling*, and Peter Rudnytsky and his editorial board's publication of the journal *American Imago*, which bring literary and psychoanalytic theorizing together. Of course, this entire effort starts with Freud's "Creative Artists and Daydreaming."

22. See a collection of essays on compassion that resonate eerily with the clinical enterprise: Lauren Berland, *Compassion: The Culture and Politics of an Emotion*.

23. Anne Hudson Jones, "Literature and Medicine: Traditions and Innovations."

24. See Andrew DuBois's "Close Reading: An Introduction" in Frank Lentricchia and Andrew DuBois, eds., *Close Reading: The Reader* for an overview of the endurance of close reading since New Criticism.

25. See Tod Chambers's discussion of the framing of ethics cases in *The Fiction of Bioethics*, 17–19.

26. See Sandra Gilbert and Susan Gubar's *Madwoman in the Attic* and Rachel Blau Duplessis's *Writing beyond the Ending* for powerful examples of the dividends of attending

to that which is not said. See Toril Moi, ed., *What Is a Woman? and Other Essays* and *Sexual/Textual Politics: Feminist Literary Theory* (including essays by Helene Cixous and Luce Irigaray) and Rita Felski, *Literature after Feminism* for recent publications in feminist theory.

27. Percy Lubbock, *The Craft of Fiction*, 3.

28. See Jonathan Culler, *Structuralist Poetics* and Ross Chambers, *Story and Situation* for scholarship in the field of poetics or the study of genre.

29. See Marie-Laure Ryan, *Narrative as Virtual Reality: Immersion and Interactivity in Literature and Electronic Media* and Marleen Barr and Carl Freedman, eds., "Science Fiction and Literary Studies: The Next Millennium," a special topic section of a recent *PMLA* for introductions of new genres.

30. See Suzanne Poirier and Daniel Brauner, "The Voices of the Medical Record" and Rita Charon, "The Life-Long Error, or John Marcher the Proleptic."

31. T. Hugh Crawford, "The Politics of Narrative Form."

32. Cynthia Ozick, *Metaphor and Memory*; George Lakoff and Mark Johnson, *Metaphors We Live By*; James Boyd White, *When Words Lose Their Meaning*.

33. See James F. Mayfield, "Memory and Imagination in William Maxwell's *So Long, See You Tomorrow*" for a fine examination of this novel's temporal scaffolding.

34. Jean Stafford, "The Interior Castle," 199–200.

35. Richard McCann, "The Resurrectionist," 101.

36. Rita Charon, "Time and Ethics," in *Stories Matter*, edited by Rita Charon and Martha Montello, 59–68.

37. Peter Brooks, *Reading for the Plot: Design and Intention in Narrative*, 19.

38. Henry James, "The Art of Fiction," 63.

39. Frank Kermode, *The Sense of an Ending: Studies in the Theory of Fiction*, 39.

40. Frank Kermode, *The Genesis of Secrecy*, 145.

41. See Roland Barthes, *The Pleasures of the Text*, for the most articulate defense of these pleasures.

42. Henry James, *The New York Edition*, 19:xx–xxi.

43. Judith Butler, *Bodies That Matter*, xi.

7 ▣ ATTENTION, REPRESENTATION, AND AFFILIATION

Many of us in narrative medicine have learned how writing in nontechnical language about our patients helps us to *perceive* them, to interpret what they do, to acknowledge our own emotional responses to their plight, and to cohere all that we receive about them. Many health care professionals and educators have been attracted to narrative writing as a road toward empathy and reflection in clinical work.[1] More and more clinical settings offer trainees and health care professionals opportunities for reflective writing. Nursing students keep reflective journals as they proceed through clinical training.[2] First-year medical students are asked to write about their feelings in dissecting the human body.[3] Preclinical students in courses on the doctor-patient relationship write about their patients' lives.[4] Medical students are encouraged to write fiction or poetry to foster sensitivity and humane care.[5] Students and residents write of "critical incidents" to understand their own experiences.[6] House officers write naturalistic descriptions of what they learn about their patients while making house calls.[7] Physicians write of the meaningful experiences in their practice to process their clinical work.[8] Doctors, nurses, and social workers together write in narrative oncology sessions about their care of in-patients on the hospital units they staff.[9]

These practices share a theoretical orientation that values *narrating* as an avenue toward consciousness, engagement, responsibility, and ethicality. The reasons we write are not only to express what we have learned about clinical work to others. Anterior to this goal—as I learned from Luz many years ago—is the goal to fulfill our clinical duty toward patients. It is through writing that we can *know*, most fundamentally, what might be the case with a patient and our relationship with the patient. If we can understand clearly the passages that link the confrontation with a suffering person with the representation of that experience and the subsequent reflection on the meaning of it, we can conceptualize roads toward the eventual goals of narrative medicine—extending empathy and effective care toward the patients we serve and building community with colleagues with whom we do our work.[10]

In developing this form of medical practice, I find myself thinking about the heart. As I sit in the office with a patient, I am doing two contradictory and simultaneous things. I am using my brain in a muscular, ordering way—diagnosing, interpreting, generating hypotheses that suggest meaning, making things happen. This is the systolic work of doctoring—thrusting, emplotting, guiding action. At almost the same time or alternating with this systolic work is the diastolic work—relaxing, absorbing, making room within myself for an oceanic acceptance of what the patient offers. In the diastolic position, I wait, I pay attention, I fill with the presence of the patient. The systolic and diastolic movements of the heart together constitute cardiac function, by which the heart *acts*, and dysfunction of either is catastrophic.

▦ ATTENTION

Any effort to provide health care begins by bestowing attention on the patient. We sit in our offices, our cubicles in the ER, or our side of the green curtain separating our hospitalized patient from another suffering stranger, doing what we can to *attend* to the person who is sick. Even before we trigger the cascade of events that culminates in diagnosis and treatment, we bear witness to the patient in his or her plight. Whether we treat post-traumatic stress disorder or crescendo angina, we must begin our care by listening to the patient's account of what has occurred and confirming our reception of the report.

The state of attention is complex, demanding, and difficult to achieve. A topic of growing interest among clinicians, psychoanalysts, writers, and philosophers, attention connotes the emptying of self so as to become an instrument for receiving the meaning of another.[11] The recent movement toward mindfulness in medicine has articulated the need for a state of focused attention that requires the clinician to actively mute inner distractions to concentrate the full power of presence on the patient.[12] Such contemplative practices as Zen or Tibetan Buddhism, Sufism, Transcendental Meditation, and various forms of yoga are all avenues toward purity, concentration, and insight.[13] In the words of the philosopher Simone Weil, who in turn has studied the practices of religious mystics and meditators, "Extreme attention is what constitutes the creative faculty in man. . . . Attention alone, that attention which is so full that the I disappears, is required of me."[14]

We clinicians donate ourselves as meaning-making vessels to the patient who tells of his or her situation; we act almost as ventriloquists to give voice to that which the patient emits. I put it that way because the patient cannot always tell, in logical or organized language, that which must be told. Instead, these messages come to us through the patient's words, silences, gestures, facial expressions, and bodily postures as well as physical findings, diagnostic images, and laboratory measurements, and it is our task to cohere these different and sometimes contradictory sources of information so as to create at least provisional meaning.

One of the most memorable depictions of clinical attention is found in Henry James's late novel *The Wings of the Dove*. Young, ill, and quite alone in the world, Milly Theale seeks treatment from the doctor, Sir Luke Strett. The narrator describes what Milly goes through as Sir Luke listens to her: "So crystal-clean the great empty cup of attention that he set between them on the table. . . . His large, settled face, though firm, was not, as she had thought at first, hard; he looked, in the oddest manner, to her fancy, half like a general and half like a bishop. . . . She had established, in other words, in this time-saving way, a relation with it; and the relation was the special trophy that, for the hour, she bore off. It was like an absolute possession, a new resource altogether, something done up in the softest silk and tucked away under the arm of memory."[15]

James knew, somehow, that to perform healing of another, one has to empty oneself of thought, distraction, and goals and to donate oneself to the other. Sir Luke *suspends* himself in order to hear Milly out. Not only does James posit the relation between Sir Luke and Milly as essential to the healing situation but he also construes it as mutually embodied—his face, her arm of memory. That this novelist—whom many take as virginal, celibate, distant from his own body—realized the corporeality of this attentive state helps us clinicians understand how fortunate we are to be able to include the bodies of our patients in our deliberations about their health.

In a remarkable essay on generative empathy, the psychoanalyst Roy Schafer writes, "Generative empathy may be defined as the inner experience of sharing in and comprehending the momentary psychological state of another person, . . . experiencing in some fashion the feelings of another person."[16] Earlier in the same essay, he cites Christine Olden who writes that "the subject temporarily gives up his own ego for that of the object" (344). Do we not feel exhilarated when we can achieve this empty attention, when we can place ourselves at the disposal of the other, letting the other talk *through* us, finding the words in which to say that which cannot be said? As an amphora, resonating with the wind, puts sound to the presence of the moving air, the listener transduces the words of the speaker into meaning.

This suspension of the self is poorly understood, certainly by medical doctors. It is not to suggest that one abandon one's clinical judgment or fund of medical knowledge when faced with a patient, nor yet that one withhold one's authentic self from the therapeutic connection. Quite the opposite. One wants to put all that one knows at the disposal of each patient, individually, in an act of fitting generosity and humility. More: one wants to join, with the patient, as a whole presence, deploying all one's human gifts of intuition, empathy, and ability to bear witness to each patient one sees.[17] At the same time, one wants to diminish one's own private concerns toward giving pride of place to the patient's concerns. "The patient," in the memorable Law Number 4 of the House of God, "is the one with the disease."[18] The Christian existentialist philosopher Gabriel Marcel articulates most forcefully and clearly the concepts of attention most helpful to clinical practice. He writes about presence and availability (*disponibilité*):

It is an undeniable fact, though it is hard to describe in intelligible terms, that there are some people who reveal themselves as "present"—that is to say, at our disposal—when we are in pain or in need to confide in someone, while there are other people who do not give us this feeling. . . . The truth is that there is a way of listening which is a way of giving. . . . Presence is something which reveals itself immediately and unmistakably in a look, a smile, an intonation or a handshake. . . .

The person who is at my disposal is the one who is capable of being with me with the whole of himself when I am in need; while the one who is not at my disposal seems merely to offer me a temporary loan raised on his resources. For the one I am a presence; for the other I am an object.[19]

The religious scholar Ralph Harper writes that "often we are so encumbered with our fragmented and shaky souls, that we may be closed to presence when it is offered, and totally unable to give our whole attention, the gift of ourselves as a whole, to anyone else."[20] Despite the seeming contradiction or ambiguity of this available and yet suspended state of the self in attention, the doctor or nurse or social worker who achieves it *knows* it, as do his or her patients, who can take comfort from the radiance and elevation of being accepted as a mystery, a singularity, a self.

Attention is achieved not only in rare times of exhilaration. There is another, more ongoing, form of attention, best described by the philosopher and novelist Iris Murdoch. Unlike the Anglo-American and continental moral philosophers of the early twentieth century, who deemed as "philosophical" activity only choices made rationally and juridically at decisive nodes in one's moral career, Murdoch confirmed attention, defined as "a just and loving gaze directed upon an individual reality . . . [which] is a result of moral imagination and moral effort," as equally worthy of serious philosophical consideration.[21] In the effort to reintroduce the inner life into philosophical discourse and to locate human freedom interiorly and humbly, Murdoch suggested that "the exercise of freedom is a small piecemeal business . . . and not a grandiose leaping about unimpeded at important moments" and that "the task of attention goes on all the time, and at apparently empty and everyday moments we are 'looking,' making those little peering efforts of imagination which have such important cumulative results" (36, 42). The stance of tonic attention—the habit of mind of an openness and readiness to absorb what we see—contributes to the day-in, day-out work of medicine by giving clinicians constantly refreshed knowledge of the patient and giving the patient an attuned and ready-to-be-surprised doctor.

This great empty cup of attention—both James's focused and Murdoch's diffused movements—has profound implications for narrative medicine, for it is the method through which we clinicians can enact our professional duty. To attend gravely and silently, absorbing diastolically that which the other says, connotes, displays, performs, and *means* is required of effective diagnostic and therapeutic work. By emptying the self and by accepting the patient's perspectives and stance, the clinician can allow himself or herself to be *filled* with the patient's own particular suffering, thereby getting to glimpse the sufferer's needs and desires, as it were, from the inside.

When we achieve this state of diastolic attention, we are available to our patients' call. We are summoned by our patients' suffering, their needs, their plight, their authentic selves. The French philosopher Emmanuel Lévinas provides perhaps the most rigorous and helpful frameworks within which to consider the presence of another person who requires clinical attention. Lévinas's work is guided by his concept of the face and the duties incurred by virtue of one's authentic contact with and response to it: "The way in which the other presents himself, exceeding *the idea of the other in me*, we here name face."[22] Lévinas's very grounds for philosophy start with ethics—before knowledge, before being—as explained most profoundly by one's responsibilities to (and one's being summoned by) the face of the other: "[T]he presence before a face, my orientation toward the Other, can lose the avidity proper to the gaze only by turning into generosity, incapable of approaching the other with empty hands. This relationship established . . . is the relationship of conversation. . . . This *mode* does not consist in figuring as a theme under my gaze, in spreading itself forth as a set of qualities forming an image. . . . *It expresses itself* (50–51)."

When one responds authentically to another, entering what Lévinas calls the "conversation," the beholder possesses "a world I can bestow as a gift on the Other—that is, as a presence before a face" (50). When we are called forth, in the Lévinasian sense, by the other's face in a clinical setting, we are called forth to join patients in the fear and pain of illness or nearness to death. At the same time, our bestowing of the gift of attention, or presence, incurs in us both responsibilities toward the other and transformations within the self: "[T]he ethical relationship which subtends discourse is not a species of consciousness whose ray emanates from the I; it puts the I in question. This putting in question emanates from the other" (195). The *I* who is so summoned, who is put into question, is the authentic *I*. The self who hears the call is the genuine self.

We are finding that narrative training and practice may help one achieve this state of attention, letting us both *hear* and *answer* the summons. Close reading, as described in the last chapter, stimulates the skills required of attention as might the reflective writing that the remainder of this chapter describes. Harper's study of presence pivots on the novels of Proust, whom he reads with the understanding that Proust "tells more than he himself intended or knew. An open-minded reading—itself an example of presence—can have enormous rewards" (5) We allow ourselves as readers to be taken up by the author or the text; we donate ourselves—our cognitive machinery, our affective responsiveness, our powers of interpretation, our memories of other texts—to the demands of form and of plot. As Norman Holland, Peter Brooks, and other psychoanalytically oriented literary theorists have suggested, this process simultaneously clarifies and reveals the self—its characteristic modes of coping with tension, its dispositions toward meaning-making—while it can lead to substantial personal change. By developing the capacity for attention, narrative training may not only give doctors, nurses, and social workers the means to hear patients more accurately and comprehend their situations more fully but also, as a powerful dividend, may help them in their search for personal meaning.

▣ Representation

There seems to be a powerful, reciprocal connection between this state of attention and the representation that takes place in the process of narrative writing. We are finding in our narrative medicine practice that the clinician must *represent* what he or she has witnessed. In many different settings—narrative oncology writing seminars for nurses and doctors and social workers who staff the in-patient oncology unit, Parallel Chart sessions with medical students who are invited to write "off the hospital chart" about their care of patients, and primary care residency sessions in which house officers write naturalistic descriptions of house calls they have paid to patients—we give clinicians permission to write in ordinary language about what they observe and undergo in the care of patients. Without extensive training or practice, clinicians are able to produce complex and moving descriptions of their patients and their work with them.

There is a tremendous and varied conceptual literature on the theory and practice of representation. From the fields of philosophy, cognitive psychology, aesthetics, literary studies, creative writing, and psychoanalysis, vast amounts have been written about the actual creative processes involved in perceiving or imagining and then rendering a situation or state of affairs, either "real" or invented, in language. Let me but gesture toward this whole continent of thinking about representation with a few citations from Henry James's prefaces and notebooks, in which he details his own processes of "showing" that which he witnesses.

In the preface to *The Ambassadors,* James writes, "Art deals with what we see, it must first contribute full-handed that ingredient; it plucks its material, otherwise expressed, in the garden of life. . . . But it has no sooner done this than it has to take account of a *process* . . . that of the expression, the literal squeezing-out, of value."[23] That which is represented *comes from* something seen, experienced, perceived, James argues, rather than from "pure" invention. Like the dreamer, the creative artist—or the doctor or nurse writing about a clinical encounter—does not sit in his or her garret, with eyes closed, making things up. Too impressionable to *not* reflect impressions, the imagination metabolizes its associated memories and sensations and perceptions, giving them new form but *originating* somewhere, at some level, from that which has been undergone. To describe the expressive process as a "squeezing-out of value" suggests that the artist does not simply tell what he or she sees but actively generates from the perceptions their rare value, using the word "expression" in its biological sense, much as one expresses milk from a nipple or secretions from a gland. James knew, that is to say, about systole! This sentence foresees Walter Benjamin's powerful description of the storyteller, emphasizing that the meaning is "expressed" from the teller as well as from the subject: "Storytelling . . . sinks the thing [being represented] into the life of the storyteller, in order to bring it out of him again. Thus traces of the storyteller cling to the story the way the handprints of the potter cling to the clay vessel."[24]

Those who theorize about the creation of visual representations have much to contribute to our beginning examination of representational writing in the clinical setting. Such scholars as John Berger and Susan Sontag, for example, dig deeply into the interior and aesthetic ramifications of *seeing* and representing visual images for others to see.[25] Without citing James's comment but no doubt having read it, Roland Barthes pays tribute to this notion of expression in *Camera Lucida,* his jubilant treatise on photographic representation. Although he distinguishes photographic representation from textual representation, he retains James's awareness that the value of a representation resides within the object being represented: "It seems that in Latin 'photography' would be said 'imago lucis opera expressa'; which is to say: image revealed, 'extracted,' 'mounted,' 'expressed' (like the juice of a lemon) by the action of light."[26] Barthes's comments help us to clarify the *actions* of representation that make it so powerful a tool in medicine: it is by virtue of the "action of light" that the image appears—be it visible light that darkens silver grains in developing film or the light of attention that radiates the subject.

It may be the case that all acts of attention—whether or not performed by gifted artists—culminate in form. We in narrative medicine are convinced that attention will not be achieved and will not work without the obligatory corollary of representation. It is a commonplace to say that no perception occurs without representation, even if it is on the back of the retina or in the occipital cortex. The neurologist Antonio Damasio describes the act of perception as that which generates knowledge of the world, "the knowledge that materializes when you confront an object, construct a neural pattern for it, and discover automatically that the now-salient image of the object is formed in your perspective, belongs to you, and that you can even act on it."[27] Consciousness, in Damasio's terms, proceeds through image-making, which is another way to say that attention demands representation. Beyond the corporeal step of neurally inscribing perceptions, the actual aesthetic practice of conferring form—in words or in visual media—may be required for the attention to be applied and to lead to therapeutic affiliation.

The contemporary writer who perhaps sheds most light on these processes of representation is the phenomenologist Paul Ricoeur. In his authoritative three-volume work *Time and Narrative,* Ricoeur sets forth a hermeneutical investigation of the ways by which human beings can comprehend their own experience in the world while they can comprehend—through the intermediary of text—the experiences of others.[28] I am drawn particularly to Ricoeur's tripartite framework of mimesis. *Mimesis,* of course, is the Greek term for representation, or imitation, that Aristotle uses in *Poetics* to describe the means by which form is donated to action to create plot. Following Aristotle's usage, Ricoeur defines mimetic activity as "the active process of imitating or representing something . . . in the dynamic sense of making a representation, a transposition into representative works" (1:33). Ricoeur sticks to Aristotle's precepts that mimesis is accomplished with textual tools—plot, character, language, thought, spectacle, and melody—which, by extension to contemporary discourse, suggest metaphor, genre, meter, allusion, and other aspects of poetic form. Not merely copy or replica, Aristotle's (and Ricoeur's) mimesis "is an activity and one that teaches us something" (1:236, n. 8). Mimesis creates something through its praxis, something that was not there before its act.

In a way that slowly becomes extraordinarily radiant and explanatory, Ricoeur separates mimesis into three stages: $mimesis_1$, $mimesis_2$, and $mimesis_3$. I had no idea, on first reading this rather arcane formulation, how useful the three-staged plan would become for narrative medicine. The mimetic act, suggests Ricoeur, contains within itself three movements, both sequential and simultaneous, each of which is required for the spiral toward creative understanding to occur. $Mimesis_1$ refers to the "preunderstanding" of human action with which one beholds the world. The beholder brings to that which is beheld categories of thought—in semantics, symbols, and temporality—that endow the perceived with the *potential* that meaning may emerge from it, and even more fundamentally, that understandable event or action can be configured from it. This preunderstanding is posited on a shared realization—shared by the entire human community of potential makers and receivers of mimeses—of what might deliver meaning. This complex process is the reverse, or the "inside-out," of emplotment, in that it is the process through which human beings recognize incipient plot when they come across it. Not unlike what I have been calling *attention*, $mimesis_1$ brings the human agent freshly and openly in front of whatever is to be beheld so as to free from it its meaning.

$Mimesis_2$ refers to the act of composition itself, the creative practice of configuring events or states of affairs into something "tellable" or representable. Through this operation, form is conferred onto raw experience, therefore making it seeable or receivable. Within form, of course, are contained all such textual devices as metaphor, diction, genre, allusion, and temporal scaffolding. Aristotle's *muthos*, or emplotment, is contained within this movement of mimesis, for the author bestows a shape, an order, and therefore a *meaning* onto that which is witnessed, dragging it up from the meaninglessness of coincidence or randomness toward the significance of emplotted story. If Ricoeur's $mimesis_1$ corresponds to my diastolic "attention," $mimesis_2$ corresponds to my systolic "representation."

Ricoeur's final movement, $mimesis_3$, refers to the consequences, for the reader, of receiving what another composes. "It is in the hearer or the reader that the traversal of mimesis reaches its fulfillment" (1:71). $Mimesis_3$ is the actual action—the cardiac function, if you will—engendered by the beholding and the representing, *for these two stages spiral toward actual change in the world*. $Mimesis_3$ "marks the intersection of the world of the text and the world of the hearer or reader, the intersection, therefore, of the world configured by the poem and the world wherein real action occurs and unfolds its specific temporality" (1:71). $Mimesis_2$, or representation, mediates between the beholding of $mimesis_1$ and the action of $mimesis_3$, enabling people to *do* things or to *change* by virtue of either having produced representations of what they see or having read others' representations. Looking ahead to this chapter's discussion of affiliation, $mimesis_3$ gives us terms with which to establish the fact that actual clinical actions—of therapeutic engagement and building of collegial community—are the inevitable and powerful dividends of achieving attention and representation.

When health professionals write, in whatever genre and diction they choose, about clinical experiences, they, as a matter of course, discover aspects of the experience that, until the writing, were not evident to them. "We have but to think a moment of such a matter as the play of *representational* values, those that make it a part, and an important part, of our taking offered things in that we should take them as aspects and visibilities—take them to the utmost as appearances, images, figures, objects, so many important, so many contributive items of the furniture of the world—in order to feel immediately the effect of such a condition at every turn of our adventure and every point of the representative surface."[29] This is from James's preface to *The Golden Bowl* just a little before the magnificent pronouncement, "[T]o 'put' things is very exactly and responsibly and interminably to do them" (23:xxiv). Action, for James—and, by extension, for me and, perhaps, for this narrative effort within health care—amounts to representing what one sees.

Routinely, we hear our clinician-writers say, "Yes, now that I have written that description, I understand what I thought or felt about this patient." It is by now routine. As we try to conceptualize what occurs *by virtue of the writing,* we believe that representing the clinical experience is a critical positional step. Once these things we live through are represented—not only in words but in genre, metaphor, time, diction, narrative situation, and structure—they can be examined from all sides. By conferring form on formless experience, the writer can display and appreciate all dimensions or facets of the situation. He or she can walk around the representation, seeing aspects around its back or over to its side that were, until form was bestowed, unavailable to the writer. With the shift in the subject position possible by virtue of writing, the writer can see himself or herself from afar or from the point of view of another actor in the scene.

Better than just talking about these things in a support group or venting session, the actual writing endows the reflections with lasting form and, therefore, gives them existence. They become "things"—I find myself thinking of texts as pagodas or pavilions or edifices of some kind—that can be beheld and inhabited by the writer and by his or her readers. My writers are very proud of what they write. We realize that they are getting better and better *as* writers, able with greater and greater power to capture their experience in language that can convey it to others. If they can capture it with greater force and accuracy, it means that they are perceiving it more accurately and more fully as it occurs. The writing not only helps them answer the call of the patient's suffering but helps them hear it. This is very radical. And so, I feel bold enough to say that representing these events enables us to attend to them.

Acts of representation combine complex processes of perception, neural handling, accruing of associated impressions, and then imaginative filling out, rounding out, *developing* that which is seen into something created anew. As the philosopher Martin Buber makes clear, these states—both embodied and spiritual—partake of art: "This is the eternal source of art: a man is faced by a form which desires to be made through him into a work. . . . I can neither experience nor describe the form which meets me, but only body it forth. And

. . . I behold it, splendid in the radiance of what confronts me."[30] Another formulation of these ideas comes from psychoanalytic theory. The writer Guy Allen reminds us of the playfulness of narrative writing for his college composition students: "Personal narratives are objects of play because they exist in a space between the student's world and the outer world. . . . Winnicott would call them 'transitional phenomena'—things that mediate the potential space between inner and outer, things which operate in 'the third area' between self and other."[31] Writing, Allen suggests, functions to free the writer from self-consciousness and, therefore, restriction into one's own subject position, enabling him or her to range beyond the self-space, like the infant with the security of the "good-enough mother" in the background, into that mediating boundary-space that bridges self with other. By no means a Xerox reproduction or neutrally given "reality," acts of representation proceed from the subject who sees, the object seen, the perspectives of view, the aesthetic "endometrium" into which this fertilized view nests, and the audience for whom the representation is being prepared.

While one person attends, the other represents, and while one person represents, the other attends. These are reciprocal and collaborative processes—no attention without representation, no representation without attention—that embroil attender and representer in situations of penetration, surrender, and mutual need and trust. And, of course, he or she who attends one moment will represent the next, making intersecting spirals within self and between self and other. These textual practices beckon us toward intersubjective relation—even with an author long dead, as in my case with James, or, more saliently here, between a sick person and a clinician committed to serve. Ricoeur's spiral of mimesis indeed culminates in action, in function, in transformative *contact* of one with another, banishing aloneness, refusing to abandon, demonstrating love.

▣ Clinical Representation: Hospital Charts

In probing these new forms of reflective clinical writing, it helps to acknowledge the enduring place of writing in clinical care. Clinicians have always written their way through every day. Whether the writing is done in fountain pen ink in the paper chart, in computer memos for online notes, or in spoken language dictated for another to transcribe, the writing doctor or nurse or social worker not only saves but also creates his or her clinical impressions, not only marks but also chooses his or her clinical actions. We have had the experience of reading our own handwriting as we move from impression to plan—"So I see I'm worried enough about his hypertension to start him on a second medicine. I'm concerned enough this might be PE to order a VQ." The plan is formulated not before being written down, but in the actual act of writing.

Close examination of how we have been doing these things may be repaid in greater power over our continued acts of attention and representation in today's practice. Before examining the third term of my triad of attention, representation, and affiliation, let us look briefly at two genres of clinical writing—hospital charts and private office records—to pose questions of form and consequence. How do these clinical representations illuminate interior aspects of the writer and the subject, and how might they inflect the actual practice of health care?

Hospital charts—in the United States anyway—share common forms, whether the hospital is in Boston, Atlanta, or Missoula. Any hospital chart you open will have the patient's name, date of birth, and hospital number stamped on each page's upper right-hand corner. The chart itself is a chronological daily record of the patient's condition, written by many different authors, each of whom records the date (and sometimes the time) and identifies himself or herself at the top of the note in a prescribed fashion—Intern Progress Note, Medicine Attending, Ethics Consultation, Physical Therapy, ENT. The temporal order of the notes is impeccably respected: one cannot write in the spaces between previously written notes, even if there is plenty of room. Indeed, one must strike through in ink empty sections of pages, preventing a later author from writing in that space. The notes themselves are iterative, repeating in the first few lines the age, admitting diagnosis, and situation of the patient, "61-year-old woman with MS, neurogenic bladder, recent ICU admission for urosepsis admitted with fever, dysuria, and change in mental status." Each note will repeat almost exactly these same words, perhaps as proof that each author has read prior entries, understands the patient's situation, and endorses the current interpretation of it.

There are comforting stabilities to charts. Surgeons usually illustrate their notes with anatomical pictures diagramming the point of maximal pain. Ophthalmologists write in a hand unreadable to the non-ophthalmologist. Neurologists tend to use roman numerals and Latin phrases. Most notes start with a clinical summary and then describe the events of the day or the hospitalization, represent the findings of the physical examination, report the results of diagnostic tests, formulate an assessment, and outline a plan. Because there can be many, many different physicians and nurses and therapists caring for an individual patient, all must read the chart in order to know the findings and impressions and plans of the others. Except in extraordinary circumstances when a case is presented publicly and discussed, reading the chart generally substitutes for conversation among caregivers.

When third-year medical students struggle to master the complexities of what gets included in a hospital note—how to structure the sentences, how to array the words on the page—many do not know that they are mastering the wisdom and habit of almost a century of Western medicine. Until 1916, each hospital ward had a recording log in which were written the events of the day for all patients on that ward. It was at my hospital, Presbyterian Hospital in the City of New York, that the brilliant idea of giving each patient a book of his or her own—the unit chart—arose.[32] Having an individual chart for each patient enabled the early hospitals to keep track of and evaluate the medical care provided by each doctor, and today's charts fulfill a similar evaluative function. What started early in the century as an effort to improve the quality of hospital care has by now become a central medical activity—"Did you write your notes?" one intern will ask the other to know how close she is to being able to go home—and a required element in the multiprofessional care of the hospitalized patient.

When we pay close attention to the hospital chart, we see that it is, indeed, a strange document.[33] Whatever the specialty of the writer, his or her chart note carries information in its form as well as in its content. As is true for novels, plays, or poetry, the news one gets from a hospital note is transmitted by the words written as well as by the formal characteristics in which it is written. Written almost entirely in the present and future tense, the chart is also written in either the passive or the imperative voice, "Abdominal film and lactate to be followed, rehydrate gently, consider tapping belly." Most of the chart is written by an effaced narrator, that is, by a speaker who mutes his or her own voice. Instead of writing, "I pushed 80 mg of Lasix," the doctor writes, "80 mg of Lasix was pushed." The differences among different individual authors are thereby minimized, even though differences among groups of writers—surgeons, neurologists, nurses—are enforced.

These implicit generic rules of writing in the medical chart mean that the implied author of a note is not an individual doctor or nurse but rather a representative from a specific discipline. When the internal medicine attending physician writes, "Follow anion gap, may need to tap belly," he or she portrays the future actions of the entire group of internists caring for this patient over the days or weeks or months of hospitalization. (During a long hospitalization in a teaching hospital with periodic changes in the membership of ward teams, there can be cumulatively more than 20 internists caring for an individual patient.) Each individual author writes as if representing the point of view of a collection of individuals that acts as if it is one individual, emphasizing the group's collective knowledge but muting the individual's actions and accountability.

By virtue of being trained to write in the style appropriate to the genre of the chart, doctors learn to suppress their own authorial voice, their own *I*. At a time when doctors valued detachment as the ideal clinical stance, the effacement of the personal point of view achieved by saying "80 mg of Lasix was pushed" was perhaps considered dutiful. By now, however, we have learned enough about the rhetorical power of form and the clinical consequences of detachment to question the wisdom of such effacement.[34] If, indeed, doctors' interpretation of the problems confronted by their patients and their resultant behavior toward them are shaped, in part, by the language and forms in which they speak about, write about, and think about these problems, then it may be fruitful to look very critically at these genres and to make choices about how we want our doctors and nurses and social workers to be writing about us.[35]

The first step in this effort is to study various clinical texts so as to understand how they work. I was given typescripts of a hospital ward log from Roosevelt Hospital in the 1880s. Here is an excerpt from a hospital admission from August 31, 1884, titled Cancer of Lung, Haemoptysis:

TJM, 24   New York   Single   [Streetcar] Conductor

PH: Father died of pneumonia, mother poisoned by mistake. Has had scarlet fever, intermittent. Denies syphilis. Drinks very little. Has had numerous hemorrhages, the first one seven years ago and the last two years ago, varying from a cup to a quart. Had night sweats.

Present Sickness: At 8:15 last night, while on his car, had a coughing spell immediately followed by a sweet taste in his mouth and bled from his mouth some 20 minutes. Took gallic acid which had good effect.

On Admission: Patient walked in bleeding profusely from the mouth. Pulse strong, at first rapid, later slowed down. Ord. Ergot, tannic acid solution.

Sept 1:   Feels better this AM. Ord. Ergot

Sept 3:   Very weak and short of breath, still spits blood clots.

Sept 4:   Very much weaker. Infusion Digitalis. Growing cyanotic, still raising blood.

Sept 5:   Patient gradually sank at 8 AM. No radial pulse. Temperature 105 and at 9:15, quietly died.

We read the formal dignity of this prose, we recognize the formats we use today, and we witness more than 100 years later this death that connects us with the lost young man and with the sad doctor who tried to save him. The story of this young trolley conductor is told in a genre very familiar to any doctor trained since the end of the nineteenth century. The case is reported with sections titled PH [Past History], Present Sickness, On Admission—much like today's Past Medical History, History of Present Illness, and Chief Complaint. And so, in addition to learning about this unfortunate conductor who dies by bleeding from the lungs, doctor-readers simultaneously feel an earthy, eerie connection to the doctor writing more than a century ago—and by extension to all doctors who think and write and reason in these special collective ways.

More than 100 years later, doctors still write similarly in their hospital charts. With Institutional Review Board permission, I cite excerpts from a recent hospital chart chronicling an unremarkable hospitalization of an elderly man with end-stage metastatic cancer who dies in his sleep.[36]

Medical Senior Resident   Admitting Note   1 AM   10/22

73 year old male with diagnosis poorly differentiated ?squamous cell cancer, head and neck, seen by Ear, Nose, and Throat service @ —— Medical Center, recommended radiation therapy but patient deferred, has not had treatment. Tumor appears to extend to neck, nasopharynx, left tonsil. In anticipation of nutritional needs, percutaneous enterogastrostomy [i.e., a feeding tube] tube placed 10/6/xx, gastric biopsy revealed (?adeno) carcinoma, poorly differentiated, chest/abdomen/pelvis CAT scan shows metastases to lymph nodes, skin nodules, bilateral adrenal masses. Presents with pain on swallowing, decreased intake by mouth, weight loss 30 pounds/3 months. Complains of pain increased at neck . . .

Social History: Married lives with wife. Has stepchildren, no children of own. Lives NY most of life, army service, born Ohio.

Exam   140/70   pulse 100   Temperature 99^2

General: Elderly Black man, lying on side, looks uncomfortable.

Head, Eyes, Ears, Nose, Throat: large infiltrative soft tissue mass; involving entire
jaw, left neck . . . left external ear canal with whitish exudate external canal interior, too painful to visualize. . . .

Lowe

This elderly man is admitted to the hospital because of a mass in his neck and
face, preventing him from swallowing. He has lost a lot of weight and is in great
pain. Upon a routine procedure to place a feeding tube, it was discovered that
this tumor originates in the stomach and not in the neck. This amazing discovery is hardly noted by the writers of the chart, who flatten this and all other
sources of mystery in this case.

The patient becomes acutely depressed and suicidal upon learning that he
has cancer, and a psychiatrist is asked to evaluate him and recommend treatment. The psychiatrist learns that the patient has a history of schizophrenia and
was hospitalized for psychiatric treatment during World War II. He also learns
that the patient has been increasingly depressed over the past few months, with
loss of pleasure, difficulty sleeping, decreased appetite, and decreased hope. The
psychiatrist orders that the windows in the patient's hospital room be locked to
prevent his jumping to his death. He orders several different psychoactive medications to be administered and a private duty attendant to sit by the patient's
bedside to prevent the patient from harming himself.

The psychiatrist approaches the care of this patient in much the way that the
internists, surgeons, and otolaryngologists approach it—with medical diagnoses
and physical treatments. The reality of the patient's suffering reaches one person
on the health care team—the private duty attendant (PDA) who sits by his bed
every day because of the risk that the patient will hurt himself. The least well
educated person on the team, this attendant is perhaps closest in life experience
and background to the patient and is able, like Tolstoy's Gerasim in "The Death
of Ivan Ilych," to bridge the divides between the sick and the well by attending
to and even representing what this gravely ill man says:

10/28/xx   Psych note

Pt reports improved mood, increased sleep. Denies any further thoughts about jumping out window. However, PDA reports pt speaks frequently of death and wish to suffer no more. Continues to appear depressed—though less so. Tolerating psychiatric
meds.

And again two days later:

10/30/xx   Psych note.   Above noted.

Pt complains of dry throat. Otherwise reports that his mood is improved. Appears
less dysphoric. Sleep improved. Wants to eat. Denies suicidal ideation. PDA reports
that patient sang song about death all day 10/29.

There are problems deciding what to do for the patient. His wife does not want to accept heroic care on his behalf, nor is she financially able to pay for nursing home care. All possible treatments are deemed futile, and the patient is declared DNR. On the last day of the patient's hospitalization, the following notes are recorded:

11/17/xx 9:45 AM   Intern Progress Note

S: Patient drowsy + lethargic this AM . . .

A/P: Pt is a 73 year old man with metastatic Gastric adenocarcinoma to the head, neck + brain. Patient with persistent bleeding from an ulcerated gastric lesion. Now with poor oxygen saturation, receiving radiation treatment. Pt stable . . .

Murray 4507

And yet an hour later, the medical junior resident is "called to see patient":

11/17/97   Medical Junior Resident Event Note

10:45 AM   Called to see patient found without respirations + pulseless by PDA + RN. Patient lying in bed with non-rebreather face mask unresponsive to verbal/noxious stimuli. No chest movements; on exam: no heart sounds; no air movement; no pulses.

Patient declared dead @ 10:39 AM today. Pt was DNR. Wife notified.

Perella 8327

What we see in this very brief stretch of text from the hospital chart is how overwhelmingly dense has become the instrumental aspect of our clinical representations. Because of the administrative and legal uses to which these charts are put, perhaps the writers are not free to express their own realizations about what the patient endures. This contemporary chart has none of the gravity of the chart from 1884, although the patient is as ill as the trolley conductor who bled to death. If one looks closely, one sees evidence that those who cared for this elderly man were moved by his suffering. For example, the admitting medical resident describes the patient's left ear as "too painful to visualize," a phrase that may contain within it merely an explanation that the doctor was unable to insert the otoscope into the patient's external ear canal because of the undue pain it caused. The phrase may, at the same time, signal a more global "pain" experienced by this young doctor upon witnessing the plight of this poor, elderly, mentally ill gentleman soon to die.

In this chart and the countless others like it, a string of medical reporters describe one aspect of the biological illness of the patient—the neck surgeon reports on the neck, the gastroenterologist reports on the stomach, the psychiatrist reports on the depression. When I read this entire chart covering a nearly monthlong hospitalization, its full weight of suffering, uncertainty, conflict, and sadness overwhelmed me. Not by reading one or two entries but by being engulfed by all that befell this gentleman and his wife, I could piece together the situation as it was obliquely and fragmentarily reported by the dozens of health care professionals who wrote in his chart. I needed to bring to the chart my readerly powers of interpretation and imagination, stitching together diverse pieces of evidence from different notes to build a sense of the patient's isolation, panic, and sense of having been abandoned. Were I actually caring for this patient, these hypotheses generated by the words of my colleagues would have prompted me, I hope anyway, to try to assuage the patient's loneliness and to accompany him in his fear.

However, I feel quite confident that I am the only person to have read this entire chart, and it is only by virtue of the iterative, relentless story of illness that I can appreciate the gravity of the suffering represented. Because I have learned to be a close reader, I can follow the plight of this man and his wife, the urgency of their need, and the affective response of his caregivers to their suffering. I do this despite and not by virtue of the formulaic, jargon-laden, and abbreviation-ridden prose in which we today couch clinical representations. It should not be so hard to get the news of a patient's situation from our charts. It should not require a Ph.D. in English to decode the complex secrets that lurk in our so-called progress notes. As we help one another develop the skills in close reading necessary to crack the codes in conventional medical charts, we might also develop more direct and transparent ways of representing the full range of what we doctors, nurses, and social workers come to know about our patients and ourselves.

▣ CLINICAL REPRESENTATIONS: OFFICE CHARTS

Hospital charts are, by definition, read by many readers who now include not only other health professionals but also lawyers, hospital administrators, so-called quality assurors and risk managers, insurance companies, and billing clerks. Sadly, the hospital chart is being lost as an instrument of reflection because it has been burdened with nonclinical functions. Because health professionals are no longer allowed to write in the chart about their disagreements or their uncertainties lest such revelations have legal consequences, the chart becomes less and less useful to those actually caring for patients. But private office records may afford more honest rumination on patient care. Doctors who care for patients in private practice keep personal files on them, written only by themselves and read only by themselves. These records may be more likely than the hospital chart to reflect the individual and personal thoughts and feelings of the attending physician, even though regulating bodies and insurance companies examine private office charts routinely. Instead of the heteroglossic, or multi-tongued, text of the hospital chart—written by dozens of health professionals but structured to minimize the idiosyncratic voice of any one physician—the office chart privileges and gives voice to one doctor's understanding of and treatment for a particular patient's clinical situation.

My father, George Charon, was a general practitioner in Providence, Rhode Island, caring for the French Canadian population who worked in the mills there. I have drawers full of his handwritten office charts, in his blue black ink, under my desk at home. As I read through a drawer of yellow charts, I vicariously relive my father's office hours. He sees a 25-year-old married woman for the first time on 8/23/73. "I delivered her 25 years ago," is the first line of the chart, with a notation of the name and address of the patient's mother. She has been "sick 3 yrs—no medical care—separated 3 yrs from husband—afraid of Drs—very unhappy—away from husb who makes life very miserable for her— She yells at daughter for no reason. 160/100!! Should have Hdur. Very anxious and depressed (was thinking of suicide)." He sees her weekly and starts her on an antidepressant and a diuretic for the blood pressure. She is able to return to work after three weeks. She continues to see him in the office regularly and consults him by telephone as well. And then, with the date specifying only "1974," my *mother,* who worked as receptionist/nursing assistant for my father, writes in the chart, "She sent us a Christmas card."

What emerges here is a synthesis of the instrumental and the reflective, in which the attention and the representation mutually support and nourish one another. At the same time—often in the same run-on sentence—that the blood pressure medicines are being started, the patient's emotional state is registered. The connection between the instrumental and the reflective in the patient's own life is intuited, as when marital difficulties intensify the symptoms of depression. The doctor's own engagement in the ongoing life of the patient is everywhere evident, both in the level of perception achieved of the patient's life and the intermittent inclusion of the doctor's own private life. On April 26, 1973, my father writes in the chart of a difficult patient with terrible vascular disease and out-of-control diabetes, "Today is Michele's 15th birthday!" He marks my sister's birthday right there in the middle of Mme R's glucose readings.

Other charts reveal a tenderness and deep commitment to the well-being of his patients. My father sees a couple in the 1960s. They are unhappy, fractious with one another, stumped. He takes the medical history, concentrates on their emotional strains, listens as they take turns complaining about their in-laws.

12/19 Treated recently at home for acute pharyngitis with Madriban tabs: throat is good today—Now: emotional tension and friction with his wife: who was present: Both give history of unhappiness at home when young. Now friction over unfriendliness with relations—he blames her for upsetting peace—she not altogether admitting guilt. Relationship between 2 is poor now.

Encouraged: stressed guilt on each party because of existing emotional instability on both sides: Enc: re keeping family unit—save it. Rx: Equamil both qid 1st wk, tid 2nd week, bid 3rd week then once. $5.

Over the next months and years, different family members are treated for sore throats, poor appetite, boils, puncture wounds, a fractured toe, cough, and wheezing. The husband quits one job, has money troubles (at one point, there is a notation in the chart, "I owe him .40 but he owes me 9.00"), goes into business for himself with a food truck of some kind. The family situation is followed as the context for the many health problems of them all. "2/27: All kinds of arguments with relations and wife. Out of control. Encour: You will be OK again. Adv walking 1 hr, milk q 2 hrs prn, vitamin tid." The occasional acts of "encouragement" amount to a modest psychotherapy. He is not dispensing the recommendations of a psychiatrist. He refers his patients quite a bit to the mental health clinic or to private psychiatrists. But what he does in his acts of encouragement is to join the patients, somehow, after having listened with what seems like great precision and regard.

As I read these charts, the practical task of learning how doctors write about their patients is suffused with the discovery of the kind of doctor my father was. It was never evident that he knew these sad, dark, angry, pessimistic, grave things about life, about the ordinary malignancies in families. The reason for him to write these things in patients' medical records must have been that he conceptualized health to include emotional health, marital stability, and sexual gratification. His medical charts are simultaneously and transparently stories of individual patients' illnesses, of an individual practitioner, of the ways of a culture, of privacy, of woe, of one person accompanying another through the darkness.

This very brief examination of medical charts suggests that some forms of writing about patients may contribute to the effort to comprehend patients' experiences and, as a dividend, the writer's own while others may, through formal means, constrain the vision of such unity. My father wrote about his patients, his own family, and himself in forms that achieved a modest unity of body, mind, and spirit. By reasons of form, audience, and function, he was able to write about his patients in ways that *helped* him to appreciate the unities instead of ways, as seen in the hospital chart reproduced above, that obscure the unities within patient and among all witnesses to his ordeal.

AFFILIATION

Let me recapitulate the argument about the relation between such acts of representation and the states of attention and affiliation that surround them. States of attention exist in reciprocal relationship with acts of representation in clinical practice. Not unlike the systole and diastole of the heart, these states, although "opposites" in direction or intent, require one another in ordinary, day-in, day-out clinical practice. All involved in the transaction—patients, families, clinicians—take their turns attending and representing. While one represents, the other attends, and then they may revolve into the complementary role. Doctors, nurses, and social workers do not always achieve Simone Weil's or Henry James's ideal and complete states of attention. Nor do they often have the time and skill to produce careful, thick descriptions of patients that qualify as rich, singular representations of all they behold and undergo in practice. Nonetheless, they try for these things. They try, as best they can, to listen to their patients and clients. They represent what they see and think in writing, one way or another, each and every time they see a patient professionally.

Narrative medicine—and its cousins literature-and-medicine, relationship-centered care, patient-centered care, and the like—has developed means of encouraging clinicians to represent more fully what they learn about patients and about themselves. This new kind of writing is reflective or creative. It is not bound by the conventions of the hospital chart. It allows for the "I" of the writing subject. It does not belong in the hospital chart. What I have called the "Parallel Chart" is an example of this kind of narrative activity—writing done in nontechnical language that captures the personal and metaphorical dimensions of meaning, for both the sick person and those caring for the sick person.

Like any effective creative writing, the reflective writing of narrative medicine understands the play of imagination, the richness of the unconscious within reach through language, and the resonance of the writerly vessel in giving voice to the subject. Unlike the studied altruism of professionalism—a consciously chosen and regulated replacement of greed by the patient's best interests—the bounty of narrative medicine unfolds through the surrender of oneself to be used as a creative instrument for the representation of the other.

Writing narratively about a patient forces the clinician to dwell in that patient's presence. In describing a clinical encounter with a patient, I have to sit silently with my memory of having been with her. The descriptions of the patient and of myself usually include very powerful interior dimensions—the biological interior of the patient's body, the emotional interior of the patient, and my own emotional interior. Finally, there is the interior of the two of us. The portrait is the portrait of a dyad. The patient/clinician dyad is doing the work, and both are critical to the work that *only these two people can do*.

I find that after I have written such a story, I am more able than had I not done so to notice things on subsequent visits. By virtue of the writing, I become invested in the patient's singular situation and am more likely to remember what occurred on earlier visits and to grasp the significance of actions, words, or feelings. This memory includes all kinds of knowledge—medication dosages, results of diagnostic tests, recent deaths in the patient's family, the patient's fears. One embarks, with the patient, on a search.

Having represented the patient, in what I recognize now as a spiral toward affiliation, I see that I am more able to attend to her the next time I am with her. We are able—mutually—to achieve presence. Gabriel Marcel describes the state of presence in *Mystery of Being*: "When somebody's presence does really make itself felt, it can refresh my inner being; it reveals me to myself, it makes me more fully myself than I should be if I were not exposed to its impact."[37] What a healing state—for the patient and the clinician—to have achieved, this communion that, through intersubjective affiliation, makes evident not only facts of illness but also aspects of self.

And so we turn the corner toward the third movement in narrative medicine's practical triad after attention and representation—*affiliation*. These narrative practices, we see now, authorize a new kind of affiliation between clinician and patient and among clinicians themselves. The spirals of attention and representation, as I have described them above and as sharpened by Ricoeur's formulation of mimesis, culminate in *contact*. The psychoanalyst Donald Moss writes about contact in the analytic setting: "Contact, taken to its limit, is . . . the sense that no matter what is about to be said, access to the object will not be lost. Without the belief in the safety of such contact, we are burdened with the threat that sectors of mind, if spoken, will lead to abandonment."[38] We in the clinical practice of, say, internal medicine or midwifery or pain medicine forget or perhaps never know how threatening is the loss of contact for sick people, how lowering the worry that some things *spoken* will disrupt the channels, will sever the connection with the listener. How can the doctor stand to hear about the pus? or the interminable pain? or the migraine that—despite all the pills and injections and hypnosis and botox—returns? How can the primipara *say* to the midwife that she fears that she is carrying a monster? or that she does not feel capable, after all this trouble conceiving, of mothering? Dr. Moss helps us in our effort by counterposing *abandonment* with *safety*. Achieving safety and refusing to abandon—not normalizing a high LDL, not reaching an HbA$_1$C of less than 6, not landing a BMI between 18 and 24—are the goals of clinical care. These other things will follow, we are convinced, once the clinician and the patient are in contact, in all the belief and safety and nonabandonment of Dr. Moss's elegant formulation.

Acts of attention and representation culminate in action. I can *do* things for my patients as a consequence of these narrative actions, achieved dutifully and skillfully. I *reach* my colleagues and teammates more systematically and person- ally and consequentially by virtue of hearing what they write about their clini- cal work and their hearing what I write about mine. All of us who read and write in clinical settings are finding that our practices build community— within medical school classes, among team members on hospital units, in the neighborhood health center between pediatric residents and community health workers. We build community—even though we had no idea we would! What seemed at the start to be a happy side effect of narrative training we now see is its primal drive: *our shared narrative acts enable us to affiliate into effective dyads of care with individual patients and into cohesive professional collectives with colleagues.*

Narrative medicine is beginning to capture and articulate the processes whereby reading and writing benefit doctors and patients. Provisionally, we can adopt a Ricoeurean model of mimesis, in all its complexity and depth, to help us to think through the triad of attention, representation, and affiliation. Medicine being as practical an enterprise as it is, we could not be satisfied with our theo- rizing if it didn't lead somewhere, if it didn't have demonstrable and replicable outcomes. Affiliations are the outcomes of narrative work—healing affiliations with patients and collegial affiliations with our fellow nurses, doctors, and social workers.

Were it not for the affiliative results of narrative medicine, it could not be sanctioned in our busy practices. I devote the remaining chapters of this book to a detailed catalog of the consequences of practicing narrative medicine and of the kinds of affiliations that result from rigorous and sustained acts of attention and representation in the clinical setting. These affiliations include mentoring communities with students, individual partnerships with patients, professional collectives with colleagues, and community networks with members of the lay public. The next chapter outlines, in very practical terms, what happens in a narrative medicine teaching session—what to expect, how to prepare, what to say in response to clinicians' reading aloud from their writing. The final section on the dividends of narrative medicine delineate, again in what I hope are very down-to-earth terms, the practical outcomes of practicing narrative medicine in the office, on the wards, and in the community.

We live through victories and defeats with our patients; we are moved by these events as they happen; we incur ethical duties toward them; and we become different people ourselves because of them. By attending to them and by representing them, we incorporate ourselves into them, becoming through mimesis not only observers but participants in an infinitely complex and generative world.

NOTES

1. See Charles Anderson's special issue of *Literature and Medicine* on writing and healing, Gillie Bolton's *Therapeutic Potential of Creative Writing*, and my "Narrative Road to Empathy."

2. C. Skott, "Caring Narratives and the Strategy of Presence: Narrative Communication in Nursing Practice and Research."

3. Jack Coulehan, "The First Patient: Reflections and Stories about the Anatomy Cadaver" and Douglas Reifler, "'I Actually Don't Mind the Bone Saw': Narratives of Gross Anatomy."

4. Marcia Day Childress, "Of Symbols and Silence: Using Narrative and Its Interpretation to Foster Physician Understanding" and Patricia Marshall and John O'Keefe, "Medical Students' First-person Narratives of a Patient's Story of AIDS."

5. David Hatem and Emily Ferrara, "Becoming a Doctor: Fostering Humane Caregivers through Creative Writing" and Suzanne Poirier, William Ahrens, and Daniel J. Brauner, "Songs of Innocence and Experience: Students' Poems about their Medical Education."

6. William Branch, R. J. Pels, Robert Lawrence, and Ronald Arky, "Becoming a Doctor: Critical-incident Reports from Third-year Medical Students" and D. W. Brady, G. Corbie-Smith, William T. Branch, "'What's Important to You?' The Use of Narratives to Promote Self-Reflection and to Understand the Experiences of Medical Residents."

7. Eileen Moroney, "Home Is Where the Residents Visit."

8. C. R. Horowitz, Anthony Suchman, William T. Branch, Richard M. Frankel, "What Do Doctors Find Meaningful about Their Work?"; Jeffrey Borkan, Shmuel Reis, D. Steinmetz, Jack H. Medalie, eds. *Patients and Doctors: Life-Changing Stories from Primary Care*; and B. B. Dan, Rosemary Young, *A Piece of My Mind: A Collection of Essays from the Journal of the American Medical Association*.

9. Joan Klein, "Narrative Oncology."

10. I again acknowledge my tremendous debt in what follows in this chapter to the National Endowment for the Humanities Study Group of faculty from Columbia University who have met throughout 2004 and will continue to work together in 2005 in the Program in Narrative Medicine. The members of the group are Maura Spiegel, Rebecca Garden, and Tara McGann of English; David Plante of creative writing; Sayantani DasGupta of pediatrics; Craig Irvine of family medicine and philosophy; Eric Marcus of the Psychoanalytic Institute and psychiatry; and Patricia Stanley of the Health Advocacy

Program at Sarah Lawrence College. Our guests have included David Morris, Anne Hunsaker Hawkins, Charles Anderson, Joanne Trautmann Banks, and Marsha Hurst.

11. See Sharon Cameron, "The Practice of Attention: Simone Weil's Performance of Impersonality" and *Beautiful Work: A Meditation on Pain;* Simone Weil, *Waiting for God;* and Roy Schafer, "Generative Empathy in the Treatment Situation" for some strands of scholarship and clinical work in this developing field.

12. The work of such clinicians as Julia Connelly and Ronald Epstein introduced internal medicine and family medicine to mindfulness as a method of attunement that can be practically and time-effectively adopted in a busy clinical office. See Julia Connelly, "Being in the Present Moment" and Ronald Epstein, "Mindful Practice."

13. See Daniel Goleman, *The Meditative Mind: The Varieties of Meditative Experience* for a useful summary of meditative paths and the psychology and outcomes of meditation.

14. Simone Weil, "Attention and Will," in *Gravity and Grace,* 170–72.

15. Henry James, *Wings of the Dove,* in *New York Edition,* 19:231.

16. Roy Schafer, "Generative Empathy," 345. Subsequent page references to this work appear in parentheses in the text.

17. See Richard Zaner, "Power and Hope in the Clinical Encounter: A Meditation on Vulnerability" for a moving discussion of the presence, *ex-stasis* (being pulled beyond oneself by another), and the evocation of a moral sense by the routines of clinical work.

18. Sam Shem, *House of God,* 72.

19. Gabriel Marcel, *Philosophy of Existence,* 25–26.

20. Ralph Harper, *On Presence,* 42. Subsequent page references to this work appear in parentheses in the text.

21. Iris Murdoch, "The Idea of Perfection" in *The Sovereignty of Good,* 33, 36. Subsequent page references to this work appear in parentheses in the text.

22. Emmanuel Lévinas, *Totality and Infinity,* 50. Subsequent page references to this work appear in parentheses in the text.

23. Henry James, *New York Edition,* 21:ix–x.

24. Walter Benjamin, "The Storyteller," in *Illuminations,* 91–92.

25. See John Berger, *Ways of Seeing* and Susan Sontag, *Regarding the Pain of Others* and *On Photography.*

26. Roland Barthes, *Camera Lucida,* 81.

27. Antonio Damasio, *The Feeling of What Happens,* 126.

28. Paul Ricoeur, *Time and Narrative.* Page numbers appear in parentheses in the text.

29. Henry James, *New York Edition,* 23:xxiii. Subsequent page numbers appear in parentheses in the text.

30. Martin Buber, *I and Thou,* 9–10.

31. Guy Allen, "The 'Good-Enough' Teacher and the Authentic Student." We owe Professor Allen a tremendous debt of gratitude for bringing Winnicott's formulations to bear on the practice of narrative writing in health care settings.

32. Stanley Joel Reiser, "Creating Form out of Mass: The Development of the Medical Record."

33. See a growing strand of textual research on hospital charts, including Suzanne Poirier and Daniel Brauner, "The Voices of the Medical Record"; Joanne Trautmann Banks and Anne Hunsaker Hawkins, eds., "The Art of the Case History"; and my "Life-Long Error, or John Marcher the Proleptic."

34. Jodi Halpern, in *From Detached Concern to Empathy,* contributed an enormous gift to clinical practice by examining for us all the pernicious roads that led to valorizing clinical detachment and the methods we might adopt now to correct this false turn.

35. See Thomas Laqueur's "Bodies, Details, and the Humanitarian Narrative" for an explication of the social source and narrative cousins of the clinical note.

36. This textual study of hospital charts, "Linguistic Analysis of Hospital Charts," was approved by the Institutional Review Board of the College of Physicians and Surgeons of Columbia University on June 1, 1997. All names, dates, and identifying data on patient and health care professionals have been changed for reasons of confidentiality. I have taken the liberty here of spelling out abbreviations and symbols in the rendered hospital chart notes in the text, because the actual text is unduly impenetrable. For example, the actual chart text of the first section reproduced here is the following:

> 73 yo ♂ w/dx poorly differentiated ?squamous cell CA H+N, seen by ENT svc @
> —— MC, rec XRT but pt deferred, has not had tx. Tumor appears to extend to
> neck, nasopharynx, L tonsil. In anticipation of nutritional needs, PEG tube placed
> 10/6/xx, gastric bx→ (?adeno) CA poorly diff, chest/abd /pelvis CT shows mets to
> LN's, skin nodules, B adrenal masses. Presents w/dysphagia, ↓po intake, wt loss
> 30#/3 mos. C/o pain↑ @ neck . . .

More extensive excerpts from this chart, with all the ungainly abbreviations and symbols, were published in my "Life-Long Error, or John Marcher the Proleptic."

37. Gabriel Marcel, *Mystery of Being*, 1:205.

38. Donald Moss, *Hating in the First Person Plural: Psychoanalytic Essays on Racism, Homophobia, Misogyny, and Terror*, xx.

8 ▣ THE PARALLEL CHART

To bring to life the conceptual frameworks of narrative writing and to demonstrate the pedagogic methods we have developed and tested in coaching narrative writing in clinical settings, I want to bring to you a mise-en-scène of an actual writing session in the hospital. In lieu of including a CD-rom or DVD of a teaching session, I will try to offer a virtual transcript of what might occur in a teaching session.

Five medical students sit in my office in Presbyterian Hospital. They are third-year clerks on the internal medicine clerkship, each of them assigned to a ward team, admitting patients every fourth night, rounding, writing in hospital charts, and—within the limits of their experience—being doctors for their patients. I am their preceptor, a designation that requires that I meet with the group three times a week for one and a half hours at a time for the five weeks of their clerkship at Presbyterian. Like my internist colleagues who function as preceptors, I ask my students to present cases at our preceptor sessions and assign them topics to research and teach to one another on such diseases as breast cancer or atrial fibrillation or painless jaundice.

Unlike my colleagues, I also ask them to write about their patients in ordinary language. Years ago, I found myself unhappy that my students did not have a routine method with which to consider their patients' experiences of illness or to examine what they themselves undergo in caring for patients. We were very effectively teaching students about biological disease processes, and we were systematically training them to do lumbar punctures and to present cases at attending rounds, but we were not being conscientious in helping them to develop their interior lives as doctors. Nor were we modeling methods of recognizing what patients and families go through at the hands of illness and, indeed, at our own hands in the hospital.

In 1993 I invented a teaching tool I called the "Parallel Chart," and I have been using it since. It is a very simple device. I tell my students,

> Every day, you write in the hospital chart about each of your patients. You know exactly what to write there and the form in which to write it. You write about your patient's current complaints, the results of the physical exam, laboratory

findings, opinions of consultants, and the plan. If your patient dying of prostate cancer reminds you of your grandfather, who died of that disease last summer, and each time you go into the patient's room, you weep for your grandfather, you cannot write that in the hospital chart. We will not let you. And yet it has to be written somewhere. You write it in the Parallel Chart.

These are the only instructions the students get. I ask them to write at least one entry in the Parallel Chart each week and to be prepared to read aloud what they write to their classmates and me in preceptor session. I devote one of our three sessions each week to the students' reading aloud what they have written in the Parallel Chart. From the start, students have written powerfully about their deep attachment to patients, their awe at patients' courage, their sense of helplessness in the face of disease, their rage at disease's unfairness, the shame and humiliation they experience as medical students, and the memories and associations triggered by their work. They have found comfort in hearing one another read Parallel Chart entries, commenting often that they no longer feel alone in their mournfulness or sadness or guilt.

From the beginning of the Parallel Chart, I have distinguished it from support groups, venting sessions, or group therapy. Although I firmly believe that students derive emotional benefit from their writing and reading (a belief that rests, in part, on what the students tell me), their emotional well-being is not the Parallel Chart's primary goal. Instead, the goals are to enable them to recognize more fully what their patients endure and to examine explicitly their own journeys through medicine. This textual work is a practical and, I believe, essential part of medical training, designed to increase the students' capacity for effective clinical work.

I have come to make these distinctions for practical reasons. The death knell of any innovation in medicine or medical education is for it to be labeled "touchy-feely" or "soft." Such interventions as informal support groups do not usually last in medical school. To attend them signals weakness or neediness to some students, and those who need them most will not attend. Reflective writing in medicine is not tailored to repair psychiatric illness or to provide mental health support. It is not to be reserved for those students who are unwell or find it hard to cope with training. Instead, it should be thought of as a mainstream, ongoing part of the training of clinicians.

My warrant for requiring and supervising this work is that I am a doctor trained in literary studies. I am not a mental health professional, and I have not been trained to run group therapy sessions. (I make sure to tell this to the students as we begin our sessions to dispel fears that I will be probing their inner thoughts or diagnosing their psychiatric lesions.) The skills I bring to the work are textual ones—I am a good reader. I know what people try to do with language. I think I am getting good at following a story's narrative thread, figural language, narrative shifts, and the like. I do not think, it must be said quickly, that one needs doctoral training in literary studies in order to do this well. Nor must one be a physician oneself to do this, although one does need a modicum of familiarity with and sympathy toward the clinical enterprise. I coached several of my internist colleagues at Columbia to conduct Parallel Chart sessions very effectively. The coaching they needed was, in effect, contained in this book's previous chapters on reading and writing.

I make further distinctions. I tell students that the Parallel Chart is not a diary. Writing Parallel Chart entries is not the same as writing a letter to your sister. Instead, it is part of clinical training. The writing I want is indexed to a particular patient. It is not a general exploration of one's life and times. It is, instead, narrative writing in the service of the care of a particular patient. The requirement that the students read aloud what they write in the Parallel Chart signals the proper level of disclosure for this exercise. Only once in what is now more than 10 years of doing this work have I had to stop a student from reading his Parallel Chart entry because he seemed to me to be disclosing unduly private material about himself.

In the course of writing about patients, of course, students write a great deal about themselves. The patient's biography is always braided with the student's autobiography. Among the most lasting lessons of my Parallel Chart work is how central and *exposed* is the doctor's self in the care of patients. As we brood about patients and how best to care for them, our own memories and associations and dispositions come to the fore. Students recognize this presence of self very forcefully while writing their own Parallel Charts and reading and listening to one another's.

Some students resist writing. Those students assigned to me in June of their third year—after eleven months of the hardest work they had ever done—were just too exhausted to contemplate the emotional demands of this activity. "Dr. Charon, you want us to do what?" I had to accept the observation that narrative writing places a significant demand on the student, and that teachers should be discrete about knowing when they can expect students to join in it. Other resistance is individual. A woman student, an athlete, contradicted my suggestion that writing helps us to reflect on our experience. She has never found writing useful, she stated vehemently; instead, writing is an unpleasant chore for her. "When I want to think about things, I go for a five-mile run, and when I get back, I find that things have gotten sorted out in my mind." I said to her, "Fine. When you get back from a five-mile run, please make a list of the things that have gone through your mind. That will be your Parallel Chart entry." She did that dutifully, and she produced fragments that, at the end of each list, became unified. I told her she had invented a literary genre. Here is an example:

> Not a good patient for you—not interesting
> —not communicative
> noncommunicative?
> "Do you know this ♂"
> A twinkle of the eye, a shake of the head, a sly glance
> quality
>
> ESRD + Hct of 44, explain the paradox, Lillian—this
> is interesting

> Hmm . . . Ah PCKD, autosomal dominant, chromosome—an
> > interesting physical exam, an interesting family hx
> "Did your father have this condition? Does your son?"
>
> Rounds—an interesting patient, a lovely family, the
> > son from DC
> Between a rock + a hard place—GI bleed or stroke
> The son wants to talk about quality of life
> Autosomal dominant, chromosome, 50% probability
> Does he have it? Does he know?

On the last Parallel Chart session, this student brought copies for all her classmates of Dylan Thomas's poem "Do Not Go Gentle into That Good Night," because she wanted her colleagues all to have it, to have the truth of those words, along with her own creation:

DO NOT GO GENTLE INTO THAT GOOD NIGHT

> We want everything done.
> > Do not go gentle into that good night.
> The nurses don't think she needs pain medicine
> > Do not go gentle.
> Tell your husband to stop torturing me.
> > Do not go gentle into that good night.
> You're a liar, you're not taking care of him. Forget the DNR
> > Do not go gentle.
> If only they could rage.

▨ PEDAGOGIC PROCESS

For the hour-and-a-half session devoted to Parallel Chart, my students each bring something they have written about one of their patients. I ask that they limit the length to no more than a page so that each student will have time to read aloud what he or she has written. Because we are trying to teach students to be attuned listeners to stories (their patients will not bring them written text when they talk to them in the office), I have not gotten into the practice of asking students to make copies of their entry to distribute to the group. So when students read aloud what they have written, we all listen very intently. I generally take lots of notes as the writer reads to guide my own thoughts and to help me in making textual comments afterward. The students give me the papers on which they have written at the end of the session. I handwrite comments on the papers and return them to the students the following session, thereby opening a private dialogue with each writer on his or her texts.

Over the years, I have learned what kinds of responses are most fruitful in

Parallel Chart sessions. Since developing the method for third-year medical students, I have introduced it in a broad range of teaching settings—working with nurses and social workers on in-patient hospital units, holding intensive workshops with physicians of many specialties at professional meetings, coaching interns and residents to write about their out-patients. In all settings and with learners at all levels, I have found myself being guided by the same principles and following roughly the same process:

Honor the text. The goal of our writing is to deepen writers' abilities to capture perceptions and to represent them fully. It is the textual act—and not initially the clinical behavior or the emotions that arise from the situation—that must be foregrounded. My initial comments usually relate to genre, temporality, metaphors, narrative situation, or structure of what has been written. (I have seen writing groups lose steam when a well-meaning but nontextually trained clinician-facilitator responds to a piece of writing by saying, "Gee, I'm sorry that happened to you," or "That reminds me of a patient of mine who . . .") I teach my reading drill to each group of students and encourage them to be attuned to frame, form, time, plot, and desire as they hear one another's stories.

Ask the writer to read the words. Inexperienced writers are apt to try to talk about their writing instead of reading it. I insist on hearing the words as they appear on the page, because so much of what can be derived from the exercise is derived from seeing *how* the text is built.

Listen for each writer's style. Not all writers know that they have a style and a voice. Make comments on previous pieces of writing by the author as the reading process unfolds. Let the continuity—and the singularity—of each writer's writing over time be revealed.

Invite the listeners to respond to the text. Writers need readers who can reveal what the writer himself or herself cannot see in the created text. Writers are most helped, I have come to believe, by learning what others hear or read in their words. I have found three simple questions to be helpful as listeners respond to a text read aloud: What do you see? What do you hear? What do you want to learn more about? These questions allow the listeners to give beneficial feedback to the writer while engaging each listener in an individual dialogic process of discovery. That each listener sees and hears and is curious about something different (and often contradictory) demonstrates the ambiguity and pluripotency built into any text we create; what a powerful lesson to learn that there is no one "right" reading possible, that possible readings have little to do with conscious authorial intention, but that each contradicting interpretation *adds to* the truth of the work.

Praise something about the writing. Because our students or clinicians are often inexperienced as writers, it has seemed to me important to give much positive feedback in listening to their texts. There is always something skilled in a piece of writing, and I am committed to praising aloud the elements that reflect skill.

Let me try to re-create a Parallel Chart session, providing a metanarrative gloss on the process of the group. I will change what details I must in the texts so as to protect the privacy of patients and of student-writers. (Because some of these texts were written many years ago, I cannot solicit consent from the patients and so have altered clinical details to render them unrecognizable). I will also take the liberty of selecting Parallel Chart texts written over the past several years of teaching, mixing up students from different years into a virtual group so as to reproduce here some of the major elements of the pedagogic process. There are Parallel Charts written by five third-year medical students included here—three men, two women; three white, one Asian, one African; three science majors, one English, one history. No student objects to writing in or reading from the Parallel Chart. These students have known one another since their first day of medical school and have worked closely together on the wards for many months.

▨ DAVID

David reads from his Parallel Chart:

> SC is a 79-year-old Black female with CHF, a host of medical problems, and a poor prognosis. There's not much for our team to offer her. We'll keep her symptoms under control and we'll assess how long she has to live but we really won't accomplish amazing medical things in her life. But what we've done is to give her a sense that we're here, that we'll stand by her. And that alone has made all the difference in her world. She's afraid but she's calm. She's worried but appreciative and trusting. She is accepting the decline at the end of life with great dignity.
>
> *She's* the kind of person I want to be when I'm facing my own frailty and decay. *I want to be like her* when I'm dying. I want my heart to be as *soft* as hers is when I'm through this life. I find myself frequently daydreaming about how this woman copes with the debilitation and despair. I want to learn from this woman. I want to listen to her. I want to understand her. I'm blessed to have the time I do have to be with her and take care of her.

David reads slowly and earnestly. When he comes to the end of his reading, I begin the discussion by calling attention to the structure and the narrative voice of his story. There are two paragraphs. The first paragraph is written in the first person plural, the second in the first person singular. It strikes me that David has noticed the difference between the collective work of medicine and the individual work of medicine—the "we" and the "I."

With his teammates, as represented in the first paragraph, he stands by the patient. With them, he offers medical care to the patient and, together, they accompany her through her heart failure. The diagnosing, treating, prognosing, and standing by her are done collectively in medicine's sociality. I wondered, as I heard the first paragraph, whether David, like the patient, was calmed by his teammates, his worry helped by his appreciation and trust for what his teammates knew. This hint of identification between patient and student becomes confirmed in the next paragraph.

The second paragraph shifts voice and stance. If the first paragraph begins in a very familiar-sounding medical diction—"SC is a 79-year-old Black female with CHF"—the second paragraph begins with a personal link made between the patient and the writer. "*She's* the kind of person I want to be when I'm facing my own frailty and decay" is almost shocking in its intimacy. Here is a white man, Ivy League college graduate, sturdy in his evident good health, in his mid-twenties making a powerful interior connection with an old black woman, ill, poor, not well educated. He accepts her as his model for living. He endorses her goodness, her softness as his ideal *at the very end, when it matters*. The heart that fails her near death is strong—in its softness—as his model in dying. Of course, this paragraph cannot be written in the plural, for this part of his relation with her is privately intersubjective. It is between her and him, two singular human beings, alone together.

I ask next about the plot of the story. What happens in the course of the story itself? The diagnosing and prognosing have been accomplished already once the story opens or will be accomplished in the future; they are reported on in the first paragraph but they are not the action of the story. What happens in the present of the story is that the speaker *wants* something and *finds* himself doing something. He wants to be like SC, to learn from her, to listen to her, and to understand her. He finds himself daydreaming about her. The story is *about* desire—the desire to be near her, to absorb her wisdom, and to experience vicariously, in the daydream, her living through the debilitation and despair. It is a remarkable portrait of a very daring act of transparency. Where did David get the courage to open himself to such realizations, such yearnings? To want to be like someone so very unlike himself, the difference most urgently in the fact that she is very ill and soon to die, takes the brave realization that he himself will die. David accepts his own mortality in the course of these two paragraphs with something like SC's dignity.

The last line accomplishes important metaphoric work. "I'm blessed to have the time I do have to be with her and take care of her" transposes the work of medicine onto the plane of spirituality. David's patient becomes the occasion of grace, his care of his patient sacramental. A spiritual humility is present here on the busy ward, through the agency of a careful doctor and a courageous patient.

The other students were struck with David's gratitude toward his patient and his work. They, too, had experienced this sense of medicine as a privilege, *giving* them things they had no idea would be forthcoming from it. They wondered whether David's patient knew what a powerful role she played for him, and we talked for some time about how to convey to our patients our admiration and love for them. We all felt grateful for David's having given us a mood of reverence and, even in the face of death, a sense of shared serenity.

▣ Nancy

Nancy reads next.

> My intern looked stressed as she rushed out of one of her patients' rooms. I was at the nurses' station talking about one of my patients with the senior resident. She broke into our conversation and said to the senior, "Can you come with me?" They rushed back into the patient's room and I and the other students on our team trailed behind them, hoping we could learn something or be of help. As I came into the room, my intern was putting an O_2 mask on the patient and my senior was auscultating her heart. He took his stethoscope off of his ears and said to the patient's husband, "Can you leave for a moment, sir?" The husband looked confused. He stood and stared and finally walked away looking back over his shoulder. "She's dead," my senior said. "Take off the mask." My intern hesitated. She felt for a pulse. "She's DNR," he said. My intern slipped off the mask and sighed heavily. She looked at her watch. "9:20," she said. "What do we tell her husband?" she asked. "We tell him that she has passed away," said our senior. We all stood for a moment. I looked at the patient as the intern drew her cover over her face. Her jaundiced and edematous face showed no distress.
>
> We slowly filed out of the room. The other med students and I headed for the nurses' station in silence. Our senior's voice faded behind us. We then heard the loud and sad protests of the patient's husband filling the hall. Everyone at the nurses' station stopped and looked. "Poor man," I thought. He had signed her DNR form just 2 days earlier. He had seen her wax and wane for the last few weeks but this morning he thought "she was asleep."
>
> My intern returned to the nurses' station. "She had been married for sixty years," she said. I felt lonely for him. My senior resident returned to the nurses' station within a few minutes and we continued to round. The patient and her husband were no longer our issue. I looked down the hall and saw the nurse with her arm around the patient's husband's shoulder. My intern turned to me and said, "Let's call this in and write the death note."

I hoped immediately that this writer and her auditors noticed what she had accomplished in this elegantly structured story. It approaches, it seemed to me on hearing it, the narratorial control that Hemingway models in his Nick Adams stories. The focalization remains unerringly with the narrator—"my" intern, "our" resident, the "other med students and I." This is amazing in view of the production of the story—we all could see that Nancy was reading her story from a piece of hospital chart Continuation Sheet, scribbled in ink with some crossing out and messy insertions. Clearly a rush job, this was not carefully crafted and worked over but, instead, a fresh and brilliant first draft! All the more impressive, then, was the control of point of view to her own eyes, reporting events only within her vision and in her ken.

We readers are given this student's cinematic view of these events in a telegraphic, quickly evolving scenario. The first paragraph begins with a blur of activity: the intern rushing, breaking into conversation, doctors rushing back into the patient's room. Our focalizer, however, trails behind them, conveying her sense of insecurity or confusion or, if nothing else, lack of agency, "hoping we could learn something or be of help." We readers are given the ensuing scenes exactly as they came to the narrator, leading us to feel very close to her in this experience.

What she witnesses and gives to us is the scene of death. The rushing activity gives way to a grave tableau: the resident bent over the patient's silent chest, the husband forlorn as he is banished from the room, the intern reaching hesitantly for the absent pulse, the student watching the draping of the corpse. 9:20 marks the present and the end of this elderly woman's life.

Despite the serious nature of the events being portrayed, the writer does not flag in her control. "Off camera" events are described with only their sound track. Everyone at the usually frantic nurses' station stops and looks at the sound of the sad protests of the grieving husband. And then the reader gets an interior glimpse of the narrator's feelings. "'Poor man', I thought. . . . I felt lonely for him." The reality of this moment seems to reach the student. Reminded by the intern of the 60-year marriage, the student seems suffused with pity for this man, embarking at 9:20 A.M. on a life alone. That the nurses and not the doctors are the ones entrusted with his care only intensifies the medical student's sense of having been encapsulated away from the immediacy of the experience. Her job is to "call this in and write the death note" and not to embrace this poor old man whose life has just irrevocably changed.

When I asked the listening students what they heard in Nancy's story, they agreed that the story conveyed sadness, forlornness, and silence. Even though there was dialogue and action in the scene, its overall mood is one of distance, as if we are sensing the events through a dense fog. And perhaps this is the most urgent truth that Nancy conveys in her story, again not necessarily by the words or the plot but in how it is given: her experience as the third-year medical student separates her from the experience of this unfortunate man. She is at an unbridgeable distance from him, his confusion, his vigil for the last few weeks, and now his acute suffering. (Perhaps they are united textually in their shared confusion, both the student and the husband wandering trailingly in the wake of everyone else's purposive certainty.) She is encapsulated into her own inexperience, her responsibilities—such as they are—to the professional tasks of medicine, leaving the nurses to accomplish the *more real* and more human duties toward the survivor.

Nancy's writing opened up for our group a troubling sadness—that patients undergo authentic losses while we doctors (less so nurses) sometimes, in comparison, seem to undergo shadow experiences. When I asked the group to reflect on the *desire* apparent in this story, according to my reading drill, some thought that Nancy seemed to yearn to be free from the hermetic fog, to be *present* with this husband or even with this dying woman, who died out of sight, alone herself now after 60 years of marriage. The silence and the stillness of the grave tableau presented by the author signaled for us a danger. That the author, within this story, was unable to pierce through the fog and was not able to attain agency, either with the patient herself or with the husband, at least signals a yearning, a need, and a preparedness for presence and action in the future. Indeed, the next Parallel Chart entry that Nancy wrote reported how she diagnosed an acute abdomen all by herself early on a Saturday morning, getting the surgeons to the bedside of an elderly woman and soon to the OR, having recognized a surgical emergency. It was a tremendous celebration of the student's clinical judgment and bravery, in telling contrast (and perhaps not unrelated) to the silent passivity of the earlier scene.

▥ TOLULOPE

Tolulope, a Nigerian who moved to this country as a teenager, had been assigned to the oncology service for his medicine clerkship and was caring for very ill and dying patients. However, he wrote in his Parallel Chart about a "boarder," a patient who did not have cancer but who was admitted to oncology because there was no room for him elsewhere. As often happens when patients are particularly complex or demanding, the student wrote about this patient more than once. Over two Parallel Chart entries, Tolu described his attempts to care for this young man with AIDS:

> I have had moments of extreme sadness when thinking about the prognosis of some of my oncology patients. I have had to question some of my deeply ingrained beliefs. I have even questioned what my role in medicine is going to be and why I am in medicine in the first place. . . . I have learned that curing a patient is not the only thing medicine is about. . . . I have worked with an excellent intern and resident who . . . have taught me a lot about how to deal with patients to make them feel better. . . . I have seen them express emotions of sadness and happiness evoked by patients.
>
> Yesterday while on call, I was sent down to the ER to meet an HIV+ man who was getting admitted to my service for work-up of severe diarrhea. . . . LD was in his early 30s, he was first told he had HIV in 1990, but refused to take any of the drugs for his infection. In 1997, he developed PCP pneumonia. At this time he was treated and convinced to start taking HAART. He did so until some time in 1999 when he met a girl who soon became his girlfriend. (When I asked him why he stopped [HAART], he said he did not want her to know he had HIV.) His girlfriend is now HIV+ (it is unclear if she contracted the virus from him) and he has a child with her who was born 2 weeks prior to the time I met him and who is still in the NICU for complications. (I don't know the child's HIV status, but I know that the mom did not take the appropriate prophylaxis during pregnancy). He is an immigrant . . . who has not worked in a long time and who is on welfare and has Medicaid.
>
> As I learned more and more about this patient, I noticed that I was getting angry or maybe even furious. . . . Interestingly, the fact that I was so aware of feeling furious allowed me to put my feelings aside and deal with the patient ap-

propriately. I think he is very unaware of the consequences his behavior has on himself and his family. . . . He has basically brought a child into this world who has little chance of making it. . . . As an immigrant myself, I feel he gives all immigrants a bad name.

There is no possible way I can have empathy (being aware of, being sensitive to, and vicariously experiencing the feelings, thoughts, and experience of another) for him. . . . My imagination is not so vivid as to allow me to see myself in his shoes. . . . For me to imagine myself in his shoes, I basically have to imagine myself to be someone I hate, someone who is the total opposite of me now. It is basically impossible. So I have spent a lot of time thinking of what emotion led me to want to help this patient. I came up with pity (sympathetic sorrow for one suffering). I really felt sorry for this guy. This was a man who in his 30s has AIDS, a newborn child, major denial about his condition but realizes he is sick. He is probably aware of his deterioration and knows the end is near. . . . I feel sorry for him, not empathy but pity. That is what makes me want to help him.

The students understood the significance of Tolu's writing. They had all been wrestling with the *realities* of what they had learned in the abstract about empathy and clinical relationships. They often felt the distances that separated them from their patients and grappled with the difficulties of bridging these differences. Tolu's paragraphs enact that struggle. Interior and affective, the plot depicts a slow and active shift of the student's point of view toward recognition of this patient's situation. As they heard this text, the other students were able to appreciate Tolu's accomplishment in *reaching* this patient despite the fury engendered by the patient's behavior.

This text is at the same time an expertly written clinical summary of a complex disease course and an affectively dense double portrait of an unfortunate patient and of his doctor, who is moved to anger and pity on the patient's behalf. One of the elements that enables the text to perform its dual tasks is its deployment of several distinct registers, which either coexist or are heard in quick succession. The opening paragraph voices mournful reflection on the recent clinical past and questions, in an ontological self-examination, the beliefs and the motives that led the writer to choose medicine. The second paragraph cuts away from a private, interior register toward a distanced narrator recounting fast-paced clinical events in the emergency room. Jarring by comparison, this hospital register is brittle, staccato, and impersonal, banishing the first-person narrator almost entirely to parenthetical expression. The text then returns to an interior realm, this time not in an autobiographical self-examination but an intersubjective one, probing the relation between the writer and his new patient. This final realm synthesizes the cognitive understanding of certain emotions with a private realization of the meaning of the emotions engendered by the care of this patient.

Tolu agreed that having written this Parallel Chart entry enabled him to understand what it represented. He had not noticed prior to writing how he had set aside his fury so as to care for the patient. Nor did he parse his own emotions toward the patient until writing. Looking up definitions of the words "empathy" and "pity," he expected of himself the same clarity in anatomizing his feelings that he did in presenting the clinical events. As a result of representing both the patient's actions and his own responses, he uncovered the dualities of this care—two immigrants, one unaware and the other aware, one ill and the other committed to caring for him. What impressed the listeners of Tolu's story was the exacting demand the writer placed upon himself to visualize, comprehend, and claim his own slow movement toward this patient, reflecting in the gravity of his prose the weight of his own professional duty. We all agreed that Tolu had, after all, achieved empathy for his patient, for his pity enabled him to see the events from the patient's perspective, not only recognizing the stated aspects of the situation but also even imagining the patient's fears for his future.

Bijan

Bijan next read from his text. He was helping to take care of a 65-year-old man with idiopathic pulmonary fibrosis, a debilitating lung disease whose only definitive treatment is lung transplantation. This patient had been on the list to receive a lung transplant for the past nine years, but he had not had the good fortune to receive one of the rare donated organs. The student has just learned that the patient has been taken off the list because of his age.

> My mind began to wander as I put down the phone and started writing in the chart. . . . I had just finished talking to Mr. Encarnacion's pulmonologist, Dr. M, about why Mr. Encarnacion recently had been taken off "the list" for a lung transplant and a new life. Dr. M had rather matter-of-factly informed me that the age "cut-off" for lung transplants was around 60, and that Mr. Encarnacion, being 65, *became* ineligible because his age boded poorly with respect to prognosis. . . .
>
> Irrespective of the reason for taking Mr. Encarnacion off the list, what I was faced with was that he *had* been taken off of it, and was now left without the only known cure for his inexorably progressive disease. And as I had started writing my note, the word "cut-off" had stared up at me from the crisp white page below. A funny word, I thought; did Dr. M even realize the twisted pun within his own phrasing? To him—in fairness, to the rationalist—the cut-off was an austere, unprejudiced number that signified that the risks for transplant outweighed the benefits. But to me, the "cut-off" was a concept that conjured up the image of a vivid dream of falling off a rocky cliff. . . . This "cut-off," little black letters with the trace of an ink smudge, signified to me the cutting off of a life. Due to the simplicity of one designated number, all Mr. Encarnacion's hopes for the last nine years were effectively now extinguished, and he was being left to die.
>
> I couldn't help but think how Mr. Encarnacion had dealt with the news when he had first found out, and how I would deal with such news if I ever were

on the receiving end. How in the world had he gotten to the point where he could tell me with a wry smile that barely crept out from behind his green oxygen mask, "I used to be strong like a bull. That will never again be possible." Had he cried when he found out? Had he been strangely relieved that his wait in uncertainty was over? Or had he simply taken things in stride, knowing all along that hope was futile? At the time, I didn't have even the ability to guess. I figure now that I could have asked him—I could easily have mustered up the courage to get up and walk down the hall, past my own fears that made the hallway so uninviting, and over the threshold of his room. . . . He would have answered me calmly and I would have been crushed by visions of my own mortality and fleeting, fragile existence; I would have left the room an enlightened and broken student.

But I never went into his room; I finished my note and went to lunch because I just didn't have the strength to confront the inevitability of my own death—possibly, hopefully, many years ahead of me. At that moment, it was way too close; so close that I couldn't face Mr. Encarnacion's acceptance of his fate; it was just too eerie, much too unnatural, and very very frightening.

There are many "I's" here: the I who writes in the Parallel Chart, the I at the nurses' station trying to write a note in the chart, the I of a few days ago talking with Mr. Encarnacion, and, of course, the I of Bijan sitting with us in the room, reading what he had written. Noting the verb tenses that mark the story's temporal scaffolding lets the reader appreciate the complex unfolding of the many separate sets of events: the past perfect participial "I had just finished talking" is distinguished from the simple past of "My mind began to wander." Within the first two sentences, the reader or listener realizes that these time periods are laid like transparencies over one another. It is not until the end of the text that we realize how far forward in the life of the author this transparency reaches.

What impresses me about this piece of writing is the way in which the author has gained access to the *connections* among these different I's, in effect harnessing the power of the autobiographical process. From the remove of his current position, he inspects his thoughts, feelings, and actions of the immediate past and of the slightly more remote past. By representing himself as he sits writing his note, he recaptures—or probably captures for the first time—the complex emotions and realizations that emerge in the scene. He *finds* that it is his fear of his mortality that prevents him from entering the patient's room. This discovery is based not just on the plot of the event but also on how it is told. For example, the use of the word "cut-off" is complex and instructive. It becomes a fetish in the story—an object, smudged on the page—as well as a metaphor connecting the nightmare of "falling off a rocky cliff" to the concept of the age limit for medical treatment.

As the reader juggles the many time periods simultaneously in mind—the putting down of the phone and the wandering of the mind—more remote events in both past and future intrude. The patient says in an unspecified past, "I used to be strong like bull," and the narrator imagines the conditional future of "I would have been crushed." Finally, in what the writer hopes is the remote future but is now visible by virtue of his narrative creation is the time of his own death.

One week after the student wrote this essay and read it to his classmates, he visited Mr. Encarnacion with me. During our visit to the bedside (I was there to observe him conducting a clinical interview and contributed nothing to the actual conversation), the student asked the patient and his wife how they had felt when Dr. M told them that Mr. Encarnacion was no longer a candidate for lung transplantation. Both the patient and his wife wept on hearing the student's question. They spoke at length about their children and grandchildren, and they expressed with great eloquence their trust in God and acceptance of their earthly fate. From then on, Bijan was the most trusted member of the medical team for the Encarnacions, who relied on his advice and guidance in making all future medical decisions.

Months later, the student was asked to comment on his writing in the Parallel Chart:

> In one or two cases, I wrote about something I had seen that did not "feel right"; as I wrote, I realized that this was something that was actually bothering me without my realizing it. . . .
>
> After writing down my thoughts for each chart entry, I developed them— trying to find themes and organizing my thoughts to make each chart entry able to "have a meaning" and to be able to stand on its own as a writing sample (and not just as a piece of paper with thoughts written down on it). As this happened, I realized that my thoughts became more structured, and that what had previously simply been an expression of "not feeling right" was now able to be translated into something more meaningful. *In other words, I attempted to transform feelings into organized themes.* As a result of this I was able to find that what really made me feel uncomfortable about Mr. Encarnacion and his ordeal was the fact that I found it difficult to confront my own weaknesses and mortality. I do not think that I would have been able to discover this had I simply written down my thoughts and left them there without editing directed at finding a meaning within what I had written. Likewise, I certainly would not have been able to discover this had I simply spoken about the topic. . . .
>
> I think that this self-discovery enabled me to improve upon how I dealt with individual patients; becoming more comfortable with my own feelings enabled me to focus on the problems of the patient. For example, when we broached the subject of death with Mr. Encarnacion, I was certain of how I felt about it and was able to concentrate my efforts on attempting to make Mr. Encarnacion feel better. [Italics in original.]

Able to report on the activities of his past self's wandering mind, this writer used the practice of autobiographical writing to overhear the language of his prior experiencing self. By writing and editing the resultant text, the student becomes his own reader and interpreter, using the autobiographical gap as an invitation to reflect on the self. That the student credits his writing and rewriting with the insight and wherewithal to do what needs to be done clinically—to talk with the patient and his family about this serious development in his health—gives us great heart that narrative training has practical consequences for the student or health care professional.

◨ NELL

Nell was the last student to read from her Parallel Chart.

> One day last week, during hour two and a half of rounding, I saw a young man walking down the hospital hallway towards me. The seven of us on my team were standing in a circle, the two interns, the two attendings, the resident and my fellow student; I was the only one facing his direction. He was unassuming, of average height and build, with wavy brown hair, green eyes and glasses. He had no shoes on, only gleaming white socks. He kept trying to catch my eye, like he knew me, as he walked towards us down the hall. He had a mischievous smile on his face. When he was only two feet from the group, he winked at me. Quickly. Joyously. As if we were in on some great joke together. I don't know if it was my sleep deprivation or the blood rushing from my brain after standing so long, but I thought to myself what if this young man, who seems to want to let me in on his prank, was God? The idea filled me with joy. It was revitalizing. What a strange thought to have! Why would I think that, I asked myself? First, this is exactly where God would want to hang out, in a hospital amongst the sick and the dying and amongst those always around the sick and the dying. And this is exactly how God would want to appear, as a patient, though one inexplicably cheerful in the face of suffering. And why not? He's in on the joke that the rest of us aren't. Finally, God would definitely not want to wear shoes. I can't picture God in shoes.
>
> I was hoping that God would visit some of my patients. Let them in on what was so funny. I hoped he would stop by the room of my 35-year-old patient with CF, now three years older than she ever should have been. God could put on His contact isolation precautions and go in for a chat, put His socked feet up on the windowsill. He could explain why a 35-year-old woman is in the hospital, drowning. Why she is the youngest person on the floor by forty years. Why she is counting the rest of her life in months.
>
> After God told that patient His joke, maybe he could move down the hall and look in on another patient of mine. His ALS has left him trapped in a coffin that once was his body, no longer able to eat, to urinate, to move and almost to breathe. Any day and that will be gone too. He can understand though, his mind is still there. He would want to know God's joke, I think he would appreciate it. If it's a good day, my patient might be able to wink back at Him.
>
> And last of all, I hope God comes back my way and lets me in on the secret. Maybe then I can know how to handle pain and sickness on a daily basis, how to welcome death in the second case and accept it in the first. How to sit with suffering, anger and regret without wanting to avoid it and save myself. The secret

must be how to sacrifice the idea of justice for peace, how to substitute science for fear.

But God doesn't stop to tell me the joke, Not just yet. He only smiles mysteriously, winks and shuffles off down the hallway.

We sat like stunned steer when Nell finished reading. For what felt like minutes, no one said anything. Nell had nailed the underlying savagery of disease, its meaninglessness, its random cruelty so that we all felt exposed as charlatans. Unlike David's reverent summoning of the language of spirituality in the first text we had heard that day, Nell's evocation of God undermined every shred of comfort anyone ever got from faith; it ridiculed the impulse toward the search for meaning in medicine.

I felt I had to find a way to make sense of the heightened experience of the absurd that this impressively skilled piece of writing had subjected us all to. It had taken courage to envision it and to write it; it had commandeered courage of all of us to hear it. Nell was by now in tears sitting in her habitual seat in the far corner of my office. Dressed as she usually was in pastels, pearls at her neck, an elegant if somewhat fragile-looking young woman who had impressed me with her grasp of—and wonder at—the basic science foundations of medicine, she had just revealed to us an until-then hidden recognition of the brutality with which we are surrounded.

My recourse, then, to commenting on the formal elements of her writing accomplished more than its typical goals of showing the writer and the readers the "inside" meaning of a piece of writing. This time, it was our lifeline back to the world of coherence. And yet, even now in retrospect, I can recognize that my comments on genre and metaphor were not only instructive but were the most responsible responses to this writing and, more important, to this young writer.

I began with a few words about irony. When an author says the opposite from what he or she means, the dislocation sets up two levels within the text: the said is false, the unsaid opposite of what is said is true. Irony is resorted to in situations in which the true cannot be said directly. The most savage convention in writing, irony confers distance on the author, who often selects it when nearing a truth that is too painful to say. Nell's selection of this mode of writing signified that she was attempting to represent something so hot, so provocative, so potentially destructive that it had to be done in reverse.

But this writing is not simple irony. Its elaborate comic fantasy of God in socks contributes an element of surreality, transporting the reader to a highly unstable world where nothing can be trusted to be what it appears to be. Is there a young man on the ward without shoes? Is Nell really having a near-syncopal experience of altered mental status? We had heard Nell's erudite presentations of these two patients in earlier preceptor sessions, detailing the pathophysiology of their diseases, the rationale of treatment, the medical prognoses, the diagnostic tests, the physical findings. How empty of meaning these former discussions of disease now revealed themselves to be. How beside the point for both these patients, who are, indeed, simply waiting to die.

The portrait of God as jokester strips him of all mercy. Ruthless, his glee vilifies whatever little effort we might make toward acceptance or consolation. The text amounts to a renunciation of God, of faith, of a commitment to meaning in human life. This cosmos has been abandoned by its maker, who now gloats at the plight of his hapless subjects.

I realized that another reading was possible of this text, although my initial impulse was to dismiss this gentler reading as self-protective. Nonetheless, I thought it might help the group to wonder aloud whether God in socks might be not ironic but providential. Maybe, I mused, there *is* some cosmic order ultimately available to us to behold. Maybe Nell's vision means that God, for whatever reasons, cannot reveal the meaning of our experience of illness and death, and yet maybe *he* knows what it all means. Instead of gloating at his victims, in this interpretation God is entreating us to be patient with him while holding out the hope—with the humility of his shoeless approach—that we will eventually be able to perceive the benevolence and sense of what to us seems cruel and unfair.

Two sentences in the text bear extended inspection for the good of the writer. "I was the only one facing his direction." This student has been abandoned, perhaps by the power of her vision, to *see* all this alone. The other members of her team are deep into their pathophysiological and management decisions about all 15 or 20 patients on the service. They are oblivious to the brutality of what Nell sees. They are blinded by their own little, perhaps meaningless, tasks to the big savage picture. The other sentence that calls for urgent attention sums up the student's course of action in the face of her discovery. "The secret must be how to sacrifice the idea of justice for peace, how to substitute science for fear." Perhaps the student can be encouraged to substitute other things besides the science for the fear. Indeed, the science helps, but one of the dividends of Nell's writing in her Parallel Chart was to hear her classmates and me gently suggest that other things work to counter the fear—generosity, benevolence, maybe simply being a witness for patients in their dread.

I had noticed even before this session that Nell seemed particularly distressed by the Parallel Chart sessions. She was often tearful, either in reading her own texts or listening and commenting on her classmates. I had asked her in private whether the reflective writing put too great an emotional burden on her. "Is this too much for you?" I asked her very directly. She answered quickly that the Parallel Chart writing was the best part of this clerkship for her. She found it extremely helpful to write about her experiences and to hear the group's response. "I send my Parallel Chart entries to my mother," she said. "For the first time in medical school, I feel that she knows what I am going through." I realized then that her having written about God in socks did not *create* the brutality, did not lead to the renunciation. But, by virtue of the writing, Nell was no longer alone with her apocalyptic vision.

My most immediate concern as the session neared its end was to ensure that the group recovered from Nell's brutal vision, and the most coherent way to do that was to bring us back to David's transparent humility with which we had started. His attachment to his dying patient had set us up for the savagery of Nell's repudiation of meaning within illness but might also have provided us with an alternative ending to her text. Maybe trust and appreciation have a place next to the science and the fear. Maybe standing by patients in their illnesses *matters* for them and, also of consequence, matters for us.

▨ SUMMING UP

Our hour and a half was almost up. Each student in the group had had a chance to read aloud to classmates from his or her Parallel Chart and to hear and enter into a discussion of the forms, the plots, the moods, and the implications of one another's texts. We had shared an intertextual experience over the course of the session that itself required comment.

It helps, I have observed, to sum up at the end of a session with comments on some similarities among the texts. I assembled these texts myself into the virtual Parallel Chart session presented in this chapter, so I cannot report on what was actually said in the wake of these five readings. And yet, had they been read together, I can predict that we would have talked at the end about the nearness of death, the problem of agency, and the safe harbor provided to students by their reflective states of interiority.

All these texts treat death. This is not unusual in the writing of third-year medical students, who are for the first time themselves face-to-face with their patients' mortality, and the good ones find themselves simultaneously face-to-face with their own. Bijan's "cut-off" was not unlike Nancy's dense fog, both of them severing connection with patients, with the future, with themselves in the effort to address their patients' dying. Tolu's pity toward his HIV+ patient and David's daydreamed experience of SC placed them both at the side of a seriously ill or dying patient. By virtue of their clinical tasks, all of these students had to envision, even briefly, their own ends.

In several of these texts, the students found themselves, temporarily anyway, without agency. Nancy trails slowly after her team, excluded from the ability to comfort the bereaved husband by the role-realities of the ward. Bijan has to escape off the ward because he cannot immediately summon up the capacity to *act,* to reenter Mr. Encarnacion's room to talk with him about the cut-off. And it is hard to know what Nell does with her savage insight. She waits to be let in on the joke.

Several of the students find safe harbor in the rich and complex imaginative mental states in which they found themselves as a result of their narrative writing. Time and again, the writer withdrew from the fragmented or incoherent ward into a daydream, a wandering mind, a prophesy, a mystical experience of seeing God, suggesting to me the inadequacy of daily *reality* in comprehending all that they witness in their new life. Such altered mental states might be rejuvenating for these exhausted young people, challenged daily with the grimness of disease and medicine's powerlessness in the face of so much of it. Indeed, as Guy Allen suggests, the personal narrative may function as a Winnicottian playground somewhere between one's inner reality and the outer reality of the world, functioning as a safe place in which to enact in fantasy what one will then "try" in the real. As we take leave of one another at the close of Parallel Chart sessions, it is often with the sense of returning to the battlefield, but with a found serenity, perspective, and blessed reflective retreat.

The Parallel Chart session itself functions as a safe harbor for these writers, as is evident from their answers to evaluative questions about the practice. Here are some of the answers to the question, "How did you feel after writing Parallel Chart entries? After Parallel Chart sessions?" asked of third-year students using the Parallel Chart:

> I felt good after writing entries. I felt as if, by writing, I forced myself to understand what I was feeling, and forced myself to confront something I was avoiding. After sessions, I felt exhausted, deflated, comfortable, clear, fragile but with knowledge of my delicacy.

> I felt better, relieved of some anxiety and distress. Meeting with the others was very helpful also. It was a supportive atmosphere and gave me a sense of camaraderie and hope.

> Sometimes it made things more personal and harder from an emotional point of view. Other times, it was sort of liberating—it allowed me to have more empathy and also more distance.

Students often find the Parallel Chart to be beneficial. (In one series of 49 students who were randomly assigned to add Parallel Chart sessions to their medicine clerkship, 82 percent of the students found it to be beneficial, therapeutic, or cathartic.) Writers found that they understood their own emotions more clearly by virtue of writing and reading aloud of their experience. They also found that they understood their patients more fully:

> I learned how vulnerable so many patients feel. They are scared, also, and yet place so much confidence in the doctor. It made me recognize the need to be kind and careful always as so many patients are in such a vulnerable state.

> The process helped me acknowledge my role and see the patients more clearly. The process was an exercise in something I already believed—that the relationship between the patient and doctor/medical student is not a passive one and exploring my responses helped me see patients more clearly and probably be more effective.

> I wasn't aware I empathized so much with one particular patient until I wrote a Parallel Chart entry. Yes, I think I was more giving of myself, more open about my life outside of medicine.

An ongoing research effort to characterize the outcomes of Parallel Chart writing by medical students is showing that students randomized into writing groups are rated by their faculty members as more effective in conducting medical interviews, performing medical procedures, and developing therapeutic alliances with patients.[1] Students who use Parallel Chart methods report more confidence in their ability to care for seriously ill and dying patients and to disclose bad news to patients. By administering psychological scales that measure empathy and perspective-taking to students, we are generating evidence that students who write are more likely than those who do not write to improve their ability to adopt the perspectives of others. Our provisional understanding of this process is that clinically relevant narrative writing and disciplined examination of that writing in groups improves students' skills in seeing from their patients' points of view, a capacity requiring cognitive and imaginative flexibility. The ability to shift one's perspective in order to see events from others' points of view may be one critical and currently missing skill in health care professionals—and one that can be taught.

I close this chapter with an extended evaluation of the Parallel Chart written by a third-year student on her medicine rotation:

> Writing the chart entry about my . . . lady who we just diagnosed with aggressive terminal cancer was an effort, because I hadn't yet really addressed my feelings about the situation and had been keeping distant, excusing it in the rush to keep up her medical care. I felt cold and businesslike, especially after we had "the talk" with her about her prognosis. Even writing the chart entry, I felt cold, and afraid of my coldness. I was always gentle, and sweet, and careful to listen to her. But I walked away stunned that I hadn't felt more, and then rushed off to some conference.
>
> But in Parallel Chart session, when I finally got up the nerve to read about it, to tell my friends the story of this . . . lady, and my fear about her death and my death and my work, it all hit me, and I broke down in tears. And once I had finally thought about, talked about, and cried about this situation, I was free of my fear, and was able to go back into the patient's room, and sit down with her, and ask her about her thoughts and fears. I was able to re-associate, and get back in there, and get closer to her, and care for her emotional well-being as well. That felt like a huge step. . . . I think it was priceless.

NOTE

1. The Fan Fox and Leslie R. Samuels Foundation, New York, N.Y., has funded an outcomes research project at Columbia University to test the hypotheses that writing in the Parallel Chart improves medical students' empathy, perspective-taking, and clinical performance of interpersonal tasks. Both quantitative and qualitative measures were taken of a group of experimental students randomly assigned to write in the Parallel Chart and control students who underwent the medicine clerkship at the same time as the experimental group without the Parallel Chart training. Quantitative results are as noted above. The research team is currently engaged in the detailed content analysis of qualitative data. Research results will be published in the appropriate medical literature upon completion of the study. We are also engaged in the effort to replicate the study at another academic medical center.

PART IV

Dividends of Narrative Medicine

9 ▣ BEARING WITNESS

A 46-year-old Dominican man visits me for the first time, having been assigned to my patient panel by his Medicaid Managed Care plan. He has been suffering from shortness of breath and chest pain, and he fears for his heart. I say to him at the start of our first visit, "I will be your doctor, and so I have to learn a great deal about your body and your health and your life. Please tell me what you think I should know about your situation." And then I do my best to not say a word, to not write in his medical chart, but to absorb all that he emits about himself—about his health concerns, his family, his work, his fears, and his hopes. I listen not only for the content of his narrative but also for its form—its temporal course, its images, its associated subplots, its silences, where he chooses to begin in telling of himself, how he sequences symptoms with other life events. After a few minutes, the patient stops talking and begins to weep. I ask him why he cries. He says, "No one ever let me do this before."

Slowly, narrative medicine's implications for practice are becoming clear. As we clinicians develop the capacity for attention and the power of representation, and as these states spiral toward affiliation with patients and colleagues, we find that *what we do* in practice is altered. By developing narrative competence through close reading and reflective writing, we find ourselves *positioned* differently with patients, our missions in individual patient care and as members of our professions altered by our new narrative orientation and skills. Routines of patient care are fundamentally changed by virtue of our new skills, as I outline below—how we collect and record clinical information, how we develop alliances with patients over time, what, very basically, we do for patients in our care.

▣ SICKNESS OPENS DOORS

Sickness opens doors. It may not always have been the case, but today, it is more likely to be sickness than, say, the loss of faith that propels a person toward self-knowledge and clarifying of life goals and values. It is when you are sick that you have to question whom in your life you trust, how much life means to you, how much suffering you can bear. It is more likely to be the doctor than the priest or confessor who hears the answers to these questions. Illness and body state have eclipsed other life events as that which *defines* individuals to themselves, first of all, and then to those around them. Cancer survivors' groups proliferate; disability rights are the contemporary civil rights of most valence; attendance at alcoholics or narcotics or overeaters anonymous replaces church attendance for many; and we call our country *Prozac Nation*. We find our kin through our bodies—not among blood relatives but among those who share our corporeal dispositions. I recently posted a message on the narrative medicine online discussion group about how sickness seems to open doors.[1]

> It has recently occurred to me how sickness opens doors. I don't know if it is because [people] don't tend to have religious advisors or confessors these days, but when people come to see me because I am an internist, they tell of very deep, grave concerns in their lives. The situations of their physical health enable them to examine and consider their lives. [I now see with] deep regard how patients accept challenges and dividends from changes in health. We seem to be expanding our notions of how to respond to illness. The task of preparing oneself to receive others' stories of illness seems a tremendous one and a most rewarding one.

The clarity and force of the responses to my posted message impressed me. I cite a couple of responses—from an oral historian and a physician who has become a gestalt therapist.

From Mary Marshall Clark, director of the Oral History Project at Columbia University:

> I can't keep myself from responding to this message—I recently have conducted a number of oral history interviews with chaplains affiliated with the Health-Care Chaplaincy—a multifaith organization that coordinates the assignment of chaplains with most major New York hospitals. The project has also included interviews with former patients, and families of those, for example, whose children have died at Memorial Sloan Kettering, as well as doctors like Jimmie Holland who founded the field of psycho-oncology. It is true that many people, with or without religious affiliation who are facing death find the need to "narrate" their experiences as a part of the search for meaning that in some ways characterizes the essence of the human condition. The chaplains I have interviewed often find that they never speak about religion or god (for that reason they no longer use the term religion but talk about spirituality) but are simply there as receptacles for stories people need to tell. And they also find that medical professionals need to talk as much as the patients and their families. What expert listeners do, whether doctors, oral historians or in this case professional chaplains, is to open the door to hearing stories that they feel others might not be willing to hear. Indeed, as our September 11, 2001 oral history projects have taught us, this is a deeply rewarding if not unique experience.

Another reply was posted by the family physician and Gestalt therapist Barry Bub, reflecting on his training in pastoral care:

> As one of those who trained with the Healthcare, I was forced to confront my own apprehension at visiting the sick, armed with nothing but a book of psalms. With no stethoscope to confer authority, no white coat to hide behind, all psychotherapy techniques on hold and my physician identity for the most part hidden, I was totally dependant on the power of Presence and ability to listen. . . . My role was to bring a human connection, to establish an I-thou relationship that relieved some of this isolation which is the very essence of suffering. . . .
>
> This required me to listen with great care and at varying times to reflect back, to inject humor, to support silence or to offer blessing or prayer. All of this was based on what I heard and my own emotional response to the narrative. Far from being a passive receptacle, this was a very, very active process.
>
> While I displayed empathy (therapeutic validation), little was based on compassion. This, in fact, is one of the great myths of listening. Rather, I was simply doing my job, which was to listen professionally, something few physicians are trained to do. Compassion emerged from the interaction, not caused it.
>
> Finally, while I heard their narrative, they heard mine—my body language, choice of words and so forth, hence determining what they in turn chose to share.

And in a later response to clarify her use of the word "receptacle," Mary Marshall Clark wrote:

> In oral history we think of stories as gifts (we literally deposit them to the library as "gifts" on our submission forms), so I was thinking of "receiving" the stories as gifts. Additionally, I was thinking (in psychoanalytic terms) of the origins of the word, as "container" or something "that holds." I wasn't thinking of a passive vs. an active process, as in oral history we often think of silence as a presence, and talk of it as a form of "active listening" that is registered in intersubjective and non-verbal ways.

There followed a lengthy and many-voiced dialogue online—including nurses, doctors, other chaplains, and patients—about how one can receive patients' stories and how to best fulfill the role of bearing witness to sickness. The states of attention, representation, and affiliation, we agreed, contribute to our ability to bear witness to the suffering of patients and colleagues. We worked to clarify the role of the health care professional not as a passive hearer but rather as a skilled partner in building true intersubjectivity with sick people. Many of us had discovered the centrality of bearing witness in our practices. At the same time that we delivered medical care or pastoral care or physical therapy, we realized—and struggled to articulate—that we were summoned to the side of sick people to take heed of their suffering, to not let it go unnoted, to acknowledge it, and to hear them out as they told of it.

Our work in narrative medicine has led us to learn about bearing witness from oral history and trauma studies, two fields among others that, like ours, rely on attention and representation to lead to healing affiliation. Although the demands of a clinical practice devoted to the care of individual ill patients differ from the effort to let traumatized people register their experiences as public testimony, the methods developed by oral historians and trauma scholars are salient for our work. Starting with the definition of post-traumatic stress disorder in 1980 and its inclusion by the American Psychiatric Association in the DSM III, there have emerged new vocabularies and ways of thinking about trauma and its survivors.[2] Trauma studies and trauma theory grew from the practices of psychiatrists, psychoanalysts, therapists, lawyers, documentary filmmakers, autobiographers, and literary scholars who tried to understand the sequelae of trauma—including war, ethnic violence, political repression, and sexual abuse—and to treat those who had undergone it. Urgent questions surrounding the accuracy of memory and the metabolism of traumatic experience were opened up to impassioned discourse. Traumatic events on larger and larger scales came into view—the Vietnam War with the related Cambodian and Laotian atrocities, apartheid, Eastern Europe ethnic cleansings, genocide in Rwanda. In the shadows of WWI, the Holocaust, and Hiroshima, these massively scaled sufferings recapitulated the earlier unspeakable losses and the impossibility of answering to them. If all Dr. W. R. H. Rivers could do for Wilfred Sassoon was to send him back to the front, having successfully treated his shell shock, could one not do more in the face of Shoah, the atom bomb, or Khmer Rouge?

At the same time, such private traumas as childhood abuse, rape, and domestic violence became, if not more prevalent, at least more tellable, and more and more therapists and educators and clinicians found that they lacked effective responses to their patients' unburdening themselves of trauma. Not just matters of technique but of fundamental comprehensions of how human beings experience painful events were being exposed to view. In a deeply moving collaborative moment, scholars and writers and clinicians and scientists gathered, despite languages and practices that were very strange to one another, to ask, What can be done? What can be done to ease the suffering of the child who witnessed her mother's rape and murder in civil war in Rwanda? Or the soldier who perpetrated civilian casualties in Vietnam, never knowing who the enemy was? Or the Holocaust survivors still alive, who have yet to fully tell of all that they witnessed and endured?[3]

What we can learn already from oral history and trauma studies is that the work of bearing witness does not do violence to the speaker, does not *interfere* in the telling, but rather is committed to active, respectful, confirming listening. We learn from the practice of Dori Laub, a psychiatrist treating Holocaust survivors, that the survivors "needed to tell their story in order to survive. There is, in each survivor, an imperative need to *tell* and thus to come to *know* one's story, . . . to know one's buried truth in order to be able to live one's life."[4] We learn from the Cambodian healer Phaly Nuon working with women survivors of Khmer Rouge atrocities that the survivors must first remember and then forget, for then they can learn to work and to love "so that they will never have to be so lonely and so alone again."[5]

If health care professionals find themselves borrowing concepts and practices from trauma studies and oral history in the routine practice of medicine or nursing, it is because we can see one loss perhaps more powerfully in the light of another; we can recognize in catastrophic and public suffering that which is always present and needful of attention in local and private suffering. A number of doctors—Kate Scannell, Abraham Verghese, Abigail Zuger, Peter Selwyn, and Daniel Baxter—who care for people with AIDS have written about their patients' individual suffering within the frames of the global suffering this epidemic has caused.[6] The family doctor Cathy Risdon finds ways to bring human authenticity into her clinical practice by offering herself as a fresh "receiver" for a troubled teen-ager who suffers the perhaps universal burdens of adolescence.[7] The psychiatrist and pain medicine specialist Mark Sullivan treats patients with chronic pain not with nerve blocks or opiates but by encouraging them to tell, in rigorous and systematic narrating, all that surrounds the pain.[8]

Reorienting our clinical practice toward the *possibility* of bearing witness to our patients' suffering requires training and skill in listening to patients' self-narratives and in caring for the self-who-listens.[9] Not only receiving an account of trauma but also allowing the teller to see beyond it may be required for healing, for, as Dominick LaCapra notes, "the tendency for a given subject-position to overwhelm the self and become a total identity becomes pronounced in trauma, and a victim's recovery may itself depend on the attempt to reconstruct the self as more than a victim."[10] We incorporate, LaCapra reminds us, temporality and intersubjectivity into our practice through the shared effort to envision with a patient a future beyond trauma, realizing how critical are our narrative skills for our witnessing practice. We may be on the threshold of a more muscular clinical practice having made this turn toward witnessing, sharpening our understanding of empathy or compassion to include within it the "respectful, disorienting, emotional experience of the otherness of the other person: an experience that is 'straightaway ethical.'"[11] Our narrative efforts toward ethicality and intersubjectivity enable us to not just *feel* on a patient's behalf but to commit acts of particularized and efficacious recognition that lead beyond empathy to the chance to restore power or control to those who have suffered.

As curators of the body, doctors and nurses hold a special responsibility toward those who survive trauma. Geoffrey Hartman reminds us that "[p]erhaps the only way to overcome a traumatic severance of body and mind is to come back to mind through the body. We recall how voice dries up, and chokes its way out again."[12] Whether transient or terminal, all illnesses in our gaze will traumatize, will sever, will require an ethical, intersubjective effort toward reclaiming unity. In fiction as well as in practice, we can see how our response to physical illness can cross over into the generation of such noncorporeal states as hope. While Henry James's protagonist in *Wings of the Dove*, Milly Theale, lies in the palazzo dying, Sir Luke Strett returns to her side, providing care both to her and to the man, Densher, who has betrayed her:

> The facts of physical suffering, of incurable pain, of the chance grimly narrowed, had been made, at a stroke, intense, and this was to be the way [Densher] was now to feel them. The clearance of the air, in short, making vision not only

possible but inevitable, the one thing left to be thankful for was the breadth of Sir Luke's shoulders, which, should one be able to keep in line with them, might in some degree interpose. . . .

Sir Luke finally stood before him again. . . . The great man had not gone then, and an immense surrender to her immense need was so expressed in it that some effect, some help, some hope, were flagrantly part of the expression. . . . [S]ince Sir Luke *was* still there, [Milly] had been saved.[13]

The implications for health care professionals of such new roles as bearing witness and actively receiving patients' stories—and surrendering to their immense need—are enormous. If sickness opens doors to knowledge of one's self and one's values through the testimony it occasions, then the person who cares for the sick has to be prepared to midwife the life scrutiny that inevitably accompanies illness. We have to learn how to listen to the multiple registers of the body, the self, and the storyline and how to respond ethically and dutifully to what we hear. We cannot forgo this part of our task and still hope to accomplish the other parts of medicine, for the body will not bend to ministrations from someone who cannot recognize the self within it, the self exposed to the new light of day by virtue of ruptures in its surface of health.

◱ THE ACTIVE TRANSPORT OF LOVE

My own commitment to bearing witness has intensified of late by virtue of a serious illness of a close relative, who read this text and consented to my publishing it here. All along, she has been transparent in representing her interior states to me, in part so as to hear them said but also, I believe, so as to have a record of what she is going through. Her doctors did not hear all I write here for you, having signaled an unreadiness to learn about her deep experience with her illness. Because I am a doctor *and* I love her, I have a special kind of warrant to be the listener for these rocky, challenging aspects of the new self she has discovered through illness.

At age 46, Rosie (not her real name) discovered that she had a meningioma, a tumor of the lining of the brain that, although not malignant, can cause serious damage to brain and nerve tissue. Her tumor was in the part of the brain, the cerebello-pontine angle, that influences hearing, swallowing, voice, binocular vision, and balance. She went through an eight-hour neurosurgical operation less than a month after learning of the presence of the tumor. She stayed in the hospital almost a week. She was told that she might be back to work in six weeks.

This was not to be the case. Instead, Rosie has embarked on a perilous discovery of another self. As a result of the tumor itself and the surgery, she lost the hearing in her left ear. She also lost many of the functions of the brain that are so automatic that they remain out of consciousness until they are disturbed—balance, swallowing, convergence of the eyes, and speaking. What she struggles with—and what she has been able, incredibly, to put into words—is the absolutely new experience of living without these automatic abilities and having to perform each one, consciously, in order to get through a day.

"When I take a shower, I don't feel the warm water. Instead, I feel the cold water and the hot water separately." I was astonished when she said this in the weeks following her surgery. I realized that she must have lost averaging functions of the sensory brain that would, for the rest of us, smooth out the tactile sensations of different punctate elements of temperature. It is as if she went from nineteenth-century realist oil painting to pointillism overnight. Similarly, she found that she had lost certain auditory filters that she had no idea she had had: "Last night on the news, I heard the anchor saying, 'I know, I know' in the middle of the newscast. I assumed that he was talking to the voice from the control booth that comes through those earpieces they wear, but I was the only one who heard him say that." Perhaps, even with her hearing loss, her acuity with the remaining ear has become sharper and she simply heard something that others did not hear. Or perhaps an automatic sensory filter—that would have excised as meaningless this unintended and interruptive auditory tag—is disengaged, giving Rosie more intimate access to all her sensory input.

Loss of vestibular function is not a simple matter of feeling dizzy when you move. Rosie has lost the knowledge of where her body is in space. In order to walk, she has to think, consciously, of where she puts each foot. She has to decide what to do with her arms while she walks. Each motion causes a sea-swell of feeling in her head, not nausea and not dizziness but the sense that everything has gone awry. This happens whenever she moves. Damage to the eighth nerve has caused not only vestibular dysfunction but tinnitus. She describes it not as buzzing or ringing in her ears but as "screaming in my head" that accompanies her always. Doctors say there is little treatment available for tinnitus and that most patients find a way to live with it. I doubt we understand fully the burden of this chronic and, to our minds, benign symptom.

Damage to the vagus nerve and the hypoglossal nerve have caused difficulties in swallowing. Despite vigorous swallowing rehabilitation exercises, Rosie is unable to swallow even liquids without consciously relaxing the upper esophageal sphincter by tightening the abdominal muscles. If she doesn't do this, she chokes. She has found herself changing tonic behavior to adapt to this change in function. For example, she no longer tastes food as she cooks, because she would have to go through the rather complex and time-consuming procedure of opening the sphincter before putting food into her mouth, and so she has "learned" to cook without tasting as she goes.

I put learned in quotation marks, because it is exactly this process of adopting new behaviors that I want to emphasize. This new self of hers is one who does not taste as she cooks. It is an odd discontinuity. This new self of hers cannot spontaneously sprint to the front door when the bell rings. She cannot, alas, go fishing on the weekends because the stimulation of the light, the waves, the motion, the expanse of being on her beloved fishing boat is a sensory overload. She cannot enjoy a meal or read a book. She has lost about 20 percent of her preoperative weight by virtue of her difficulty with eating. I asked her if the new self were becoming more familiar or less alien to her. What she said in response was, "I remember not to taste food while I'm cooking." Which is to say: she doesn't live naturally in this new self. She continues to be struck by who she has become, looking around to realize the dimensions of strangeness she has suddenly inherited.

Nonetheless, her treatment is considered a success. The meningioma was completely removed, as well as we can tell from postoperative MRIs. The deficits she is left with are known complications of neurosurgery and, it is hoped, will improve with continued aggressive rehabilitation, glottal repair, perhaps upper esophageal sphincter dilatation, and procedures to realign the extraocular muscles. She attends vestibular rehab twice a week, swallowing therapy twice a week, physical therapy three times a week to restore function to the upper extremity muscles weakened by the surgery, and a psychological support group and individual counseling once a week apiece. This is what she does. She tries to get better. When people see her, especially after a length of time, they tell her how marvelous she looks. She accepts their compliments graciously, but usually says to herself, "If only they knew. If only they knew how foreign I feel to myself. I am not myself. I have become a different person. I will never be the person I was."

Knowing I wanted to write a narrative description of Rosie's experience enabled me to achieve a particularly careful state of attention in the conversations I record here. When my relative read what I reproduce here, she felt heard; she felt that she had been given voice in my little text. She showed what I had written to others as a marker of her experience. The simple transaction of attentive listening and then faithful representation of what had been heard deepened the bonds of affiliation between us—an enactment once again of the spirals of narrative medicine, here not in the office but at home.

By reporting "from the front" aspects of illness that none of us on this side of the divide can fathom, Rosie has taught me lessons about the self altered by disease, lessons that I have absorbed through the membranes of love. I know that her neurosurgeon and otolaryngologist do not know what I know about Rosie's recovery, and yet the case can more and more strongly be made that they would care for her more effectively if they *did* know these things. What I learned about Rosie through the active transport of love can be learned, I believe, about our patients. This is not to say that patients are to be treated as if they are family, and yet the lessons we learn in our loving relationships have their corollaries or their instances in our practice. Once we experience our capacity to witness the plight of another—through loving commitment—we have at our disposal, to use in our practice, this permeability to others' suffering, this receptivity toward the words of others, this generosity of self in the service of another self, trying to be heard.

▨ NO ONE EVER LET ME DO THIS BEFORE

My new patient, I shall call him here Mr. Ignatio Ortiz, told me a great deal about himself during that first visit, including the early death of his father to kidney disease, the death at a young age of his oldest brother also to kidney disease, the disruption of moving from the Dominican Republic to New York City as a teenager, the recent shift from construction work to part-time clerking in a clothing store because of physical inability to do strenuous work, and his current shame at being unable to support his family without accepting welfare. Throughout his account of himself, he interspersed reports of such physical symptoms as chest pain, shortness of breath, joint pain, and fatigue. I thought he seemed depressed, and his symptoms were atypical for angina. Nonetheless I scheduled a stress test, in part because I thought he might feel relieved to have proof of a healthy heart. He accepted with gratitude.

I was shocked, on dialing up the report the next week, to find he had coronary artery disease with a reversible perfusion defect in the territory of the right coronary artery. I called the cardiology clinic myself to schedule an appointment for him. (Had he been a patient with insurance more desirable than Medicaid, I would have called one of my friends in private cardiology practice, and Mr. Ortiz would have been seen the next day.) A cardiology fellow saw my patient within a week or two and started him on an antianginal protocol of beta-blockers and nitrates, holding cath in reserve should this fail.

Upon a subsequent visit to my office, Mr. Ortiz and I reviewed the events of the past months. His chest pain and shortness of breath had entirely resolved. He felt much more vigorous—and looked to me considerably less depressed and passive. In the meantime, I had published a description of our first visit in a medical journal (having changed many clinical details to render him unrecognizable) because I had been so moved by his tears and his saying that no one had ever let him tell of himself before.[14] I told him I had published my recollection of our first meeting and offered to send him a reprint of the article. When I asked if he remembered our first visit, he became very animated. "Of course I remember it," he said. "I felt great confidence in your skill as a doctor because of what you did that day. Every day since then, I pray for you." We just sat there, both of us smiling broadly, taking in our good fortune at having found one another.

What it amounted to, it seemed to me in retrospect, was that, together, we appreciated our medical transference. We both understood that our relationship had developed some ingredient that deepened it and rendered it particularly powerful. I certainly do not call the cardiology clinic myself for every patient, I must admit. He might not have attended the appointment given to him by a new doctor had we not "met" in the way we did. Since then, we have continued to follow his coronary artery disease. His sadness and shame have by no means gone away. He continues to have joint pain, fatigue, trouble with his son, bursts of intolerable but uncontrollable anger. I invite him to tell me about what he goes through. Although I *do* listen as an internist—deciding to get knee films, for example, and to start anti-inflammatory medicine for his joint pain—I listen also for his story of himself. He finds comfort and strength in the telling and finds himself remembering things from childhood and making connections among his emotions, his past, and his physical symptoms. His insight is deep, sophisticated, and brave, as I tell him.

He agreed with me that he is depressed—not suicidal, not hopeless, but discouraged, often tearful, and stumped. I told him that we can treat his depression, either with talking therapy or with antidepressant medication. He chose to begin with talking therapy. Instead of appointing him to the social worker for supportive psychotherapy, I see him myself every two weeks. I asked a colleague of mine, a medical social worker with a background in family therapy, to become my supervisor as I undertake this new blend of internal medicine and supportive talking therapy. It feels right for me to commit this work myself instead of referring Mr. Ortiz to a separate psychotherapist, because his emotional pain is intimately tied to his physical situation. It would feel disruptive of his integrity as a self-with-a-body to pull apart those two aspects of his suffering, apportioning the discouragement and depression to the social worker and keeping the chest pain and shortness of breath for myself.

I believe that what I am trying to do for Mr. Ortiz is to bear witness to his suffering while learning which aspects of it might be relieved, sharing with him the understanding that we have no idea which "causes" which. Do the fatigue and joint pain, by preventing him from doing strenuous work, contribute to his discouragement and deepen his shame? Does his clinical depression, with its element of pessimism and discouragement, trigger feelings of fatigue and intensify his awareness of his chronic pain? I work to manage his joint pain and coronary artery disease while learning about his life, his past, and the sense he now is making of it. Our work can, perhaps, help him to understand his outbursts of anger, to learn how to be a father for his teen-age son, and to work in the clothing store as best he can despite his physical limitations. The attention with which we began our work led to representation, and his reading the description of our first meeting that I published in the *New England Journal of Medicine* added a concrete proof of my investment in him. Together, these movements of attention and representation led us to heed the development of our affiliation as a mutually empowering and valuable fact of our lives that could, indeed, improve his health.

THE PRACTICE OF NARRATIVE MEDICINE

I want to describe in very practical terms what differences narrative medicine's triad of attention, representation, and affiliation make in my practice as an internist.[15] Narrative considerations influence a cascade of dimensions of typical practice: the gathering of information, the keeping of records, the making of therapeutic decisions, and the building of relationships over time. More fundamentally, narrative considerations probe what, in the end, it might *mean* to be sick and to be well. With narrative illumination, much in the landscape of the body and health changes. We see how intricate are the processes that lead to one's feeling well, one's feeling oneself, and, more saliently for health professionals, we see how much we can do for those who are ill and in our hands.

If we are to make a difference in conventional health care, we are obliged to invent new practices through which health care professionals can reach these new goals. We have to articulate what they are, how one accomplishes them, how one evaluates one's effectiveness in having done them, how one trains others to do them, and what difference to patient care they make. Medicine being the instrumental field that it is, we have to come up with the forms—in triplicate!—on which one might report that one has completed the narrative parts of one's task, not only to bill for one's time (this is the nihilistic angle) but also, in John Berger's description of country doctor John Sassall, to clerk the records for one's community of patients: "He does more than treat them when they are ill; he is the objective witness of their lives. They seldom refer to him as a witness. . . . He is in no way a final arbiter. That is why I chose the rather humble word *clerk*: the clerk of their records. . . . He keeps the records so that, from time to time, they can consult them themselves. . . . He represents them, becomes their objective (as opposed to subjective) memory . . . because he also represents some of what they know but cannot think."[16]

Gathering Information

Narrative considerations of illness challenge conventional routines of gathering clinical information. If we believe that patients' telling of the self and the body means something and that the form as well as the content matter, then we cannot learn what we must learn about and from patients by asking everyone the same set of questions. Instead, we health professionals have to equip ourselves with radically more flexible and creative skills. We have to become porous to that which patients emit about themselves in many, many channels. "Not only must the physician hear what is said but with a trained ear he or she must *listen* to the exact words that the patient uses and the sequence in which they are uttered," writes the endocrinologist and former dean of Westminster Hospital Medical School Sir Richard Bayliss. "Histories must be received, not taken."[17]

When I met Mr. Ortiz, I was using for the first time the new approach I invented for meeting a new patient. It begins simply with the invitation to "tell me what you think I should know about your situation," and is followed by a commitment to *listen* and not—at least at the start—to write or even to speak. When I first started doing this, I had to literally sit on my hands to prevent myself from writing in the chart or calling up the patient's computerized medical record. The pressures are so very ingrained to write everything down, formatting them even as they are heard into the History of Present Illness or Family History or Review of Systems. It was only when I was able to forgo the ordering imperative that I became able to absorb what patients tell me without deranging their narratives into my own form of story.

As the patient tells, I listen as hard as I can—not taking notes during this segment of the interview, not interrupting unless critical, not indicating one way or another what I consider salient or meaningful or interesting. I try my best to register the diction, the form, the images, the pace of speech. I pay attention—as I sit there at the edge of my seat, absorbing what is being given—to metaphors, idioms, accompanying gestures, as well as plot and characters represented for me by the patient. Although I know I have to collect such information as dosages of medications, dates of surgeries, allergies, smoking history, and family history, I have grown confident that these items will emerge naturally as the visit proceeds. Usually, we spend around twenty to thirty minutes on the patient's narrative of self. So far, in my experience, the patient reaches a point where he or she has said what needs to be said.

At that point, I ask the patient to change into a cotton gown so that I can perform the physical examination. While the patient changes into the gown on the other side of the curtain in my exam/consultation room, I write down as accurately as I can what the patient told me in the opening narrative. I preserve the order in which things were said, trying to use the patient's words and turns of phrase. I do my best to represent the integrity of the narrative—its tempo, its transitions, its figural language. (Perhaps I should be tape-recording these recitations and then transcribing them, but I am trying for a method that can be used routinely and speedily.) I include at the end a very brief sense of the person I have just met—not only a diagnostic portrait but also a singular rendering of the person.

Here is an example of the write-up that emerged from a new patient visit conducted in my new way:

1st AIM visit 32 yo ♀

On the eve of starting a new job as placement coordinator at St. Vincent's homeless shelter, Ms. Henri has received health insurance & desires a general doctor. She thinks of herself as well—strong, knowledgeable about her body When her L leg hurt, she saw a podiatrist who assured her it was not related to poor circulation or another chronic condition. When she developed pain in the R flank, she saw her gynecologist who thought it related to a UTI & chronically full bladder.

Difficult time over past year when laid off from job as school aide for special ed students. Got through the loss through reflection with friends, faith, prayer, & church support. Examined her own contribution to work loss. Psychology major at City College, education minor. Loves to read/think/study—eventually wants to get CSW/MSW.

Moved from Haiti when 15 yo—family here already. Worked assiduously in English + language skills.

Presents as gifted in language, resourceful in problem-solving, optimistic about the future, reflective + honest about self.

I find tremendous interest and joy in allowing myself to be bathed in a stranger's telling of self. I am stunned at how singular—how absolutely unique—are these self/body narratings. It is a charged experience for us both, as the patient takes *liberties* in telling of health or illness and I work very hard in the listening. As I listened to Ms. Henri, I felt more and more eager to hear each sentence—her speech was eloquent, evocative, and figurally dense. She conveyed very deep emotions while she described tough experiences, able, it seemed to me as I heard her, to merge her past difficulties with the lessons she had absorbed from them. In effect, she was such a skilled storyteller that I heard both the girl she had been and the woman she was now. I could see her as she saw herself—able, confident, powerful in helping others, understanding of others' pain. And this vision of her, in effect in her own mind's eye, gave me a rich sense of her hopes. I could bear witness to her *future self,* in an odd way. Not only to be free from physical disease, her health goals for herself became magnified or deepened into life goals.

This is one simple way to shift the balance of the ordinary office practice of medicine toward narrativity. Linguistic research in the development of doctor-patient relationships suggests that warmth and intimacy between doctor and patient tend not to build over time, but rather achieve whatever levels they will achieve in the first meeting.[18] The first visit with a new patient is critical, then, in establishing *where this dyad can go.* How deep into the self can this partnership go? How *useful* to the patient might this new relationship become? It is one thing to have a phone number to call when one has the flu or gets a back spasm. It is quite another to feel that one has a resource, much as Milly Theale does upon her first meeting with Sir Luke Strett. Through the disciplined development of attention and representation in routine practice, I think I am beginning to offer fresh resources to my medical patients.

At first, I reserved this interviewing method for meeting new patients. As I saw what a difference it made in my *attitude* as well as in the patient's seeming comfort with telling about illness, I have adopted it with all my visits, however long I have been the patient's doctor. I find that the practice doesn't take any longer than the write-as-you-go method and that, by adopting this simple narrative corrective to my office visits, I am with the patients while they tell me what I must hear. As a wonderful dividend, my notes are far more telling than they used to be—perhaps not as systematically structured as once they were, but filled now with levels of truth, evocative, alive to the presence of patients, and dutiful to the honor of having heard them out.

Keeping Medical Records

I realize that patients may tell me things during office visits that they ordinarily would not have told the internist. Patients feel invited to tell me more about their lives than generally occurs in the doctor's office, and we find that mutual trust builds as a result of more careful listening and more extensive telling. Both teller and listener are seen as somehow more dutiful, more able to either reveal or contain that which has been said. Once told, these new aspects of patients' "histories" give us a wider frame within which to contemplate their lives. Patients seem surprised, at times, at where our conversations go. Tears flow, childhood events surface, and material that would otherwise have taken many visits to reach are exposed, even in a first meeting. If I alter my practice, through attention, to elicit rich, spontaneous, narratively liberated *telling* of self in the office visit, and if I learn to represent that talk in writing with some faithfulness, what do I do with what I have written? Once I know these things about my patients, even things that might not seem medically salient, what do I do with this knowledge?

The corollary to speaking differently with our patients is writing differently about them. Unlike my father in his solo office, I do not keep medical records solely for myself. My practice is within a faculty group practice of a teaching hospital, and I write in the same chart written in by the ophthalmologist, the urologist, the nutritionist, the social worker, or the surgeon. I have to balance my need to remember things about my patients with the desire to keep secrets from all the others who might read what I write. I cannot share all that I learn about my patients with the orthopedic surgeon who casts my patient's ankle when she falls on the ice, nor with the billing clerk who determines how much to bill Medicaid for her office care.

I have come slowly to appreciate that patients should be the curators of what we write about them.[19] At the conclusion of visits, I give patients a copy of my chart note, making sure that they can read my handwriting and encouraging them to add to what has been said on the next visit. It ought not be up to me to decide who should read the record of my patients' personal troubles, even if these troubles may influence their health status or medical care. Instead, these records should be in the patients' hands, and it should be up to them to decide who has permission to read particularly private aspects of their history. I would like the printer who makes up the Presbyterian Hospital charts to make up some charts for my patients. In the patient's chart, there will be room for the officially generated medical records—copies of my notes, copies of imaging and laboratory test results, copies perhaps of the notes of other health care professionals who wish to participate in our new practice. On the other side of the chart will be room to collate what patients write about themselves—their experiences, their questions, reports of their glucometer readings or blood pressure monitoring. There will be room for the reflections of family members—the daughter whose demented mother no longer remembers who she is, the father bereft by the profound disability of his premature neonate. There will be room for the Parallel Chart writing of health care professionals who write about aspects of the care of this patient that do not belong in the widely circulated hospital chart. Such a change in charting practice might enact forcefully our often-stated beliefs about privacy and confidentiality while asserting officially that the patient's voice is a critical ingredient in health care.

If Presbyterian Hospital introduced the hospital chart in 1916, perhaps it is time for the emergence of another form of record-keeping, in keeping with contemporary beliefs and ideas about what causes illness, what supports health, and what health care professionals can do for their patients. The electronic medical record has already begun to alter fundamentally how we handle medical data— how they are inscribed, how it is accessed, how it is formatted, who gets to read it. Checklists of complaints are electronically completed by patients before they attend their office visit; chart notes are being written online, prompted by highly regimented screens limiting the amount of free text that can be recorded. I love the convenience of our electronic records—results of imaging studies available immediately, lab tests displayed going back decades, even viewing

X-rays online is now possible from my office desk. In the face of today's electronic resources, we doctors and nurses and social workers can decide to continue writing about patients in ordinary language—using some of the time freed up by the electronic conveniences to add narrative depth to the instrumental data generated by machines.

Instead of complaining that the chart has become a billing ticket or an electronic wasteland of abbreviations and answers to yes/no questions, perhaps health professionals can take the opportunity of the current upheaval in medical record-keeping to introduce new, robust means of charting patients' journeys through illness and to develop responsible methods of articulating their own personal experiences as caregivers. Narrative medicine's focus on the power of language in illness and health should *amount to* something in the day-in, day-out practice of medicine. What it may well amount to, I am convinced, is a more effective merging of the instrumental and the reflective in the work of medicine, in the lives of patients and in the lives of caregivers. Such a merging will require new narrative forms in which to contain, reflect, and discover these perceptions of health and illness. If, indeed, increasing doctors' skill to represent that which is seen and heard contributes to more effective affiliations between doctor and patient, there is an imperative to put these narrative practices into routine use.

Making Therapeutic Decisions

Not only how we learn about our patients and where we write it down change in narrative medicine. The kinds of therapeutic decisions we make can be remarkably different from conventional medical decision-making as a result of narrative deepening of doctor-patient relationships.

Bruno Moralez first came to see me last fall. A recent immigrant from the Dominican Republic, he had lost his job as a painter in lower Manhattan after the World Trade Center attacks. Able to get only pick-up, part-time work, he was struggling to pay his rent and feed his family. At age 59, he felt relatively healthy, although he recently had developed some back and neck pain and feeling sluggish, gaining weight, sleeping late, and withdrawing into isolation. He had been treated once for depression, but the antidepressant had only made him sleepy. He was not interested in repeating that experience. He told me directly that what he wanted to do was to get back into physical shape. He wanted to work out in a gym or with home equipment, but he had no money to afford gym membership or free weights. He was quite adamant that this was the best way for him to treat his current symptoms. I realized that his dependence on his wife's family for help with the rent humiliated him and that by physically regaining his muscular presence, he might regain his presence as a man and husband and father.

While he sat in the office with me on our first meeting, I called a local city park that had recently opened a gym. I thought membership was free to community residents, and I happily held out to him the assurance that we could get him registered in a gym right away. I was wrong. Gym membership is only free to senior citizens. It would cost him $152 a year to join the gym. Both of us turned glum. We sat and stared at one another. And then I said, "It's okay. I'll give you $152." And I did. I left an envelope for him with that much money in cash the next day. My receptionist thought I was nuts, as did some colleagues with whom I discussed this.[20] Now, I knew that my giving him this amount of money was unusual and perhaps almost out of line. I discussed my plan with some colleagues before actually leaving the money for him, and they helped me to examine this contemplated act. What might be the consequences of giving the patient the money? What should I do to ensure that there were no unwanted sequelae? I had wondered if my patient felt unduly beholden to his wife and wife's mother who were helping to pay his rent. Would my act of paying for his gym membership also function to feminize or weaken him? Would he think himself unduly indebted to me as a result of this gift, and would that complicate our medical contract? I decided, after consulting with my colleagues, to go ahead and leave the money but to keep in mind these possible consequences of my unusual clinical intervention.

When I next saw Mr. Morales, he proudly showed me his membership card in Riverpark Gym. He looked terrific. He was working out in the gym about one and a half hours three times a week. His back and neck pain were resolved. His mood seemed vastly improved since the last visit. Without antidepressants and without formal psychotherapy, he seemed to be regaining his health, not through the conventional avenues of medicine but through his own choice of treatment and version of care. My impulsive offer of money, I decided in retrospect, had signaled very concretely that I heard and valued his assessment of his situation and what might improve it. It did not seem to have added to his humiliation about his lack of money but rather had improved his sense of strength and power in his daily life. In fact, during our second visit, he seemed happy that I had made his gym membership possible and seemed relieved that he had been able to start in on his vigorous program of physical training. I am not suggesting by this story that all doctors as a matter of course should contribute money toward their patients' nonmedical needs. Not at all. Nor have I made a practice of such donations. I recount this story as an unusual event in my practice that helped me learn an important lesson in narrative medicine's potential in clinical care.

STORIES GROW WITH TIME

I am impressed with the consequences over time, *for myself and for my patients,* of my narrative practices. The act of writing evocative, "thick" descriptions of patients, I have learned, alters rather fundamentally my own stance vis-à-vis the patient. Like my lesson long ago with Luz, the very act of imagining a patient, struggling to represent in words what he or she emits, inspecting my own teller's tale about the care of the patient, trying—if only for the sake of the story—to sharpen my impressions and to intensify my attention toward the patient have not only short-term outcomes (as seen in the piece of writing itself) but have long-lived spiraling effects over time.

Only as I wrote the description last week of the patient I called Bruno Moralez, some months after that first visit and the $152 transaction, I found myself wondering about his involvement in the World Trade Center attack. He had mentioned in passing that he lost his job as a result of the attacks, and yet I had not pursued the questions that now urgently plagued me. After having reviewed some of the recent literature in trauma studies for this chapter, I was particularly attuned to my role as witness. Had he been directly involved in the trauma of that horrible attack? Had he lost coworkers? Where was he on September 11, 2001? Could any of the relapse of his depression be a direct result of trauma?

He came in, fortuitously, last Thursday for his follow-up visit. He was still going to the gym, although he seemed to have lost some of his enthusiasm for the project. He was still out of work and seemed more discouraged about the likelihood of finding a job. Fresh from my confrontation with his situation in my imagination and filled with alarmed curiosity about his direct involvement in the attack, I hastened to say to him that I remember he used to work in lower Manhattan and that I should have asked about his own involvement in the events of that day.

He was there. He was himself caught in the horror of the attacks. As I sat in silence, letting him speak uninterruptedly for about half an hour, he told me of his ordeal. He had been in the Broad Street subway station, very close to what we now call Ground Zero. He heard a big explosion, thinking it was a gas main break, and then saw a huge section of ceiling cave in over the tracks. Police herded him and everyone else on the platform over to one section. No one knew what was happening. Cellular phones did not work. People couldn't breathe for the dust and smoke caused by the ceiling collapse. After about half an hour, police let the people exit the subway platform. The air outside was dark with smoke and dust and material falling from the towers. People were running and crying and falling in the streets. Police made everyone head eastward over the Brooklyn Bridge. Even though no one knew yet what had happened, they could see the flaming towers of the World Trade Center. When Bruno was about halfway across the bridge to Brooklyn, he looked back to Manhattan to see the second tower fall. It took until after midnight for him to walk all the way to his home in upper Manhattan to a frenzied and radiant reception from a family who, by then, assumed he had perished.

This recitation was given gravely, tearfully, sometimes in a rush of words as if pent up and sometimes interrupted by silences as words were sought. Bruno had had nightmares about the event and had relived all of this many, many times. It was not clear to me whether he had been able to tell it all clearly. What Dori Laub writes about the testimony of Holocaust survivors seemed that it might be the case here: "The emergence of the narrative which is being listened to—and heard—is, therefore, the process and the place wherein the cognizance, the 'knowing' of the event is given birth to."[21] And in my position as listener, even if I was just the general internist on a routine follow-up medical visit, I incurred the duty to witness. We were both on uncharted ground, Bruno not realizing he would be invited to tell of this ordeal and my not predicting that I would be the active recipient of his account, and yet we accomplished the goals, it seemed to us both, of that initial telling.

I can say this because of what happened next. Bruno described to me his belief in *destino*. He believes with great passion and force that God saved him from the World Trade Center attack for a reason and that he has a destiny to accomplish. Many Dominicans, Bruno told me, who worked in the World Trade Center were spared from death there, because they were fated to die on Flight 787 weeks later. His answer to my question, "But can we know our fate?" was to say simply that it is a mystery.

We left our forty-five-minute visit profoundly moved, the two of us. I felt he had received me into a sacred trust, marked with faith and courage. He took my hand in both of his, thanked me seriously for giving him the time to talk, and seemed elevated and *happy* at what had just happened. As with Mr. Ortiz, I felt this patient and I had shared an authentic intersubjective experience that we both valued and that would deepen and make all the more genuine—and even maybe more effective—the routine clinical work we would do together in the future. Once again, simple acts of attention and representation—this time with my own rereading of my written text as a pivotal step—led to improved clinical affiliation.

Another long-term patient from my practice helps me understand one of the mechanisms of this temporal evolution of narrative engagement. I wrote the following about a patient in my practice for a journal article around five years ago:[22]

Mrs. Ruby Nelson is an 82-year-old obese, diabetic, hypertensive woman with osteoarthritis who has been in my practice for around 15 years. Our early years together were marked by disagreement over little things: she insisted on brand name medicines, even when generics were just as good, and I bristled at the extra work and cost. She never took seriously the need to address her obesity. Consequently, her diabetes was ill-controlled and her degenerative knee disease disabling. One morning, as she sat on the examining table waiting for me to take her blood pressure (which was invariably alarmingly high and triggered in me anxiety, fear of reprisal, great impatience, and the felt duty to scold), she mentioned that she sang in the church choir. I don't know why, but I asked her to sing me a hymn. This woman, whose body habitus I routinely described as "morbidly obese," was transfigured into a form of stateliness and dignity as she raised her heavy head, clasped her hands, and sang in a deep dark alto about the Lord, on the banks of the river, bringing her home. From then on, I would do anything for her and she for me. A moment of epiphany indeed, those few bars of mournful powerful song transported us into a new geography of respect and value together.

Since then, she has developed cerebrovascular disease, requiring multiple hospitalizations to stave off strokes. She has remained for me, throughout her many weeks in the hospital, a figure of great dignity and spirituality. Despite the firm recommendations of the social workers and visiting nurses [to place her in a nursing home], I backed her deep desire to return to her own apartment, knowing, now, something about the power of her desires. She is now back home, anticoagulated, her blood pressure effectively controlled, TIAs for the time being absent. She continues to ask me to do her little special favors in the office, and I am always grateful that she asks.

I included this description in a lecture I gave, a very meaningful one for me—the convocation address at graduation when I was awarded my Ph.D. in English—letting this patient whom I called Mrs. Nelson speak *for* me about my work. The patient was able to stay home for many years with phalanxes of visiting nurses, home health attendants, physical therapists, and wound specialists who came to visit her at home. I was on the phone with one or another of her home care providers maybe twice a week. It was not easy, and I sometimes grew out of patience for being quarterback of this increasingly complex team.

In 2003 and 2004, the patient required multiple hospitalizations for falls, infections, and worsening diabetes. By the fourth or fifth admission in as many months, the nurses and social workers and I all finally relented and transferred Mrs. Nelson to a nursing home. I told her it might be temporary, but within myself, I knew she would die in the nursing home.

About three months after her discharge to the nursing home, her niece called me at the office. I assumed, when I heard her voice on my voice mail, that she was calling to tell me her aunt had died, and I felt the guilty pang of having abandoned this patient, to whom I had once felt such allegiance. But it was not a death call. Mrs. Nelson absolutely insisted that the nursing home discharge her back to her apartment. She refused to sign papers that would allow them to keep her in the home. My advice to her niece was *not* to back her aunt's desire to return home. I remembered how very difficult it had been the last time she was home. I felt that letting her go home was just too dangerous—she would fall again and break her hip; she would have a major bleed; she would have another stroke. And, I realized, I did not relish resuming the complex and wearing responsibilities of overseeing her home care.

Her niece thanked me most politely for my advice. But then a few days later, I found myself within blocks of the patient's nursing home. I could not help myself from paying her a visit. There she was—turban on head, sprawled in bed, gazing mutely at the ceiling, foot dressed where she had had a toe amputated. I called out her name softly and, when she first looked at me somewhat blankly, said my name. She rose. "Dr. Charon. You came to see me." We were silly with joy to be in one another's presence again. I drew a chair up to her bed and listened as she told me, with woe, what life was like for her in the home. I wanted to know specifically how life would be different for her were she to be back home. I asked what she would do in the apartment, who would help her out, how she'd spend her days.

"What would you eat at home that you can't eat here?" I asked her. She gazed into the middle distance and said, with eloquent and precise gestures of her angularly deformed arthritic hands, "I would get a piece of fish this big, and I would fry it up in the skillet, or have the girl to do it for me, and I would make some grits to go along with it." The look on her face of anticipatory pleasure reached my heart and formed my resolve. I introduced myself to the head nurse at the nurses' station, saying I had been Mrs. Nelson's internist for 23 years. If, I told her, the staff here thinks she is stable enough to be discharged home, I, as her "community physician," am happy to resume direction of her care.

Now: I would not have developed this loyalty without having written about the patient, without having spent time in my imagination with her and, by doing so, realizing how I valued the years we had spent as a dyad. I have a screw loose for her, as John Marcher says about May Bartram in "The Beast in the Jungle," and the screw loosened in the narrative acts of inventing, imagining, and finding the words to speak for her and about her. These narrative acts showed me what I did not know until I committed them: that this patient stands for something transcendent for myself, something primal for my life as a doctor, and something resolutely spiritual in my life. It is as irrational as it is clinically salient. I have a screw loose for her, and that means I will accept the slightly foolhardy clinical assignment toward fulfilling her deep wishes for her future.

Is it too foolhardy, which is to say, is my clinical judgment being deranged by my attachment to her? I think not. I will alter my clinical routines to be faithful to my new level of commitment. Mrs. Nelson did return to her home soon after my visit to the nursing home. We reinstated all aspects of her complex home care—visiting nurse, physical therapist, blood drawing at home, and extensive help from her extended family in many aspects of her health care. I have started paying monthly house calls to Mrs. Nelson. Instead of fielding phone calls from her nurse and physical therapist and niece and requiring her to make the arduous trip by ambulette to my clinic office every few months, we now gather around her bed, in her home, one Friday morning each month. We all derive real pleasure from being together, being with the heroine of the story, and doing our joint work in a more effective way. What matters here, it seems to me, is that I have been able to envision and learn of her desires and *act on them* by virtue of my narrative connection to her and by my narratively derived pride of what she and I can do together.

Like my work with Mr. Ortiz and Ms. Henri and Mr. Moralez, my work with Ruby Nelson enriches me, deepens me, lets me grow into a self I admire. My relationships with these people go beyond bureaucratic or professional relationships. By surrendering to the demands of these relationships—developing new counseling skills, giving money, or putting myself out to do house calls—I can claim a version of myself invisible without the surrender. I *find* aspects within me that I didn't know were there, and that I value. The screw loose, in fact, is a defining aspect of being a doctor, or at least of this doctor I find myself becoming. In addition to feeling clinically competent, I earn the means to feel narratively competent, able to register with some accuracy and benevolence the situations of others and the roles I play in their lives. I find myself an *agent* in my patients' lives, and this agency widens, *significantly*, my own sense of liveliness. At the funeral of another patient for whom I cared for more than 20 years, I read this line in the memorial program: "Mrs. Nellie Trent is survived by her niece

Belle Edwards, her friends Hetta White and Eddie Gorman, and her doctor Rita Charon." So that was who I was—I was a survivor, one of the bereaved.

I realize that the descriptions of my work with Mr. Ortiz, Mr. Morales, and Mrs. Nelson may sound excessive. More time than usual was taken with these patients. One case involved a sum of money; another involves time-consuming house calls. I do not want to suggest that all of us must be prepared to be engulfed by excessive demands of patient care. I don't do house calls very frequently at all; nor have I found myself impulsively giving money to patients beyond this one unusual circumstance. I do not write about many patients in my practice, but I find that writing about some of them intensifies the attention I am able to pay to *all* of them. Without extensive research of my practice of narrative medicine and that of others, I cannot yet know how much writing during a week or a month is "enough" to carry results over to a whole practice, but I believe that changes within a practice will come about by some narrative attention to a few patients.

The health care professional will never give up control or be swallowed up by attentiveness toward patients or excessive availability to fill all their needs. These aspects of care can be modulated, as we modulate all our professional actions. Different health care professionals will find themselves doing narrative medicine in different ways by virtue of individual interests and gifts and talents. I feel honored to have found some fresh approaches to routine clinical work, because these new ways of being a general internist *add* to my pleasure in being a doctor. Instead of feeling costly of time or overstepping of professional limits, the practices I describe here have renewed me and given me added joy. I hope I have not described any aspects of my practice as if I were being sacrificial or selfless. Quite the opposite: these new approaches to medicine have given me tremendous pleasure and lift, for which I feel extraordinarily grateful.

BUILDING COMMUNITY

Bearing witness requires community. Bearing witness to the suffering of individuals creates community—in Holocaust survivor interviews, September 11, 2001 memorials, or caring for Mrs. Nelson in her home. If narrative medicine includes the duty to bear witness to individual patients' suffering, we find ourselves naturally drawn to identify and join with the communities in which the suffering and potential healing might occur. The turn toward oral history and trauma studies for inspiration gives us the dividend of focusing on the communities that nourish our patients' sense of self, of belonging, and of future, for it is in these communities that a return to wholeness or health happens. Mr. Ortiz laments the loss of his roots in the Dominican culture and country. Bruno Morales suffers in concert with the thousands who died at the World Trade Center. Ruby Nelson yearns not only for her bed in her Harlem apartment but to be encircled by her family and neighbors and friends.

Bearing witness to suffering helps us to overcome some of illness's pernicious divides. The divides I outlined in chapter 2—relation to mortality, contexts of illness, beliefs about causality, and the emotions of shame, blame, and fear— culminate in isolating patients from those who care for them.[23] These divides separate us from our patients and require explicit bridges in order for effective care to proceed. The outcomes of bearing witness, as proposed in this chapter, can bridge the divides. We can, with health-related dividends, make contact with the communities in which our patients dwell. This contact will lead us to take account of patients' contexts of illness, their beliefs about illness's source, their fear and hopes, and what they make of dying. If pastoral care connects suffering individuals with communities of faith and trauma care connects individual trauma survivors with communities of survivors and witnesses, then narrative medicine can connect patients and their caregivers with their natural communities of care. Communities of *presence*, these are sometimes as modest and local as the five women standing together in Mrs. Nelson's bedroom—her nurse, physical therapist, niece, neighbor, and internist. We formed a community of care that itself took on the duties not only of registering the suffering but ameliorating it. Such communities of presence, I feel, are widespread within our current practices, if only we will search them out.

As my own practice of narrative medicine develops, it is nourished by trends in other forms of health care, notably social work and psychiatry, called narrative therapy or narrative psychology. From family therapy and anthropology and social psychiatry, there has evolved a nexus of treatment that centers on narrativity and storytelling.[24] Two loci for this work are in Adelaide, South Australia, under the guidance of the family therapist Michael White and in Auckland, New Zealand, where the family therapist David Epston practices. In books and essays, White and Epston have unfolded a theoretical position and a growing body of practical experience to guide the social worker or psychotherapist in narrative approaches to treatment.[25] "Meaning," they write, "is derived through the structuring of experience into stories, and . . . the performance of these stories is constitutive of lives and relationships."[26] Grounded conceptually in the work of such anthropologists as Victor Turner and Gregory Bateson and the formulations of power and knowledge of Michel Foucault, White and Epston use letter-writing, family storytelling sessions, detailed written notes shared with clients, and certificates celebrating the accomplishments of milestones to help clients not only record but also create change within their lives. The enduring contributions of narrative therapy are the focus on community witnessing and the importance of social ritual in healing.

The differences between narrative therapy and narrative medicine are evident, and yet the goals are similar, the difficulties in conventional approaches parallel, and the richness of narrative theory and practice immediately applicable. I report in chapter 11 some of our efforts to build community among health care professionals in health care institutions and the neighborhoods they serve. These wider circles of affiliation amplify the local affiliations considered in this chapter between individual patient and doctor. Narrative theory and practice hold out the promise of a set of solutions to the hobbling isolation and divisions that currently plague and weaken our medicine. Through the efforts of diverse clinicians—family therapists, chaplains, trauma psychologists, and visiting nurses—we can see practical means to improve the effectiveness of care we now offer. Recognizing, hearing out, receiving, and honoring the stories of illness may give doctors and nurses and social workers new tools with which to make contact with patients and to ease the suffering of disease.

▣ TRAINING FOR NARRATIVE MEDICINE

It is not enough to suggest that health care professionals have to bear witness to their patients' suffering, on top of everything else they do. We cannot impose on tremendously overworked and overburdened health care professionals to do that which they were never trained to do. I believe that doctors, nurses, and social workers *want* to be able to provide narratively robust, authentic care to the ill, and yet they have currently neither the resources nor the time nor the expertise to accomplish what, ideally, they should be able to do for each patient in the face of illness.

Many clinicians feel ill equipped to bear witness to patients through attention and representation in practice. The impulse to roll up our sleeves and *do* something is irresistible and, sadly, attentive listening does not feel enough like clinical action. Fortunately, we in medicine have begun to learn from the work of colleagues in pastoral care, oral history, trauma studies, and psychoanalysis how to hear about these aspects of illness. We don't have to reinvent or rediscover practices that our colleagues can teach us—what we do have to do is to humbly establish collegial contact with them.

The theoretical foundations of narrative medicine have come to foreground witnessing models from clinical fields other than medicine whose practitioners have been committed to *hearing patients out,* to being the active receptacles for patients' stories of suffering. Training, some of it quite unorthodox, is becoming available to doctors, nurses, and social workers who want to buttress their skills to bear witness to their patients. The Kenneth B. Schwartz Center in Boston sponsors a yearlong intensive training program in pastoral care skills for medical personnel.[27] The American Academy on Physician and Patient sponsors weeklong intensive courses in medical interviewing and frequent shorter courses in interviewing skills, developing therapeutic relationships, and supporting reflection and well-being for health care professionals themselves.[28] Rachel Remen has created the Institute for Well-Being at the Commonweal Center where health care professionals—whether "impaired" or not—can gather for retreats, courses, and lifelong learning in self-care.[29] We at Columbia are currently designing an intensive yearlong Certificate Program in Narrative Medicine and are planning to offer short workshops throughout the year in narrative skills in health care. Training in oral history, mindfulness, creative writing, and psychoanalytic practice; individual supervision from mental health professionals; and degree programs in literature, creative writing, and qualitative social sciences are additional ways that health care professionals are *searching* for means to improve practice and fulfill witnessing duties toward patients. Such developments as relationship-centered care and patient-centered care share narrative medicine's commitment to bearing witness and authenticity.[30]

Narrative medicine can open doors, as sickness does, toward the search for meaning in routine clinical practice. We will continue to learn from colleagues in related fields how to fulfill the duties we incur by virtue of bearing witness to the suffering of our patients. In part, we learn what we need to know through the active transport of love, letting our practice be informed by our own lives and families and accepting that it is not unprofessional to bring into practice lessons we learn at home. We will develop very practical revisions of clinical routines in the light of what we now know about attention, representation, and affiliation. If we can fortify our clinical training with narrative training, we will find ourselves transforming our practice, enabling those who suffer to be heard and making our care of them more effective.

NOTES

1. http://www.narrativemedicine.org has, on its home page, instructions for joining the list and posting messages.

2. See Cathy Caruth, ed., *Trauma: Explorations in Memory* and *Unclaimed Experience: Trauma, Narrative, and History;* Shoshana Felman and Dori Laub, *Testimony: Crises of Witnessing in Literature, Psychoanalysis, and History;* Geoffrey Hartman, "On Traumatic Knowledge and Literary Studies"; Dominick LaCapra, *Representing the Holocaust: History, Theory, Trauma* and *Writing History, Writing Trauma;* Claude Lanzmann, *Shoah: An Oral History of the Holocaust;* and Pat Barker, *Regeneration* for introductions to the fields of trauma studies and theory. See *The Oral History Reader* edited by Robert Perks and Alistair Thomson for an overview of methods and theories of oral history.

3. Geoffrey Hartman, "Narrative and Beyond."

4. Dori Laub, "An Event without a Witness: Truth, Testimony, and Survival," 78.

5. See description of Phaly Nuon's community treatment center in Andrew Solomon, *The Noonday Demon*, 37.

6. Katrien De Moor, "The Doctor's Role of Witness and Companion: Medical and Literary Ethics of Care in AIDS Physicians' Memoirs."

7. Cathy Risdon and Laura Edey, "Human Doctoring: Bringing Authenticity to our Care."

8. Mark D. Sullivan, "Pain in Language: From Sentience to Sapience."

9. See Roy Schafer's complex and useful discussion of self-narratives, storylines, and self-representations in the chapter "Narratives of the Self" in *Retelling a Life*. See Dori Laub, "Bearing Witness, or the Vicissitudes of Listening" for the cost to the authentically listening witness.

10. Dominick LaCapra, *Representing the Holocaust*, 12.

11. David Morris, "How to Speak Postmodern: Medicine, Illness, and Cultural Change," 5.

12. Geoffrey Hartman, "On Traumatic Knowledge and Literary Studies," 541.

13. Henry James, *The Wings of the Dove, New York Edition*, 20:299, 302.

14. Rita Charon, "Narrative and Medicine."

15. I appreciate the observations of the writer Melanie Thernstrom and student Nora

Gross as they attended office hours with me and my patients during 2003 and 2004, helping me to distinguish and describe the narrative components of the work my patients and I did.

16. John Berger and Jean Mohr, *A Fortunate Man*, 109. See also Fred Griffin's essay on teaching *A Fortunate Man*, "The Fortunate Physician: Learning from Our Patients" to a group of internists in a narrative medicine seminar.

17. Richard Bayliss. "Pain Narratives," 75.

18. Michele Greene, personal communication.

19. This is not a new idea. See, for example, Richard Giglio et al., "Encouraging Behavior Changes by Use of Client-Held Health Records" and Arnold Golodetz, Johanna Ruess, and Raymond Milhous, "The Right to Know: Giving the Patient His Medical Record" as evidence that health care professionals have been considering the patient as curator of the record for decades. That the practice has not yet become widespread may be a measure of professionals' sense of vulnerability and fear of losing control should patients be equal partners in their care.

20. I understood I was crossing a professional boundary in offering this patient money, but I felt confident that I could assess the impact of my gesture on our ongoing clinical alliance. See Neil Farber, "Love, Boundaries, and the Patient-Physician Relationship" for a discussion of other kinds of boundary-crossing that occur in clinical practice.

21. Dori Laub, "Bearing Witness, or the Vicissitudes of Listening," 57.

22. Rita Charon, "The Seasons of the Patient-Physician Relationship," 46–47.

23. Patricia Stanley, "The Patient's Voice: A Cry in Solitude or a Call for Community."

24. See Christian Beels, *"A Different Story . . .": The Rise of Narrative in Psychotherapy* for a summary of the evolution of narrative therapy from its origins in social psychiatry and community mental health. Anthropological dimensions of health and illness illuminate the cultural and social enactments of bodily conditions, emphasizing the requirement that groups and societies collaborate in whatever treatment or healing takes place. See Cheryl Mattingly, *Healing Dramas and Clinical Plots;* Byron Good and Mary-Jo DelVecchio Good, "In the Subjunctive Mode: Epilepsy Narratives in Turkey"; Byron Good, *Medicine, Rationality, and Experience: An Anthropological Perspective;* and Arthur Kleinman, *The Illness Narratives: Suffering, Healing, and the Human Condition.*

25. See Michael White and David Epston, *Narrative Means to Therapeutic Ends* and Epston and White, *Experience, Contradiction, Narrative, and Imagination: Selected Papers of David Epston and Michael White, 1989–1991.*

26. Michael White and David Epston, *Narrative Means to Therapeutic Ends*, 27.

27. See Kenneth B. Schwartz Center website for description of the Clinical Pastoral Education Program for Health Care Professionals http://www.theschwartzcenter.org/programs.asp#pastoral.

28. AAPP website http://www.physicianpatient.org/.

29. See website for Rachel Remen's Institute for the Study of Health and Illness http://www.meaninginmedicine.org/home.html.

30. Richard Frankel, Timothy E. Quill, and Susan H. McDaniel, eds., *The Biopsychosocial Approach: Past, Present, Future;* Anthony Suchman et al., "Toward an Informal Curriculum That Teaches Professionalism"; Thomas Inui, "What Are the Sciences of Relationship-Centered Primary Care?"; Moira Stewart et al., *Patient-Centered Medicine.*

IO ▨ THE BIOETHICS OF
NARRATIVE MEDICINE

Sickness calls forth stories. Whether in the patient's "chief complaint," the intern's case presentation, the family member's saga of surgery, or the coroner's death note, patients and health professionals recognize problems, gauge progress, and lament defeat, in part, through telling about illness and having others listen. As we inspect the role of storytelling and bearing witness to narratives of illness in routine clinical practice, a specific instance of storytelling might need particularly close attention. This instance is the practice of bioethics. Not only are bioethicists called to assist at illnesses at particularly grave points in their courses—usually at the ends of life, especially the ends of contested lives—but the practice of ethics has of late been enlivened and itself contested by narrative knowledge and practice.[1] In the same way that narrative competence *alters* what the nurse or doctor does in the office or on the ward, narrative competence fundamentally shifts what the ethicist does with patients, with families, with health care professionals, and with the self.

Bioethics is no different from other aspects of clinical practice in having been found to have deep and consequential narrative roots. Those who assist individual patients to navigate the moral channels of illness have discovered that training in health law and knowledge of moral principles do not suffice to fulfill ethical duties toward the sick. They are learning that they also must equip themselves with sophisticated skills in absorbing and interpreting complex narratives of illness—the better to hear their patients, to accompany them on their journeys, and to assist them in making health care choices consonant with their values. Echoing its transformative force in other disciplines and professions, narrative practice has renewed and redefined the very enterprise of what used to be called bioethics.

▨ THE RISE OF BIOETHICS

The contemporary field of bioethics arose in the mid-1960s in response to wrongdoing and potential wrongdoing by doctors and scientists.[2] Unlike discussions in previous chapters of this book in which doctors, nurses, and social workers have been included in our considerations, the adversarial relationships to which bioethics responded were relationships specifically with doctors. The remainder of this chapter, then, focuses on the vexed ethical situations between patients and doctors. Nurses and social workers have, to a large extent, been part of the solution and not part of the problem in bioethics.

The Harvard anesthesiologist Henry Beecher blew the whistle in 1966 on doctors and biomedical scientists who were experimenting on patients without their consent.[3] Around the same time, medicine's growing technological ability to prolong life in the face of organ failure, starting with renal dialysis, triggered the public's anxious realization that doctors might be in a position to decide which of us would live and which would die. "In large part, the appearance of a new medicine that offered promise of great benefit," wrote Albert Jonsen in *The Birth of Bioethics*, "initiated the examination of medicine's conscience."[4] Medical ethics had been in existence since Hippocrates. However, until the post–World War II breakthroughs in antibiotics, steroids, chemotherapy agents, and antipsychotics, ethics had been little more than vague oaths to do no harm, rules for courtesy among professionals, and guidelines for decorum with the lay public. Many scholars who have chronicled the rise of contemporary bioethics suggest that the relentless pace of technical progress was itself an agent in the emergence of this new cadre of health care professionals, the ethicists. In a prominent anthology of bioethics readings, John Arras and Bonnie Steinbock summarize: "Clever physicians, researchers, and technicians discover newer and better ways to do things. . . . Before we know it, however, these new techniques and services begin to take on lives of their own, expanding well beyond the problems and patients for whom they were originally intended."[5] Discovery and innovation became the driving forces in a process that seemed to outstrip even the experts' ability to deploy them wisely.

With the 1972 exposure of the Tuskegee Syphilis Study, however, it was no longer possible to ascribe the moral lapses of medicine to overenthusiasm or lack of courtesy.[6] Six hundred black men in Tuskegee, Alabama, were denied treatment for syphilis, even when penicillin became available, so as to trace the natural history of the untreated infection, both during life and at autopsy. The confluence of scientific arrogance and racism catapulted the case to sustained national attention. As a result of Tuskegee and other similar events (injection of cancer cells into elderly patients at the Jewish Chronic Disease Hospital in Brooklyn in 1963 and infection of children at the Willowbrook State Hospital in 1956 with hepatitis B virus, both without consent of subjects), bioethicists of the mid-twentieth century assumed the role of protecting the patient from the doctor/scientist and intervening on the side of the patient in an adversarial relationship between doctor and patient. In the view of the philosopher H. Tristam Engelhardt, writing from the libertarian point of view, "When health care professionals and patients meet as strangers . . . disclosures and safeguards must frequently be explicit and often detailed. . . . [O]ne needs a disinterested application of the rules to protect against misunderstandings and to guard against abuses of power."[7] Hence, many of the early concerns of bioethics—informed consent, safeguarding patients' autonomy, and resource allocation—were powered by the suspicion that doctors, left to their own devices, will exploit patients or in some way harm them and that patients need defense against them.

The assumption that the doctor-patient relationship is an adversarial process seems to have governed the development of bioethics' agenda, training, professionalization, and worldview, in North America at least. The extreme focus on patient autonomy, for example, can only be understood if the doctor is seen as poised to take advantage of a patient. In a recent review of medical decision-making, Ezekiel and Linda Emanuel write, "During the last two decades or so, there has been a struggle over the patient's role in medical decision making that is often characterized as a conflict between autonomy and health, between the values of the patient and the values of the physician. Seeking to curtail physician dominance, many have advocated an ideal of greater patient control."[8] The "physician dominance" of patients need not even be ascribed to unscrupulous motives; the demands of science and research may suffice. In a chilling comment in *Birth of Bioethics* on the rise of biomedicine in the early 1960s, Jonsen writes, "Medical research was no longer simply doing something unusual in order to observe the results; it incorporated doctor and patient in a carefully designed program to produce valid knowledge by methods that put the subjects at risk" (145). Structurally, doctors and patients had found themselves at opposite poles of interest, apportioning knowledge to one side and risk to the other.

The middlemen and middlewomen who came to populate the bioethical field between doctor and patient have tended until recently to be adversarially trained in either law or juridically inflected moral philosophy. Even physicians and scientists who functioned as bioethicists had to become, in David Rothman's evocative phrase, "strangers at the bedside," committed not to the clinical enterprise but to the policing of it.[9] Rothman writes bluntly about the early rise of bioethics, "The changes that came to medicine generally came over the strenuous objections of doctors, giving the entire process an adversarial quality. . . . Outsiders crossed over into medicine to correct what they perceived as wrongs" (4, 94). These developments were seen as fundamental challenges to the until-then uncontested authority of doctors.

The combination of scientific imperative and the postmodern fragmentation of a pluralistic society culminated in the inadequacy of earlier, profession-based systems of control. Tom Beauchamp and LeRoy Walters sound an ominous note in the introduction to their bioethics text: "Prior to the 1970s, . . . [t]o consult persons outside the profession was thought not only unnecessary, but dangerous. This conception has collapsed in the face of the pressures of the modern world. Such a professional morality has been judged not adequately comprehensive, coherent, or sensitive to conflicts of interest. The birth of bioethics occurred as a result of an increasing awareness that this older ethic had become obsolete."[10] Both the doctor-patient relationship and the doctor-ethicist relationship were seen as laced with conflict, with the self-interest of the doctor/scientist putting patients and, by extension, the enterprise of medicine at risk. This risk required the intervention of bioethics so as to protect individual patients and the virtue of medicine itself.

Once the doctor-patient dyad was conceived as an adversarial one, contractual safeguards emerged to protect the one from the other. Ethical care became governed by negotiated instruments—advance directives, Institutional Review Board protocols, informed consent processes, conflict of interest disclosures. Bioethicists joined licensing boards, policy-makers, insurance company functionaries, and hospital admissions privilege overseers in building a tort-based, law-enshrining enterprise of controlling doctors and protecting patients. Now, many of these protections were needed to control the abuse of power and the avarice of some within medicine and bioscience, and medicine as a whole is safer than it otherwise would be. Nonetheless, figuring medicine as an adversarial enterprise has had hidden costs to bioethics that are only now coming into view.

Bioethics suffered a restriction of its vision and influence once it accepted—often implicitly and seemingly unconsciously—the assumption that patients must be protected from their doctors. Again, the example of autonomy is most telling. In their zeal to protect patients' autonomy, some bioethicists designated as paternalism any expression of personal opinion or clinical counsel on the part of health professionals. So as not to manipulate patients, some doctors have ended up withholding their own viewpoints from confused patients, leaving patients and families to make their treatment choices alone. Protecting patients' autonomy, in the extreme, constitutes abandonment.

But doctor-patient relationships are *not*, or at least need not be, adversarial ones. Certainly, there can be disagreement or disappointment or defeat within these dyads. There can be misunderstandings that lead to such polarized points of view that doctor and patient see different realities. There can be, and very often are, lapses in generosity and failures to be attuned to all of a patient's concerns. There is, more often than we realize, greed. There is sometimes, we hope rarely, sadism. And there are always differences of opinion on what, clinically, to do about any medical situation. But, with exceptions, the doctor-patient dyad is not hostile and exploitative, and to treat it as such limits its growth toward true caring.

⬚ THE PRIMACY OF BENEVOLENCE

I saw a middle-aged woman two days ago in my internal medicine practice.[11] She was relatively new to me—profoundly depressed, non–English speaking, with a discouraging list of ailments including atrial fibrillation with its attendant need for chronic anticoagulation and disabling back pain unresponsive to conservative management. She lived alone in an apartment in the city with no income except a little public assistance, poverty-level rent forgiveness, and state-program coverage for her medical care. In the interval since her last visit to me, I had succeeded in appointing her to a Spanish-speaking psychiatrist—no easy task in an overburdened clinic system—to replace the prior clinic that had treated her so demeaningly that she felt the worse for going and had lapsed from treatment. With the interpreter sitting with us in the office, we set about our work. Was I ever tempted to start right in on adjusting the dose of her blood thinner and to leave it at that. The woman's dense depression was so menacing, so overpowering that I had to *force* myself to dwell in her presence. I had to resist the powerful impulse to distance myself from her mood by checking her latest coagulation test results on the computer or scanning the pill bottles for their prescription renewal dates.

She didn't need me to do those mechanical things, at least not at the start of our visit. She needed me to bear witness to her despair. Although there was another doctor responsible for treating her depression, I had to acknowledge the reality of her life—its painful and suffusing darkness. I knew from a previous visit that she had recently been to Latin America for the funeral of her mother. I learned on this visit that a young cousin had just died of the complications of diabetes, raising great fears in the patient that she, too, had diabetes. As a corollary, I discovered that fears of illness, realistic and not, added to the patient's burden of depression. I also learned that she liked the new psychiatrist and that attending the twice-weekly therapy group helped her.

So I began to find some solid ground for myself in relation to her, some ground, that is to say, upon which to stand that would not cave in and drop me defenseless into the morass of her depression. I could appreciate with her our success in finding a new psychiatry clinic that seemed an improvement over the last one. I could ask her straightforwardly about her mood, the acknowledgment of her depression now possible without eliciting my panicky helplessness because we had done something practical to address it. I could listen as she mourned the deaths that seemed to have occurred all around her. I could offer, quickly and with great optimism, a blood test to prove she didn't have diabetes. At the same time, I could behold the courage she demonstrated by living in the face of her punishing depression. Despite the depression, she got dressed in the morning, she left the apartment, she kept her appointments, she took her medicines. What a commitment to life she demonstrated. I tried to voice my awe at her strength during our conversation.

And only then could I turn the corner toward the management of her heart disease and back pain, having not sought refuge in the body from the terror of the soul. As it turned out, our conversation about the blood tests and EKGs and pills was much more brisk and efficient by virtue of our having started with her life and her mood and her fears. In effect, our medical business, by being informed by her overwhelming fears about illness and death, could proceed more effectively because I now knew how desperately she feared illness, and I could offer some aspects of her ongoing treatment as a talisman for keeping well. More important in developing an effective therapeutic alliance than any technical skill was, I believe, my ability to tolerate her profound depression and not to flee from it *because, of course, to flee from her feelings is to flee from her.*

In retrospect, as I collected myself in private in preparation for the next patient, I realized with a sense of satisfaction that I had not abandoned her, however strong had been the temptation to do so. I had found a way to *be* with her so as to fulfill the duties I incurred by virtue of having heard her (or even more simply and instrumentally, the duties I incurred by virtue of having been assigned as her physician by the Medicaid bureaucracy). The satisfaction I felt was the satisfaction of an *internist*—not of an ethicist and not of a narratologist although I am those things too—in my having found a way, today anyway, to be her doctor.

I think this glimpse of my office hours helps to convey what I mean to say about the doctor-patient dyad. I mean to draw attention to the benevolence available to us to do every day, the acts of goodness we can choose to perform or to omit in our clinical transactions. Not mere kindnesses, these acts contribute directly to our clinical effectiveness, and omitting them risks clinical failure. *These* are the acts of ethical medicine—not only signing the advance directive or talking about futility in the ICU, but these private acts that require courage and clinical common sense. It felt to me that it was a privilege that, in the course of an ordinary day in practice, I was offered the chance to give this woman what I believe she needs clinically, to do so at some minor cost to myself (the extra time it took and the sinking reminder of impending doom that surrounds us all), and to emerge from our visit feeling better than I did before it.

What would happen to bioethics if the doctor-patient dyad were to be conceptualized as an occasion for such clinically relevant benevolence, if it were seen not only as a contractually governed and potentially oppositional relationship but also as an intersubjective personal relationship of vulnerability and trust? How would one practice bioethics if medical practice were understood as an enterprise in which one subject enters relation with another subject, both participants in the intersubjectivity illuminating one another's goals, hopes, desires, and fears, and contributing regard, trust, and courage?

▣ Narrative Reframes Bioethics

Over the past decade, conventional bioethics has struggled to find its way among its chosen principles and has found itself too thin to address adequately the actual value conflicts that arise in illness.[12] Although so-called principlist bioethics might be equipped to adjudicate appropriate surrogacy for the incapacitated terminally ill patient or to assess the risk to human subjects of a clinical research trial, it is ill equipped to guide an internist in caring for a depressed woman with heart disease or to help a pediatrician to talk with parents about the meaning of their two-year-old boy's autism. Because, in part, principlist bioethics arose to deal with oppositional clinical relationships, it cannot be expected to support or to augment caring relationships.

Any number of alternative approaches to addressing the ethical problems in health care—feminist ethics, communitarian ethics, liberation ethics, hermeneutical ethics, casuistry, virtue ethics, and care ethics—have altered the conceptual geography of bioethics.[13] With their foundations not in law and Anglo/Continental moral philosophy but in the particularities of individuals, the singularity of beliefs, the perspectival nature of truth, and the duties of intersubjectivity, these complexly differing approaches share a commitment to narrative truth and to the power of telling and listening. They share a realization that meaning in human life emerges not from rules given but from lived, thick experience and that determinations of right and good by necessity arise from context, perspective, culture, and time.

These approaches do not assume that patients must be protected from their doctors. Instead, they all, in somewhat different ways, locate patients and their families *near* to those who care for them. Rather than emphasizing—and therefore intensifying—the divides between patients and health professionals, these methods seek congress among human beings limited by mortality, identified by culture, revealed in language, and marked by suffering. It is not the case that some are sick and some are well but that all will die. Although these approaches emerged rather spontaneously and simultaneously around the mid-1980s, each is grounded in a narratively sophisticated theory and practice—from literary studies, liberation theology, cultural studies, feminist studies, postcolonial studies, humanistic psychology, or phenomenology—creating, if you will, a family of narrative ethics. What is now called narrative ethics has borrowed significantly from all these efforts, finding in their commonalities a core for practice.[14] It may be that we will come to adopt the term "narrative ethics" or even "the narrative ethici" (my effort to indicate the plural of "ethics") as the embracing term for these many ethical systems grounded in singularity, temporality, and intersubjectivity. Perhaps we will come eventually to see these alternative approaches—those that find principlism wanting—as a many-roomed complex of recognition, generosity, and desire within which dwell our efforts not only to judge one another's actions in the face of illness and death but to accompany one another humbly through them.

This is not the place to rehearse the differences among care ethics, communitarian ethics, and virtue ethics or to detail the particular contributions of each of these systems of ethical enquiry. In its own way and with particular strengths and capacities, each of these multiple approaches recognizes that the individual sick person enters sickness singularly, that disease in the individual person signifies uniquely, and that each death connotes the end of its life particularly. The narrative ethici share the conviction that the individual story of illness is pivotal to the person's suffering—either vis-à-vis the community or the gender or relation or the culture. Some of these practices suggest that one must tell of what one undergoes in order to understand it and that, as a consequence, the health professionals who accompany patients through illness have a responsibility to hear them out. Among the tenets of these ethics are the requirements to hear all sides, to contextualize all events, to honor all voices, and to bear witness to all who suffer. Training for such practice, it follows, is textual and interior—developing the skills of interpretation, reflective discernment, self-knowledge, and absorptive and accurate listening.[15]

Whatever may develop as the future of these many emerging ethical practices, today's bioethics is undeniably being informed by narrative theory and practice: both through the development of narrative competence in its "bio" sphere (the practice of medicine) and the through the increasing narrative commitments of its "ethics" sphere (the practice of ethics). As medicine, nursing, and other health care professions become more narratively informed and as patient care makes room for narrative medicine, the practice of bioethics will change as a consequence. Narratively trained health care professionals will have *access* to patients' and families' perspectives. They will know about their patients' beliefs and wishes regarding end of life, if only as part of what they learn of their temporality. They will more regularly enter robust intersubjective relationships with their patients, knowing with more accuracy and authenticity than other physicians do about what donates meaning in each patient's life. Through bearing witness to patients' suffering, they will recognize and perhaps participate in communities of care or communities of presence for individual patients. The ethicality of narrative medicine, that is to say, emerges directly and organically from its practice and need not have a separate "bioethics" function appended to it. That this form of medical practice is saturated with its own intrinsic ethicality will change the current practice of bioethics in as yet unclear but emerging ways.

At the same time, quite distinct from the development of narrative competence in the health professions, there are narrative forces coming to bear on the practice of ethicists themselves. The narrative turn felt throughout the culture and the academy has amplified voices within ethics that have respected stories all along. The work of the religious scholar Stanley Hauerwas, for example, has taken on new authority since the narrativist turn was noted elsewhere in the academy.[16] Richard Zaner's phenomenology has become saturated with a respect for and insistence on narrative methods and interests.[17] The lawyer-ethicist George Annas has turned to writing plays. Inspired by such seminal texts as Alasdair MacIntyre's *After Virtue* and Bernard Williams's *Moral Luck,* philosophical bioethics has been challenged to grasp the storied elements of moral thought and the irreducibility of human plights.[18] Although principlist bioethics is still taken up with autonomy, incapacity, and informed consent, some individual practitioners are coming to realize that they are *not* judges but listeners, *not* measuring capacity or next-of-kinhood but measuring the depth of loss.

Narrative bioethics has come of age in the recent past by allying with the narrative ethics of literary studies, making explicit connections, for example, with the work of Adam Zachary Newton, J. Hillis Miller, and Wayne Booth to thereby "place" this hybrid enterprise within a disciplinary narrative home.[19] The field has also matured by establishing a conceptual ground and clinical practice that can be articulated and taught. The narrativists within bioethics have been at the bedside all this time, absorbing the particular lived experiences of illness and bodily suffering and accruing clinical authority in the process. When Arthur Frank writes of generosity in the care of the sick and when he deepens his notions of thinking *with* stories to radicalize stories' influence in our lives, he demonstrates and delivers seasoned and sophisticated principles of narrative medicine that he has challenged us to grasp with him over time.[20] The critical attention that Tod Chambers pays to the clinical cases written by bioethicists derives from his power as a literary scholar who works in a teaching hospital, teaches bioethics to medical students and doctors, and not only gazes at clinical problems with the eye of a reader but also is called upon to solve them.[21] His study suggests that ethics—and medicine—needs literary studies and narrative competence, that it cannot continue to do its work without them.

Within narrative bioethics, we find a respect for what I have come to call the three movements of narrative medicine—attention, representation, and affiliation. Richard Zaner exemplifies narrative attention to the patients and families he cares for, coming to realize slowly through a life in bioethics that his role is to be "someone to listen as the simple act of telling does its powerful, magically cleansing work. . . . Maybe there's some sorcery in the telling; all the more, then, in the act of listening, of *letting people be*."[22] What moves me more than his descriptions of what patients and their families told him is how he, himself, now must tell, in version after version, these clinical stories, enacting the need to represent fully and accurately all that he has absorbed through his states of attention. Zaner tells the same stories many times over years and decades (not unlike my chronic "telling" of Mrs. Nelson's story). His duty to represent that which he beholds never ends, it seems, for each representation fuels another turn in the spiral toward fresh attention, new sightings, new duties, and new stories.

Art Frank deepens our understanding of attention until it is seen as a gifting of the self that demands no reward but itself: "Generosity begins in *welcome*: a hospitality that offers whatever the host has that would meet the need of the guest. . . . [It] signifies the opening the self to others. . . . To guests who suffer, the host's welcome is an initial promise of consolation" (2). If anything, Frank goes beyond representation to suggest that stories become part of ourselves. Not only do we read them and write them, but they "settle into our awareness and become habits of thought, tacitly guiding our actions" (7). In a neurobiological metaphor of great power, Frank helps us to greet our stories as friendly memes, as mind-expanding frames, as self-making exemplars.

The affiliative movement of narrative medicine is more and more urgently sought by narrative ethics. In calling for a community-based ethic of health care, the philosopher Micah Hester notes, "The more complex and threatening the experience [of ailments] for the patient, the more it tears at the fabric of that person's life. And conversely, *the more an ailment tears at the fabric of our relationships, the more severely it is experienced*," elevating the building of community and preservation of the fabric of patients' relationships to a position of primacy within health care's mission.[23] Even bioethicists who may not *know* they are narrative ethicists have joined our efforts through their realization of the affiliative primacy of ethical interventions. The influential lawyer and ethicist Nancy Dubler has shifted her clinical practice toward mediation, realizing that the dilemmas of bioethics require "a setting in which cultural values can be voiced and honored, in which differing patterns in language and communication can be identified and bridged, and in which the voices of patients and families from traditionally disempowered groups can be amplified."[24] However these ethicists arrived at their narrative stance—through philosophy, through religious studies, through personal illness, through law—they are united in their determination to bridge the divides in health care and in their quest for the affiliations of healing communities.

The place of narrative in medicine and in ethics can be illuminated by recognizing the place of narrative in life (and, pari passu, this move helps us to recognize how medicine and ethics are but instances of life). In writing about the Iranian Islamic revolution and its attendant losses of freedom, especially for Iranian women, the literary scholar Azar Nafisi explains how fiction sustained her and her students through ordeals of repression.[25] Nafisi kept alive empathy, the imagination, and courage by teaching such works as *Pride and Prejudice* and "Daisy Miller," works that require their readers to inhabit alien spheres and to adopt and respect contradictory points of view, works whose protagonists develop the courage to choose freedom. Fiction's critical and irreplaceable consequences are to force readers to recognize the storied shape of reality, to understand in the most basic way that we create meaning by weaving the fragments of life into plot, and that one *must* choose one's plots. We make it up; in the most primal and primitive and primary way, we make it up. We do not "capture" the truth that exists around us through scientific measurements or through controlled experiments. We do not represent that which is external to us detachedly and objectively and replicably. No. Instead, we incorporate our sensations and perceptions and desires and ideas into a form that we first tell to ourselves and then might tell to others. Identity itself—one's sense of being a self—arises from the crib narratives infants tell, the entries we hide in our adolescent diaries, the associations we voice to our analysts, and the accounts we give of ourselves when befriended, when ill, when accused, when reflecting, or when imagining.[26] These stories we tell merge with those we hear—in fiction, in fairy tales, in family legends, in sacred texts—in great banks of plot, great plots of grounds for knowing, for rooting, for cultivating the self.[27] Telling and listening to stories seem as organically necessary as are the respiration of oxygen and the circulation of blood to establish and maintain a self by metabolizing into it that which is nonself and then contributing products of the self back into that alien domain, thereby making it home.

The narrative features of medicine that we examine throughout this book are, indeed, salient to the practice of the bioethicist. To solve, at least provisionally, the ethical conflicts that arise in health care, the ethicist needs the means to probe, honor, represent, and live in the face of temporality, singularity, intersubjectivity, causality/contingency, and ethicality. What is lacking in bioethics as well as in clinical practice is precisely the mode of vision made possible through sophisticated narrative practice, especially in relation to these five broad areas.

6 GARDEN SOUTH

Let us pay a visit to 6 Garden South, the hospital floor on which some months ago I was ward attending, caring with my residents and medical students for severely ill patients admitted to Presbyterian Hospital with terminal cancer, end-stage renal failure, heart failure, liver failure, failure to thrive. Throughout the month, we came across—and used narrative ways to live with—serious ethical conflicts.

Mrs. B. was admitted for terminal care of Stage 4 breast cancer.[28] Only 48 years old, she wanted badly to live, and yet the oncologists had nothing left to try. The resident complained that the patient's unrealistic sons wanted "everything done." The sons' obdurate demands for intensive medical care inflamed the resident's searing guilt that there was nothing more to do, and so he was very angry at them. "We need an ethics consult," he declared angrily, as if the ethicist could be called in as an attack dog. I gently suggested that he ask the social worker to convene a family meeting to clarify the goals of care. The next day, the social worker sat with both sons, their wives, the resident, the intern, and the medical student caring for the patient. With the safety of the social worker's presence, my resident was able to put into words the hopelessness of continuing treatment. He emphasized his commitment to the patient's freedom from pain and discomfort. The sons, it almost goes without saying, were exquisitely aware that their mother was dying. Their insistence that the doctor "do everything" was just the only means available to them, up until then, to register their undying loyalty and unswerving commitment to the well-being of their mother. Once my resident asked them to join with him in acknowledging that the end was near, they could surrender their stance of hostility and blame and could begin their long road of mourning.

Mr. A., a middle-aged man with a long history of alcoholism, was admitted to hospital in liver failure. Another resident and intern adeptly deployed powerful diuretics, tapped fluid from the patient's abdomen, and replenished nutrients often deficient in alcoholics. And yet the patient sank further and further into encephalopathy and coma. His mother was at his bedside, rocking and praying, even when the patient could no longer hear her. My resident and intern did not flinch, even in the face of the suspicion that their rather aggressive treatment had made matters worse, from consulting with the liver specialists, thinking through the deranged physiology involved in end-stage liver failure, and devising new approaches when the standard ones failed. What impressed me was that they did not give up. Every morning at rounds, they meticulously reported all the patient's ins and outs, the results of his blood tests and scans. One morning, he woke up. He had been more than a week in deep coma with all the earmarks of an irreversible vegetative state, and yet he rose. As I spoke with him that first morning, I said something in my little broken Spanish that I hoped translated to "Thank God you're alive!" And the patient winked. He winked! Imagine had we given up.

A woman was admitted emergently from a nearby dialysis center with fever and evidence of bacterial sepsis, probably from an infected dialysis access graft. Another woman suffered complications from needed surgery, resulting in pulmonary and neurological compromise. These two cases made our team brood on the dangers of medicine as we know it. My young doctors were forced to ask themselves, "Are patients better off with us or without us?" When a complication occurs, however well understood and accepted its risk, one cannot help but feel responsible. The residents and interns caring for both these patients had to

display enormous tact and professionalism to convey the clinical truth to the patients and their families while dealing with their own confusing calculus of
benefit and risk.

What did my team learn about bioethics? We learned that the words one
says—like "do everything"—can have multiple contradictory meanings and
that ethical medicine requires an active intersubjective process, working
against a gradient of complacency or convention or detachment, to discover the
meaning of words. We learned about duty—duty in the face of self-inflicted
disease, duty in the face of our own shortcomings, duty in the face of the inevitable complications of our yet-primitive medicine. Such duties are not prescribed by oversight committees or specialty boards but are discerned, over
time, through a life lived humbly around illness and the consequences of trying to intervene in it. Surrendering neither to nihilism nor to deceit, my house
officers fulfilled the ethical duties that accrue to their knowledge, to their loyalty toward their young science, and to their constancy in the care of individual patients.

Over the course of the month, we became all the more able to behold the singular, the mystery, the marvel. Why did Mr. A. wake up? We'll never know.
And yet, we can celebrate, as miracle, his resurrection. We can learn from his
course how to do even better with the next case of end-stage liver failure, while
we can let ourselves *wonder* what happened as he slowly awakened, from how
far away he traveled to open his eyes and then to wink. "I had a guy," my intern
will say years from now, "who was encephalopathic even longer than your guy
but he woke up. Keep giving him lactulose; diurese him gently, don't give up."
We all learned about the savage contingency implicit in our work—in the occurrence of aggressive breast cancer, in the success or failure of diuresing or tapping the alcoholic, in the ways that we and our patients responded to the sickness all around us. As they told me stories at attending rounds—"This is the
fourth CPMC admission for this 54-year-old chronic alcoholic with a history of
DTs, positive family history of alcoholism, and multiple failed attempts at
detox"—making sense in our own little way of the events of others' lives, we
understood the capricious nature of our emplotment, and we recognized the ar-
tificial process by which, for our sakes alone, we impose on the contingent our
sense-making plots, realizing full well that as new pathophysiological explanations replace the faulty ones we live with now, the stories with which we tell of
what befalls our patients will change along with them.

On 6 Garden South, we did not address the ethicality of our clinical situations
separately from their temporality or causality or contingency or singularity or
intersubjectivity. *It happens all at once.* The ethical dimension is one facet of a
narratively competent medicine that occurs *while* the intersubjectively linked
participants (some well, some ill) behold the singularity of one another and their
situations, while they fathom where in the arc from birth to death they might be
now, while they search for causes amid the random and the unfair. What human
beings owe to one another is not excisable, as a discrete concern, from the whole
texture of how they reach one another, how they place themselves in time, how
they emplot the events that occur to them, how they tolerate ambiguity or un-

certainty, or how they recognize the absolute uniqueness of one another (and, in reflection, of themselves too), how they hear one another out. As a result of all these things, they perform for one another acts of goodness, their benevolence the full enactment of their science, of their justice, of their art.

We begin, then, to contemplate the consequences of choosing a new plot within which to consider medicine and its ethics. If ethics recognizes medicine not as an adversarial process but rather as an ongoing intersubjective commitment in the face of vulnerability and trust, what becomes of its practice?

▣ THE PRACTICE OF NARRATIVE BIOETHICS

To practice such ethics requires that practitioners, be they health care professionals to begin with or not, must be prepared to offer the self as a therapeutic instrument. The ethicist must enter the clinical situation, willing to suffer in the process. If another kind of ethicist could fulfill his or her duty by hearing, in the safety of a conference room, the report of a patient's predicament and somehow making judgments from afar about the proper action to pursue, the narrative bioethicist must sit by the patient, lean forward toward the person who suffers, and offer the self as an occasion for the other to tell and therefore comprehend the events of illness. This ethicist does his or her work by absorbing and containing the singular patient's plight, soliciting others' perspectives on the situation, being the flask in which these differing points of view can mingle toward equilibrium. Not all things dissolve, and so solutions are not the only end points craved by this ethics. Instead, we choose to live with the tensions of all things being said, all things being heard, sedimenting toward stillness. What the person practicing narrative bioethics knows for sure is that he or she will be transformed by contributing benevolence and courage to another person's plight. Revolutionary, consequential narrative once again enacts its truth that nothing remains unchanged by story.

Let me close by reproducing for you a story written by a medical student in her Parallel Chart during her third year of medical school.

> Altagracia. I am obsessed with her first name. . . . I imbue her name with spiritual, romantic, and mysterious overtones.
>
> "Yo se que yo voy a morir en el hospital." I know that I am going to die in the hospital. Clutching her wrinkled face, which droops on the left, with her tendinous, wasted hands with papery dry purple skin, she looked at me through her claw-like fingers. She's childlike, hidden.
>
> Failure to thrive. She won't eat. She kicks, she hits, she clutches and bends your fingers. No, you can't open her eyes to shine a light, and you can't open her mouth. She's hiding from me, deep inside her body.
>
> Slowly, she's dying. . . . Her brain is 79 years old, infarcted, probably demented, but I want to believe that there is a complicated, dignified sadness in her mind that she is sequestering from the world. She lies in bed lamenting, suf-

fering, crouching on her side, mourning mysterious and not so mysterious losses of her life.

We all shuffle into her room and peer at her. "Hola, hola," I call softly. She swats her arms and covers her face. I keep thinking about her premonition, "Yo soy que yo voy a morir en el hospital." Did I really hear her say that? Did I imagine that she could speak? The attending spoke. "We need to peg her and place her."

Altagracia, graceful and seemingly out of touch, pretends we aren't there.

This beautiful clinical act of beholding the human mystery of this woman with humility and absorptive grace *means* something—for the student/writer and also, perhaps, for the patient. By writing this description of Altagracia, my student takes the measure of her regard, her loyalty to the patient, and her hopes for her own and her patient's futures. She exposes her own desires—to believe in the patient's dignity, to grant her her mystery, to distinguish herself from the insensitive attending physician, the only one in the story consigned to the past tense. The author's muscular imagination "fills in" that which dementia has erased, enabling her to treat her patient with reverence. My student does not mislead herself to think she now knows more than she used to know about this patient who is virtually out of reach; she has instead accomplished the modest task of allowing for the possibility that there is a coherence to this waning human life.

By searching for (or by being open to) and choosing the words, the images, the time course, and the plot of this story, the author gives birth to a particular way of comprehending the events of this hospitalization. This patient, whom the attending physician dismisses as a transfer to a nursing home once a stomach tube (or PEG) is placed, emerges by virtue of the writing as a mysterious, powerful, complicated woman whose difficult behavior can be interpreted as complexly determined and connotative. She of the highest grace is the heroine and not the victim of her story, knowing that which others do not know, hiding in her wasted husk a life of great ambition. By having apprehended such a vision of the patient, the student can more naturally care for her with benevolence and, therefore, effectiveness.

These ethics that are teachable through narrative training are within-medicine ethics, not without-medicine bioethics. This ethics is not one that one can "contract out," that one can surrender to another to perform. Nor is it applied only when certain topics arise—futility of treatment, for example, or protection of human research subjects. Governing clinical actions at all time, narrative medicine's bioethics endows the practitioner with an enduring awareness of the vulnerability and the trust of self and other. A narrative medicine bioethics saturates the doctor, nurse, social worker, or ethicist with the sensibility and the skill to recognize and to fulfill the duties incurred by intersubjective nearness, by mutual singularity, by knowledge of causes and contingency, and by the sense that time, by its nature, runs out. If sickness calls forth stories, then healing calls forth a benevolent willingness to be subject to them, subjects of them, and subjected to their transformative power.

NOTES

1. See Hilde Nelson, ed., *Stories and Their Limits* and Rita Charon and Martha Montello, eds., *Stories Matter* for introductions to the field of narrative ethics.

2. The term "bioethics" was coined around the same time by two people. Sargent Shriver came up with the word to denote the new ethics-for-medicine institute being established by the Kennedy family at Georgetown University. What Shriver meant by the term was the rather instrumental application of legal and philosophical principles to solve dilemmas in medical research and practice. The physician Van Rensselaer Potter also created the word, but in his hands it denoted a "science for survival," that is, an environmentally inclusive effort to live, as humans, in concert with the universe with a recognition that the biological life interacts with the moral life. Evidently, the first definition ascended, although the second may be emerging from the cosmic shadows. See Robert Martensen, "Thought Styles among the Medical Humanities: Past, Present, and Near-term Future."

3. Henry Beecher, "Ethics and Clinical Research."

4. Albert R. Jonsen, *The Birth of Bioethics*, 11. Subsequent page references to this work appear in parentheses in the text.

5. John Arras, Bonnie Steinbock, and Alex John London, "Moral Reasoning in the Medical Context," in *Ethical Issues in Modern Medicine*, edited by John Arras and Bonnie Steinbock, 3.

6. Jean Heller, "Syphilis Victims in US Study Went Untreated for 40 Years."

7. H. Tristam Engelhardt Jr., *The Foundations of Bioethics*, 299.

8. Ezekiel J. Emanuel and Linda L. Emanuel, "Four Models of the Physician-Patient Relationship," 2221.

9. David Rothman, *Strangers at the Bedside*. Page references to this work appear in parentheses in the text.

10. Tom L. Beauchamp and LeRoy Walters, *Contemporary Issues in Bioethics*, 1.

11. I have merged the descriptions of several patients I saw during one morning in practice to make my point, and so I have not elicited consent to publish this description, as it does not actually "belong" to any one of the several men and women who are part of this portrait.

12. Edwin R. Dubose, Ronald P. Hamel, Laurence J. O'Connell, eds., *A Matter of Principles? Ferment in U.S. Bioethics*.

13. For some seminal texts in this vast territory, see Mary Urban Walker, *Moral Understandings: A Feminist Study in Ethics*; Helen B. Holmes and Laura Purdy, eds., *Feminist Perspectives in Medical Ethics*; Nel Noddings, *Caring: A Feminist Approach to Ethics and Moral Education*; Joan Tronto, *Moral Boundaries: A Political Argument for an Ethic of Care*; Edmund Pellegrino and David Thomasma, *For the Patient's Good: The Restoration of Beneficence in Health Care*; Alasdair Macintyre, *After Virtue: A Study in Moral Theory*; Albert Jonsen and Stephen Toulmin, *The Abuse of Casuistry*.

14. See David Morris's chapter "Conclusion: Narrative Bioethics" in *Illness and Culture in the Postmodern Age*, 247–78, for a brilliant and wide-ranging assessment of the state of the field at the turn of the century.

15. Jerome Bruner, *Making Stories: Law, Literature, Life*; Stanley Hauerwas and L. Gregory Jones, eds. *Why Narrative? Readings in Narrative Theology*; Theodore Sarbin, ed., *Narrative Psychology*.

16. David Burrell and Stanley Hauerwas, "From System to Story."

17. Richard Zaner, "Sisyphus without Knees: Exploring Self-Other Relationships through Illness and Disability."

18. Bernard Williams, *Moral Luck: Philosophical Papers, 1973–1980.*

19. See my discussion of the literary branch of narrative ethics in chapter 3's section on ethicality.

20. Arthur Frank, *The Renewal of Generosity: Illness, Medicine, and How to Live.* Page references to this work appear in parentheses in the text.

21. Tod Chambers, *The Fiction of Bioethics.*

22. Richard Zaner, *Conversations on the Edge,* 15.

23. Micah Hester, *Community as Healing,* 70.

24. Nancy N. Dubler and Carol B. Liebman, *Bioethics Mediation,* 218.

25. Azar Nafisi, *Reading Lolita in Tehran: A Memoir in Books.*

26. Paul John Eakin, *How Our Lives Become Stories* and Anthony Paul Kerby, *Narrative and the Self.*

27. Jerome Bruner, *Actual Minds, Possible Worlds* and Lionel Trilling, *The Liberal Imagination.*

28. These patients are unrecognizable composites of many patients my team cared for over the month.

I I ▣ A Narrative Vision for Health Care

Narrative, by its nature, is disruptive. Unlike lists or formulas, narrative is not clean, predictable, or obeisant. Narrative makes its own paths, breaks its own constraints, undercuts its own patterns. As it does in dreams or in Beckett, narrative anywhere can make new out of old, creating chaos out of linearity while, subversively, exposing underlying fresh connections among the seemingly unrelated. Not only through its ordering impulses but also through its *disordering* ones, narrative can help one see newly and for the first time something concealed, something overlaid, something buried in code.

Narrative's effect on health care is the same as it is anywhere. The divides in health care that we have been considering are like countless other divides—in education, in politics, in religion, in marriages—bridgeable by virtue of the narrative powers of telling, listening, gathering around any kind of campfire to hear one another out. We have been learning throughout our work in narrative medicine how shared narrative acts build community. The *affiliation* movement of narrative medicine's triad slowly has come into view as the ultimate goal of the spiral put into action by attention and representation. The affiliation can bond individual clinician with individual patient. It can also make room for egalitarian groupings of health care professionals and sick people, together on the ground opened up by illness. Hence, the community-building affiliative movement we examine in this chapter is of great practical and political significance in the reach for equitable, accessible, and dignified care for all.[1]

In a chapter called "Liminality and Communitas" in *The Ritual Process*, the anthropologist Victor Turner describes many social phenomena—among tribes in Africa, Native American societies, Franciscan monks, and hippies of the late 1960s—as liminal, or boundary-crossing, rites of passage that erase signs of social status while people are "in transit" between one stage and another, be it childhood to adulthood, novice to friar, or entitled college student to committed peace activist. Choosing the Latin *communitas* over the English community (the latter word seems to Turner to connote social or political groupings rather than the elemental human groupings he means to discuss), Turner signifies the communion that can exist among human beings by virtue of their commonality simply as humans. Unfragmented, freed from temporal restrictions, beyond state, undifferentiated, this communitas gives "recognition to an essential and generic human bond, without which there could be *no* society."[2] Not unlike Martin Buber's formulation of human relatedness as "the being no longer side by side . . . but *with* one another of a multitude of persons . . . a flowing from *I* to *Thou*,"[3] Turner's liminal communitas phenomena "are products," as he writes, "of 'men in their wholeness wholly attending,'" by virtue of which the wholeness of humanity is fully exposed.[4]

The seriously ill people for whom we care in clinical practice are marooned between stable states. They are no longer defined by work role, family role, or state role and not yet defined as simply awaiting death but de-differentiated by cotton hospital gowns and plastic wristbands to be side by side only with others who, too, find themselves in the limbo regions of sickness. And those of us who have elected to live our lives with the sick must "wholly attend," must be *with* them, must open ourselves to porous transit on their journeys while building collectives of our own that help to get the work done. In the face of the instability of illness and the rigidity of the health care hierarchy that has developed, perhaps as a defense against the instability, the communitas open to us through rigorous narrative work can fulfill very practical tasks. By leveling power differentials and revealing our collective missions—anterior to specific professional niches and prior to the specifics of specialty—as health care professionals, our shared narrative work has begun to help us recognize one another as equals and make explicit our commitment to effective care of one another and of our patients.

NARRATIVE ONCOLOGY

The narrative practices that have united individual health care professionals with their patients and students are being found helpful in efforts to improve professionalism in individual health care disciplines, to strengthen team effectiveness among professionals, and to address systemic inequalities and injustices within our health care systems. Some time ago, Dr. Gwen Nichols, who directs the Hematological Malignancy Program at Columbia, came to me for help. On the adult oncology in-patient unit, there had been a devastating death—a pregnant woman died of a brain tumor, and the fetus too had died. The medical resident rotating through oncology that month threatened to quit medicine. "I can't do this," she flatly stated. "This is not something I can do." Dr. Nichols realized how paltry was the support for or the recognition of the defeat and suffering undergone by members of the oncology team, and she thought that the kind of reflective writing I coached might help.

We started narrative oncology, a twice-a-month lunchtime elective writing seminar, as an effort to decrease staff burnout, to develop means of coping with the sadness and defeat of our work, and to build collegial supports among members of our interdisciplinary team. We provided sandwiches and cookies, and participants provided short prose or poems they had written about patients on the unit. (We met with hospital counsel before starting the seminar and, upon their advice, told our participants not to use patients' names, unit numbers, or any identifying details. Anything a clinician writes about identifiable patients, counsel warned, is potentially discoverable. Materials should not be preserved if they would not be helpful if presented in court.) Nurses, social workers, oncologists, fellows, residents, and students attended, anywhere from four to twenty at a time. Using the Parallel Chart format, each writer was invited to read his or her text aloud. We discussed each text's genre, narrative situation, figural language, and diction and then widened the discussion to its emotional, clinical, and professional implications.

From the start, writers brought weighty and moving materials to the seminar. By this time, I was no longer surprised at the power of the writing generated in such settings. The quality of narrative oncology poems and prose supported my growing hypothesis that even inexperienced writers can achieve a grave and elevated style with complex literary structures as they try to represent the consequential events of illness that they witness in their work. Participants were able to hear one another out with generosity and insight, the hearers *adding* fresh knowledge to what the writer discovered through writing.

Nurses, social workers, and doctors who had known and worked with each other for years discovered new aspects of one another. There were moments of discovery at all levels—from "Chemotherapy nurses do *that?*" to "I want you to be my nurse when I'm dying." Anyone who has worked in hospitals knows the vexing hierarchies that usually obtain in the hospital, how doctors and nurses tend to chronically disagree, how social workers often feel alone in their championing of the patient's personal needs and desires. A senior oncologist once read aloud at one of our sessions about how she had covered her practice one weekend, admitting a partner's patient to the hospital on a Saturday. By Monday, when the patient's doctor was back, the patient continued to seek the writer's clinical advice and support. "I was unhappy with the situation, because I did not want the responsibility without the authority." Said the nurse manager, "Now you know how nurses feel all the time." What an electrifying moment of truth for us all.

Here is a text written and read in narrative oncology by a social worker about a woman dying of Stage 4 breast cancer:

> You seem to rise from this cold, stark environment like a crocus in early spring. Deceptively fragile looking, but oh, so strong. Your delicate beauty is apparent, even in a hospital gown and with IVs running. You crumple when I delve—Yes, this has been so very trying, this cancer. You sway, take a very deep breath, re-rooting yourself. You wipe your tears and smile. "I don't cry a lot," you say, but certainly this grief is unavoidable. Your presence suggests an inner core that is, in essence, unshakeable. But how can this be? This disease is so ugly and powerful—or maybe not. Maybe your particular spirit can never be overcome. I say goodbye, and you wink—as if you know my thoughts.

We talked about the metaphor this writer chose—the crocus, the declaration of spring, the hardy miracle after the snow and frozen earth, a beginning of fruitfulness. By having recognized that image, an image that visited her quite without her will but to which she was receptive, this writer could express the meaning from her encounter, using both of James's meanings of "express" simultaneously. By virtue of this metaphor, the writer recognized the *potential* in this patient, the promise and life in her—however short the growing season to come—and the coldness and deadness of the hospital environment in contrast to her blossoming strength.

We also looked together at the narrative situation here. Who is reporting whose thoughts, who speaks, who is the *I*? The patient crumples when the social worker delves, yet the paragraph depicts the crumpling of the writer/social worker too. Who is swaying and taking the deep breath? Allegedly the patient, of course, but there is liminal travel between the teller of the words and the teller of the tale. To whom is grief unavoidable? The final line—"as if you know my thoughts"—is a dazzling ventriloquism, for the writer knows the thoughts of the patient who knows *her* thoughts! Paying attention to this border-crossing confusion helped the author by underlining the evident identification at work, signifying that she has "become" this patient emotionally and that she suffers her own grief while in the patient's presence.

A pregnant nurse wrote of a young woman dying of ovarian cancer:

> Her abdominal girth would put her at 40 weeks—GI is going to tap her today. An unhealthy 7 liters would be born later that evening.
>
> I am self-conscious of my 26-week swell, no longer hidden, when I go in to plan her discharge. She smiles and states that it looks like I have some good news—it's out there, we can go on with business. I silently thank her for putting me at ease.

Before we talked about the affective or clinical content of this text, we talked about its form. The word pregnancy is never used. Called *aporias* in literary studies, such absences within texts usually signify something of heightened importance and freight. It was too perilous to even use the word. The pregnancy appears only as the "it" in the story. We noticed the oddness and specificity of the verbs' tense and mode. "Her abdominal girth would put her at 40 weeks" and "7 liters would be born later that evening" position these events, even though known at the time of writing, in a conditional future time. Pregnancy—and death—of course *are* conditional future events, predictable, within limits, provisionally knowable. This patient was, in effect, pregnant with her own death. Inspecting something as concrete as the verb forms allowed us to recognize how vectored toward the future—the biological and emotional and familial future—was this young pregnant nurse and how, by necessity, vectored toward a terminal future was this sad young woman within view of her end. It was the clash between their lived futures that was unspeakable and that required the patient's forgiving acknowledgment.

This skilled nurse, pregnant for the first time, felt alone in her confusion about whether her fecund state will be seen as an assault by her dying young patient. By reading this text aloud to the group, she enlisted the help of senior nurses, including her supervisor, to teach her about this intersection of her life with the life and death of her patient.

Narrative oncology brings us together as equals to consider our patients and our work. I was relieved to read Victor Turner's description of liminal communitas, because it reminds us of the bridging potential of situations where social status is undermined, or at least unsettled. The group is able to consider the human cost of what they do and the long-range meaning of what they undergo in practice by virtue of the chance to work together unimpeded by social rank. These benefits accrue also by virtue of the rigorous development of the skills of attending to and representing clinical work. This is not only a psychologically comforting support group. It may indeed be experienced as psychologically comforting, but because it builds skills in attention and representation, giving the participants new accuracy with which to view and comprehend their daily realities, it brings them together as *better able* than they were before the training to measure the costs, to recognize the realities, and to join with one another to offer what care can be given.

Our narrative work not only deepens ties among the staff of this particular oncology unit in this particular hospital but also reveals our communitas with a widely flung collective of health care professionals who, usually silently, suffer the burdens and costs of their practice. Throughout our project, we have had visitors and guests—medical students on subinternships from other schools, visiting fellows in exchange programs with other institutions, researchers and educators interested to learn about these new pedagogic methods. The next text was written by a visiting fellow.[5] I quite forget from which institution he was visiting. He was with us for a month and took advantage of the opportunity to read and write seriously with colleagues:

Frannie was 27 when I met her. She was diagnosed with chronic myelogenous leukemia at 21. She had failed interferon long ago. There was no other effective therapy available at that time. I admitted her once for symptomatic anemia and once for shortness of breath as an intern. Both times, we tuned her up and sent her out. Both times she was discharged and was inconsistent with outpatient follow-up. She was sad, resigned, tired, but a lovely girl. Grateful for our help, sick of being sick, worn out facing death.

When I admitted her as a junior resident, she had been lost to follow-up for a few weeks. She was wrecked—cachectic [skeletally thin] above the waist, massively edematous [swollen] below. She could no longer mentate. She was in blast crisis. She blasted through induction. The private doctor had never discussed do not resuscitate decisions. I coded her a couple of weeks later. The sister cursed me and praised God while I broke Frannie's ribs and shocked her heart into a normal rhythm. I sent her to the intensive care unit where she died a few hours later with strangers beating on her flail chest.

Told in the first person, this short account of the illness and death of a young woman tells its story with flat, factual sentences that seem to belie deep but unvoiced feeling. The fate of the dying woman seems interwoven with the young doctor's own coming of age, each stage in his own increasing professional mastery accompanied by deterioration of his patient's clinical status. Upon the final hospital admission, the sentence structure simplifies. "She could no longer mentate. She was in blast crisis. She blasted through induction." Even a reader who does not know what induction is can tell, from the telegraphically ordered, unadorned declarative sentences, that there is no time to waste.

Frannie's private doctor had never raised with her the issue of end-of-life decisions, and so the writer is obliged to run a resuscitative effort (a "code") on his patient when her heart stops, even though he understands that further treatment is futile. It seemed to us, as we listened, that he regretted this clinical action deeply, anguishing about events that had occurred three or four years ago as if they were fresh. In the course of the writing, the doctor is able to shift his point of view from his own to his patient's and her sister's. He describes the events from the perspective of this sick young woman and her devout sister, capturing their grief and rage at the futile cardiac arrest that is perceived by the sister as an assault. This cognitive and imaginative move, enacted in the writing itself, enabled the sad young doctor to accept the perspectives and so the judgment of his dying patient's sister. His own guilt and remorse are finally telllable by virtue of his ability to curse himself, by merging with the voice of Frannie's sister. He surrenders to her judgment, depicting his clinical actions during the cardiac arrest as not intensive care but battery. Not defensive, he seems to ask for forgiveness for his act.

We did not offer absolution to this weeping physician. We wept with him, of course, and we showed that we understood what he had done with his words, perhaps helping him to see even more clearly what he had accomplished in his narrative. We observed that he will not be the same doctor the next time he is faced with a similar situation. Frannie will live on, within his doctorly self, granting comfort to the next patient who may need, despite his wishes, to die.

Narrative oncology has met twice a month for almost three years now. New staff members join the group while some of the founding members have helped me in coaching narrative training seminars on other hospital units. The pediatric oncology staff asked for our help in starting a narrative oncology program in Babies Hospital, having learned from their colleagues in adult oncology of the usefulness of the sessions. We are currently seeking funding to document the outcomes of this narrative intervention, hypothesizing that these sessions may heighten individual professional well-being, improve team cohesiveness, and improve patient satisfaction with professional care.

To Profess Is a Narrative Act

Our work in narrative oncology began to open up for us the potential dividends of narrative medicine in wider and wider concentric circles. Not only were we developing means to teach narrative competence to medical students or to physician colleagues. These narrative paths toward clinical competence were also a practical means to bridge the considerable divides that separate and *limit the effectiveness of* the members of a vast assembly of health care professionals. By putting narrative medicine into practice in an interdisciplinary health care team setting, we slowly discovered that reading and writing together about our practice generate muscular and *lasting* affiliative bonds among us doctors, nurses, and social workers.

At the same time that individual health care professionals developed insight into their practice and strengthened specific skills of attention and representation, we also found ourselves growing in honesty, altruism, collegiality, and duty, the hallmarks of health care professionalism.[6] As we inspect and attempt to better understand our own clinical work using our new narrative practices, we find ourselves more and more deeply tied to our fellow health care professionals—and it matters less what, precisely, their professional discipline is—who, like us, struggle at the boundaries of sickness and health, work and life, other and self. What interests me is that we achieve these goals of professionalism through, if you will, the back door or, perhaps more accurately, the open door. Rather than stolid, earnest, explicit efforts to be truthful, to be dutiful, and to lessen greed, these narrative explorations lead to collegiality, authenticity, attunement to patients' best interests, and proper joy from our work as natural dividends of our growing narrative competence and the affiliations this competence affords. This process further clarifies the fact that professionalism *requires* community. It is not only solitary health care professionals who must enact altruism or accountability. It is as members of collegial communities that these traits are developed, valued, and practiced.

Our program has collaborated in developing several clinical projects at our teaching hospitals with a variety of clinical departments and health care professionals from many disciplines. In all cases, we find that narrative training methods of writing about clinical experience and sharing in some way with colleagues what has been written increase both attention and representation and yield often surprising new affiliative bonds that improve the health care we provide.

The residency program in family medicine holds narrative ethics rounds twice a month for the family medicine trainees on the wards of the Allen Pavilion, Columbia's community hospital affiliate. Interns and residents write about patients whose care presents them with ethically or emotionally complex problems and then read to one another what they have written, thereby exposing multiple perspectives on shared problems. At the same hospital, occupational therapists, geriatric nurses, and cardiologists together train internal medicine residents how to elicit patients' life history narratives as part of their required geriatrics rotation.[7] They meet with well elderly patients to speak at length about their health and their illnesses in their full life contexts. Like oral historians, the residents share the written report of the narrative session with the patient, both to check its accuracy and to return the testimony to its source.[8] At Babies Hospital, program faculty have been meeting with social workers, many of whom work with abused children, in intensive narrative writing seminars. The HIV/AIDS service asked for our help in mounting a writing workshop. In this case, several doctors, nurses, and social workers sought a structured class to work on ongoing writing projects, not necessarily related to their work with people with AIDS. A group of first-year medical students, the school of social work, and the neonatal intensive care unit have all asked for our help in starting narrative medicine training projects.

In addition to the writing workshops, we offer ongoing literature seminars in close reading. Literature@Work is a twice-monthly graduate-level seminar in fiction and poetry open to all faculty and staff at the medical center. Our writer-in-residence program has hosted such writers as Michael Ondaatje and Susan Sontag for semester-long intensive literature seminars that have convened groups of faculty and students from throughout the university for serious cross-disciplinary textual study. What distinguishes these classes from seminars on comparable texts in the English department is our willingness to inspect the personal consequences of reading, to interrogate the interior sources of interpretations, and to consider the deeply personal "messages" we accept from each text. We realize that our work at a medical center lends gravity to our own private searches for meaning in our lives. We become *identified* with our place of work as not only the payer of our salary but also as a locus that helps us to understand who we are.

The program in narrative medicine is approached by other hospitals and medical schools in New York, throughout the country, and abroad for consultation and collaboration in designing and executing programs in narrative medicine. We have had to start a Narrative Medicine Consultation Service to handle the increasing volume of such requests. We are designing Narrative Medicine Training Workshops to provide intensive training for those who wish to develop these narrative skills or to spearhead courses for their colleagues. Such endorsement helps us to appreciate the usefulness of the models we have developed at Columbia.

These teaching ventures—at Columbia and at places as diverse as Denver, Montreal, Nashville, and Philadelphia—are not sporadic shots at applying a civilizing veneer to medicine. Lessons from Columbia are, I believe, generalizable to other settings. We have made sure to engage senior and authoritative faculty and executives in our seminars, to identify the Department of Medicine as the sponsor of our courses, and to pitch the level of discourse at challenging rigor. Because we have taken these cautions, narrative medicine seminars and projects are deemed not trivial but serious, not play but work, not recreation but the real thing. Although indeed reading and writing can, in a medical center environment, be experienced as deeply replenishing and refreshing, we present these activities as mainstream parts of clinical training and not diversionary relief. As a result, we believe, narrative medicine undertakings have the capacity to shift deep cultural and intellectual patterns of our environment. Through the content of humanities teaching and through the interdisciplinary and discovery methods of our teaching, these efforts can exert a sustained, directional pressure toward egalitarianism, openness to and respect for one another's perspectives, humility, and a deep and lasting appreciation for the privileges our clinical practice confer on us: to bear witness to others' suffering and, by virtue of our presence, to lessen it.

▨ BEYOND THE PROFESSIONS

Lessons learned in the medical center led us to reach out across even wider divides. At the start, the program had targeted the professional faculty, staff, and students. The more we saw the results of shared narrative training, the more we recognized its power. Not only doctors, nurses, and social workers stand to benefit from such training. As the chart of the patient with metastatic gastric cancer reminded me, the members of the nonprofessional staff like the private duty attendant are probably closer to patients' experiences than we doctors and nurses, and as such have much to contribute toward the clinical effectiveness of us all.[9] Why couldn't our narrative groups include ward clerks, transport workers, and dietary aides alongside doctors, nurses, and social workers? We are all in the "brutally mortal environment of human health," as *Lancet* editor Richard Horton puts it in his wide-ranging indictment of contemporary medicine.[10] We are all united in the efforts to treat patients, no matter what our specific skills and responsibilities. We together have the capacity to confer dignity on the lives of the sick, and, one may argue, we *require* that all of us join in the commitment to dignified care.

Patients suffer no less from dismissive treatment at the hands of the clinic receptionist than at the hands of the senior surgeon, and they can experience great comfort through the acts of benevolence of the housekeeper as well as of the head nurse. This scene from *Difficulty Swallowing,* Matthew Geller's account of his beloved's death from acute myelogenous leukemia in 1979, is imprinted in my mind. Elley is close to death after a valiant struggle: "In the early evening I turned out the lights and lit a candle. Later, as I sat next to Elley while she slept, an old heavy black woman wearing a blue janitor's uniform came into the room. She entered quietly, without knocking, and stood at the edge of the room watching Elley. At first I didn't like her being there and staring at Elley. I asked if I could help her and she said, 'I work here and wanted to see the young woman.' These words made her coming in seem like an appropriate gesture in what now felt like a sanctuary."[11]

Our developing narrative projects have begun to intersect with the hospital's institutional planning. A senior vice president for clinical affairs at our hospital recognized the potential for staff development on a very broad scale in our methods. Not only professional education but also institution-wide growth in workplace identity and loyalty might be possible through narrative workshops. Indeed, recent research in quality improvement of health care—at, for example, the Institute for Healthcare Improvement at Harvard directed by Donald Berwick and the new Institute for Improving Clinical Care at the Association of American Medical Colleges led by David Stevens—locates our work squarely within the universe of workplace quality improvement.[12] Recent movements within the staff development field such as the narrative life history approaches, professional coaching methods, and corporate uses of creative training reflect the connections between narrative reflection and work identity and effectiveness, and help us envision engaging hospital workers more broadly in our efforts.[13]

The Committee on Quality of Health Care in America of the Institute of Medicine's recent publications *To Err Is Human* and *Crossing the Quality Chasm* articulate most forcefully health care's need to rethink its processes and principles so as to reduce error, manage waste, and improve the effectiveness of all aspects of health care. The committee proposes six overarching aims that should govern efforts to improve the health care system: "Health care should be safe, effective, patient-centered, timely, efficient, and equitable."[14] *Crossing the Quality Chasm* exhaustively outlines methods by which health care institutions, federal agencies, and individual health care professionals and patients can work toward these ideals. Both reports emphasize the systemic nature of the problems examined and their proposed solutions, requiring that we mobilize *all* who work in our health care institutions in our mission to improve their effectiveness. Whether more reports and more papers will *do* what needs to be done in our hospitals and offices is, of course, not at all clear. What we do see, nonetheless, is growing expertise in how to assess quality, how to motivate for change, and how to redirect entrenched systems toward greater effectiveness.

We believe that narrative medicine training, like narrative oncology and Parallel Charts, can make contributions to patient-centered and timely health care by providing cost-effective, integrated, and boundary-crossing methods of inspecting and valuing health care professionals' work within climates of trust and collaboration. By contributing to the well-being of individual health professionals, the cohesiveness of teams, the sustained and disciplined recognition of patients' and family's perspectives, and the circulation of knowledge and information outside of traditional silos of health care systems, narrative training can provide hospital staff with new clinical skills, personal reward, heightened stake in the mission, and the fortifying trust that their work matters. At the same time, narrative work may help to level the stratified hierarchy of the health care setting. Our growth in narrative capacities may enable us recognize damaging power relationships within our hospital and help us choose to work toward fair and equitable professional collaboration in the care of the sick.

Narrative oncology, narrative ethics rounds, the well elderly program, and our literature seminars take place in the relative homogeneity of the acute care hospital setting. We are learning that narrative medicine methods have the capacity to reach over even more gaping divides—the cultural divides between medical center personnel and community residents of our urban neighborhood. A reading group started by the pediatrician Sayantani DasGupta in a neighborhood health center helped to unite young pediatricians with community health workers who staffed a child abuse prevention program.[15] Interns and residents in internal medicine at Columbia have been paying house calls in the neighborhood to their particularly frail patients. By writing naturalistic descriptions of their home visits, these doctors are getting full benefit from their frame-shift to home as the locus of care.[16] These projects function as a blend between narrative medicine and training for cultural competence, bringing the affiliative benefits of narrative training to bear on such goals as culturally sensitive care and reducing health disparities of minority populations.[17]

There are innumerable opportunities within health care to build such bridges among health care professionals, patients, and communities and to decrease the divides inevitably present in health care. After all, illness comes to all people, and we must not relinquish the potential equalizing benefits of sickness's irrevocable losses. By identifying narrative methods as particularly effective in bridging divides among divergent groups, we hope to add to the swelling forces moving toward equitable and effective health care.

NARRATIVE ROADS TO SOCIAL JUSTICE

The affiliations made possible within health care through narrative means never end. The intimate and private communions that can occur between doctor and patient or nurse and patient are echoed and recapitulated in collegial relations between professional and student, between doctor and nurse, and in the even wider reflective *communitas* between patients in their neighborhoods and the health professionals who serve them. At all levels of health care, from individual clinical encounters to global public health efforts, deploying narrative skillfully can engender authentic knowledge of one another's needs, desires, sufferings, and strengths. Rather than submitting to the narrow and the given, narratively informed health care can *re-vision* the goals of medicine to embrace a zeal for health as well as for unity and for justice. Narrative practice is by no means a cure-all for a dangerously vexed health care system. It is a set of skills and methods that can be applied to any task, for any reason, and has its own risks and benefits in practice. And yet its methods can help us cross boundaries, inhabit one another's perspectives, and build toward effective care for all.

Narrative methods join other movements to improve health care—patient advocacy groups, health activist organizations, international health bodies, public health organizations—in conceptualizing health and health care in wider and wider frames. In the past decade, such bodies as the United Nations and the World Health Organization have conceptualized the goals of health care in terms of social justice, or rather, have measured the accomplishments and requirements of one in terms of the other. So, for example, WHO's Commission on Macroeconomics and Health set standards for states' governance—freedom from corruption, from violent conflict, and from ethnic and gender repression—as requirements for fulfilling health care missions.[18] That is, one reason to banish corruption and violence and repression is that these conditions prevent the delivery of decent health care and the attainment of health goals. The Indian economist and Nobelist Amartya Sen writes, in his influential *Development as Freedom*, that the primary and overarching goal of development is freedom—not wealth, not even self-sufficiency, but freedom—including freedom from poverty and illness.[19] "If we think of poverty as basic deprivation of the quality of life and of elementary freedoms, then ill health is an aspect of poverty. Bad health is *constitutive* of poverty. Premature mortality, escapable morbidity, undernourishment are all manifestations of poverty. I believe that *health deprivation is really the most central aspect of poverty.*"[20] The freedom from ill health thereby escapes being narrowly encapsulated as a "special interest" to merge with freedoms from all other such repressions as racism, misogyny, poverty, exploitation, and religious repression.

From radical community health projects inspired by liberation theology in Latin America to innovative prison health programs in the United States, we hear a rising insistence that health activists commit themselves to social and political equity and that *achieving health goals will follow*. The goals, that is, of achieving fair and decent health care become subsumed under goals of social justice. To assure equitable health care for all, we must work toward freedom and against exploitation. The physician-anthropologist and political activist Paul Farmer devotes his expertise as an infectious disease specialist to the care of destitute tubercular and AIDS patients in Haiti, eastern Europe, and Africa. Farmer charges that "the experiences of those who are sick and poor—and, often enough, sick because they're poor—remind us that inequalities of access and outcome constitute the chief drama of modern medicine."[21] We cannot ignore our responsibilities, as U.S. health care professionals, to address injustice, for the injustice transcends *while it includes* biological illness. Farmer continues: "[J]ust as the poor are more likely to fall sick and then be denied access to care, so too are they more likely to be the victims of human rights abuses, no matter how these are defined" (138).

Ill health comes about through randomly occurring biological disease, personal unhealthy behaviors, accidents, environmental hazards, lack of access to food and shelter and health care, natural disasters, acts of personal violence, wars, repression, and state-sponsored trauma. In all but the first category, the poor are more likely to experience ill health than are those of means.[22] If we compare the magnitude of the U.S. health effort devoted to random biological disease to all the illnesses of the other categories combined, we see that most of our health-sustaining efforts—NIH research, personal health care, the output of academic health centers, most pharmaceutical products, most surgical and medical interventions—are not directed toward the illness sequelae of poverty but toward the illnesses that afflict those of means as well as the poor.

"Structural violence," according to Farmer, is what the poor suffer from. About his patients in the Central Plateau of Haiti, he writes: "[P]olitical and economic forces have structured risk for AIDS, tuberculosis, and, indeed, most other infectious and parasitic diseases. Social forces at work there have also structured risk for most forms of extreme suffering, from hunger to torture and rape." After describing the sufferings of a Haitian woman who dies of AIDS and of a man beaten to death by Haitian soldiers because of his pro-Aristide leanings, Farmer writes: "Millions of people living in similar circumstances can expect to meet similar fates. What these victims, past and present, share are not personal or psychological attributes. They do not share culture or language or a certain race. What they share, rather, is the experience of occupying the bottom rung of the social ladder in inegalitarian societies" (30–31).

It is not a coincidence that Farmer is an anthropologist, trained in qualitative ethnographic methods. He knows what he knows about poverty and disease, in part, through his systematic and disciplined use of the personal interview and of immersion fieldwork to learn of the lives of his patients. He combines what he knows through the personal narratives of individual patients with what he calls *"historically deep"* and *"geographically broad"* knowledge of political realities, social forces, and global economic conditions (158). He frames the plight of his Haitian patients within contexts that include eighteenth-century slavery and the Western world's desire for sugar. He respects the temporal unfolding of forces that lead to current-day inequities. He attends to the causes of things, seeking the most probable way to order events into meaningful plot. And he yearns to register the desires of his patients, his beloved countries, his compatriots in his fight for just health care, and his own deep longing for things for the poor to be better. Using all the tools of narrative—from bearing witness to the trauma testimony of individual patients to emplotting the broad course of history from the points of view of the oppressed—Farmer generates and exemplifies the forms of knowledge available only through narrative ways of knowing. Statistics, epidemiology, policy statements, and scientific evidence not only cannot provide but also structurally dismiss that which those like Farmer can grow to know about health and illness and justice.

The affiliations enacted by Farmer are rich, compelling affiliations with the oppressed who suffer, with fellow health care workers, and with public health activists in global communities of agency. Through his narrative ways of knowing, not only does he *find* what he must know in order to help individual patients, but also, through practicing these ways of knowing, he assents to a community of sufferers and helpers. It is by virtue of this community that his power as an agent of change is amplified.

In another, quite different, example of the power of narrative to affiliate into community and hence to amplify power on behalf of those who suffer, the literary scholar and palliative care expert David Morris investigates the disproportionate suffering of poor patients in the United States. In an essay titled "Narrative, Ethics, and Pain," Morris presents the case of Mrs. Chavez, a pregnant Mexican American woman who was denied an epidural block during delivery because her Medicaid would not pay for it. Mrs. Chavez says, "The anesthesiologist wouldn't even come into the room until she got her money. . . . I was lying there having contractions, and they wouldn't give me an epidural. I felt like an animal."[23] Morris concludes the following: "A bioethics that addresses the international failure to provide adequate relief for pain requires something like the resources of narrative to reveal both the suffering that statistics always conceal and the complexly interwoven texture of responsibility that makes adequate relief of pain so difficult to obtain. It would need to confront the recognition that pain is not just a medical or neurological problem but implacably biocultural."[24]

The work of Farmer and Morris gives evidence that narratively obtained knowledge of the other, especially the other who has suffered pain or trauma, can serve to improve health in the widest, most global frame by harnessing narrative as a force for freedom, as Azar Nafizi did for her students in Iran. This expansive use of the power of narrative can summon for health care the singular appreciation of reality required by the complexities of illness and health. Because of the ethical duties the listener incurs by virtue of having heard personal reports of trauma or pain, the communities that result from such ways of knowing are moral communities as well as clinical communities. Our colleagues in trauma studies have taught us of the responsibility one accepts by bearing witness to another's suffering. The literary and trauma studies scholar Cathy Caruth poses the challenge to the listener: "How does one listen to what is impossible? Certainly one challenge of this listening is that it may no longer be simply a choice: to be able to listen to the impossible, that is, is also to have been *chosen* by it, *before* the possibility of mastering it with knowledge. This is its danger— the danger, as some have put it, of the trauma's 'contagion,' of the traumatization of the ones who listen. But it is also its only possibility for transmission."[25]

Such listening occurs daily in the routines of health care delivery, although not all of us who work as health care professionals recognize its importance. Whether the listener is Paul Farmer visiting a tuberculosis patient in his hut on the Central Plateau, or David Morris reading from afar the report of the indignities of the inadequate pain relief for the poor, or the oral historian interviewing and accepting the testimony of a Holocaust survivor, that listener is performing simultaneously a moral and a social task. (George Mead observes that "[o]ur morality gathers about our social conduct. It is as social beings that we are moral beings."[26]) The listener performs that task on behalf of others, including the speakers and the affiliative community that surrounds them, altering not only the individual experience being recounted but all the human agents who surround it.

Oddly, as we examine the sequelae of clinical narrative practices, we see a congruence, a curious resonance between the private and public performances of narrative medicine. What was true when Bruno Morales told me of his ordeal on September 11, 2001 is true of public hearings about the epidemic of multiply drug-resistant TB in Haiti or the reconciliation trials in Rwanda.[27] If we find ourselves going back and forth in scale or scope—from tight-shot focus on one doctor-patient relationship to wide-angle views of global health matters—it is because the principles and the practices are shared. This commonality across scale buttresses the fundamentality of narrative medicine lessons: *that healing occurs through telling, listening, and fulfilling the duties thereby incurred.*

Private trauma contributes to public inequity, and large-scale trauma confers private pain. No private individual ever stops being a part of social groups, and what hurts the individual will hurt the family, the neighborhood, the town. In corollary, anything that alters the sociality cannot but have ramifications at the individual level. George Engel's biopsychosocial model and David Morris's biocultural model help us grasp the vivid and dynamic interplay between the very small and the very large, each contributing toward the other's ills and health. To influence health, one must work at all levels at once.

There is a great deal at stake in the affiliative movements of narrative medicine. Because these affiliations take place within the spheres of illness and mortality, the *actions* our communities take together are not trivial, not disposable. They imprint the communities thereby created with traces of conscience, with declarations of values, with aspects of justice. In the light of narrative's potential contributions to justice, we must take heed of the possible dangers that inhere in the vulnerability of telling of suffering. In an essay titled "Narrating, Attending, and Empathizing," Roy Schafer cautions us to not overlook the force of power relationships within narrative work: "That [narration-attention-empathy] triad can be viewed in terms of submission to, incorporation of, or rebellion against prevailing power relations."[28] Whoever listens, from the relative refuge of health, to the ill or traumatized speaker holds a profound responsibility not to exploit, not to expropriate, not to use the other for one's own ends.

We must also remember that our moral communities, that is, those communities within which we try to articulate our moral responsibilities, can exclude as well as include. David Morris warns that moral communities "always share a dependence on exclusion"; for example, many moral communities exclude from their ranks animals or certain criminals or those, like the demented or psychotic, who are deemed not autonomous moral agents. Zaner asks indignantly, "And is it these rational agents whose job it is, in part, to turn right around and define what counts as 'moral' and therefore who gets included and has moral standing in that community? . . . Do the demented count less than the rest of us, the nondemented? Or, is that widespread, deep-lying sense of no longer counting, no longer needing to be reckoned with, expressive instead of a deep malaise within contemporary society."[29] If suffering occurs outside one's moral community, Morris continues, it may be overlooked or met with detachment, but narrative texts and skill can counter this impulse to turn away. "One important function of literature is to challenge and stretch—even to transgress—the boundaries of a moral community . . . to force us to acknowledge suffering where we normally do not see it."[30]

Listeners who bear witness as others tell of suffering are able to perform meaningful service while deriving important benefits for themselves. Zaner describes the finding that a seriously ill hospitalized patient *"evokes a moral sense"* in him that clarifies his role not only as a health care professional but also as a moral agent. "The very structural imbalance of the helper/person-helped relationship seems, paradoxically, turned on its head. An elemental moral cognizance leading to a commanding sense of responsibility is buried within this experience."[31] The states of attention described by Gabriel Marcel and Iris Murdoch that I cited in earlier chapters are here used not only for their clinical work but for their moral work and their deep and powerful work of affiliation. Paul Farmer notes that "in a world riven by inequity, medicine could be viewed as social justice work. In fact, doctors are far more fortunate than most modern professionals: we still have a sliver of hope for meaningful, dignified service to the oppressed."[32] Did we know about the dividends of our professions when we chose them, not only that they would open us to doing good work for the sick but also that they would fill us, transform us, give gifts whose value we can never estimate?

After September 11, 2001, the New York psychoanalyst Donald Moss bore witness to his many patients affected by the World Trade Center attacks while experiencing his own anguish at the events—events that threatened to silence his patients and him. "I felt both silenced and spoken for. Final judgments seemed to have been made. The covenants of civilization seemed weakened. . . . I felt no less helpless than these patients did."[33] And yet, his clinical dutifulness bore him on to try to fulfill the goals of practice: "Psychoanalytic theory promises structure and coherence, pertinence and endurance. More ambitiously, it promises an intimate, protective, nondeforming means of contact with the entire range of human possibility. . . . Can we, should we, does it matter if we try to stay in contact with whatever the terrorists might have meant, and thereby try to stay in touch with the workings of desire and rage among what some have now begun to call 'the damned of the earth'?" (328).

This meditation displays both aspects of what we have been considering: the private ability to bear witness to a person who suffers and an openness, without exclusion, to all within an expanded moral community—here, even including the terrorists responsible for the attacks—so as to achieve a *full* reckoning, a global generosity of interpretation. Not all can achieve such scope, and yet this example stands as a model and ideal for all of us in clinical practice. One attends to the private needs of the person, in pain, in one's hands while recognizing all that that person *is*—a parent, a sibling, a broker at Cantor Fitzgerald, a New Yorker, an American, a citizen of a democracy—and all that influences the fate and the potential happiness of that individual. As one *hears* one person in private, one hears behind him or her the rising voices of others, in concert and in conflict, testifying to their own suffering. The murmurings expand, form harmonies and discordances. "Not completion," as E. M. Forster said about the symphony, which he compared to the novel, "Not rounding off but opening out. When the symphony is over we feel that the notes and tunes composing it have been liberated, they have found in the rhythm of the whole their individual freedom. . . . Is there not something of it in *War and Peace?* . . . [A]s we read it, do not great chords begin to sound behind us, and when we have finished does not every item . . . lead a larger existence than was possible at the time?"[34] Like the snow general all over Ireland in James Joyce's "The Dead" that stands for a universalizing death, all that we suffer unites us, and the more deeply suffered, the more irrevocably united. We feel Turner's wholeness encircling us all, enacting the "flow from *I* to *thou*" as we reach toward one another with authenticity and generosity. As witnesses of others' pain, we expose ourselves to suffering, and so we suffer ourselves. To be equal to this grave task is our humble hope.

CODA

We inherit an unfinishable task, a practice that opens itself to unannounced and unforeseen responsibilities, one that welcomes patients whose unit numbers are not in our panels and yet to whom we owe allegiance. As we develop narrative skills to attend genuinely to others' suffering and to represent their plight accurately, we enter affiliative communities able and *required to* exert influence on behalf of the sick.

A narrative practice, ideally envisioned, might include a vastly expanded moral community that embraces duties toward individual patients, fellow professionals and students, institutions, locales, states, and nations. What I do in my internal medicine office in Washington Heights in Manhattan equips me to enter, as a citizen, into the debates about national health insurance, pharmaceutical and insurance corporation responsibilities, and health care system redesign. Indeed, we can commit ourselves to health care systems that provide safe, effective, patient-centered, timely, efficient, and equitable care for all. We can choose to include within our clinico-moral communities those inflicted with occupational injuries in underregulated plants in the United States, those infected with AIDS in sub-Saharan Africa, or any afflicted with unnecessary or undertreated illness.

Because narrative skills encourage serious communication of even the deepest fears and wildest hopes, health care professionals trained in narrative skills might support the probing, consequential conversations about health care, mercy, and justice that this country so desperately needs. We can no longer espouse a system in which conversations about meaning begin when a patient is almost dead and the family is enjoined to remove him or her from treatment. We can no longer espouse a system in which the content of the medical conversation is limited by ICD-9 codes, where it is deemed the work of the social worker to enquire about emotions and of the ethicist to enquire about values. We can no longer espouse a system that absorbs the bureaucratic costs of privatized insurance and submits to corporate control over health care spending while the numbers of uninsured people increase and individual patients' power and choice diminish.

Narrative medicine can help us find ways to activate doctors, nurses, social workers, and patients to work together to fashion an equitable, humane, and effective health care system. To do so, asserts Amartya Sen, "requires active public discussion on health care provision; it requires constant vigilance about the quality of hospital, medical, nursing services. This incentive has to be provided through the medium of public discussion and criticism."[35] We doctors, nurses, and social workers can facilitate that public discussion; we can be its spark. That we have not yet done so does not necessarily speak to a lack of courage or commitment or wisdom or resolve on the part of health professionals. It speaks to a lack of voice, an underestimation of the urgency with which the public waits to hear from us. It speaks to an ignorance of the warrant by which we can speak and, perhaps, must speak.

By what warrant do we speak? Our warrant is that we have seen pain and seen death. Our warrant is that we have witnessed the anguish of being poor and sick, of being sick and in despair, of being near death and alone. Our warrant is that we have lived through a nearness to sickness so profound, so saturating that we fear daily for our own health and that of those we love. Our warrant is the hours not slept, the family dinners missed, the nights on call of torture—not for what it cost ourselves (internship, however apocalyptic, is only one year) but for what it made us see about the plight of the ill.

By equipping ourselves with narrative competence, we are able to use the self as a therapeutic instrument—not only our cognitive grasp of human biology but our imagination, our respect for the courage of others, our awareness of our own frailty, and our willingness to forgive and be forgiven. With our narrative attunement to temporality, we mark the passage of time, providing those who live amid illness with the urgency and the patience to claim their numbered days and to see forward and backward toward their meaning, making room within our lives and the lives of our patients for the inevitable mortality that counts us human. With the narrative tools of description and diction and metaphor, we can represent—and therefore recognize and admire—singular individuals in contextualized situations, not as instances of general phenomena but as irreducible and therefore invaluable particulars. Through narrative effort, we achieve first the subject position and then, with luck, the intersubjective bond between ourselves and others, thereby inaugurating and framing the therapeutic relationship. With narrative emplotment we attempt—often against all odds—to make causal sense of random events or humbly acknowledge the contingent nature of events that have no cause, enabling us both to diagnose disease and to tolerate the uncertainty that saturates illness. With narrative acts and skills, we recognize and live up to the ethical duties incurred by having heard one another out and the indebtedness we sustain by having been heard by another. Instead of depleting us, this care replenishes us, for our suffering helps our patients to bear theirs. Its own reward, this care envelops us all with meaning, with grace, with courage, and with joy.

NOTES

1. See Paul Farmer, *Pathologies of Power;* Howard Waitzkin, *At the Front Lines of Medicine;* and Richard Horton, *Health Wars* for recent examinations of health care's social injustices and unconscionable inequities.

2. Victor Turner, *The Ritual Process,* 97.

3. Martin Buber, *Between Man and Man,* 51 (cited by Turner, *Ritual Process,* 127).

4. Victor Turner, *The Ritual Process,* 128.

5. For the sake of nonclinical readers, I have altered his text slightly by replacing the abbreviations and acronyms that peppered his paragraphs with full words and some bracketed definitions.

6. I will not rehearse here the considerable and growing literature on professionalism in medicine except to direct the beginner to Thomas Inui's monograph *A Flag in the Wind* and a special issue of *Academic Medicine,* edited by Michael Whitcomb, devoted to the topic.

7. Patricia Miller et al., "Infusing a Geriatric Intern Program with Narrative Medicine: The Columbia Cooperative Aging Program." See also N. R. Kleinfield, "Old Patients, Making Doctors Better: Myths Explode as Physicians Get to Know the Elderly." See Narrative Medicine Rounds presented by Drs. Miller and Maurer in 2004. Streaming videotape of their presentation available through archives at http://www.narrativemedicine.org

8. See Robert Perks and Alistair Thomson, eds., *The Oral History Reader* for a collection of essays on the methods of the oral historian. See especially Charles T. Morrissey, "On Oral History Interviewing" for method guidelines that require that the oral historian

send the transcript of the interview back to the interviewee for editing, elaboration, and an accuracy check.

9. This realization is the basis for Howard Brody's policy recommendations regarding such institutional ethics questions as the ideal makeup of the ethics committee. See Howard Brody, "Narrative Ethics and Institutional Impact."

10. Richard Horton, *Health Wars,* 501.

11. Matthew Geller, *Difficulty Swallowing,* unpaginated, on page dated April 16, 1979.

12. See Donald M. Berwick, A. Blanton Godfrey, and Jane Roessner, *Curing Health Care;* Donald M. Berwick, *Escape Fire: Designs for the Future of Health Care;* Molla S. Donaldson and Julie J. Mohr, *Exploring Innovation and Quality Improvement in Health Care Micro-Systems: A Cross-Case Analysis* for some introductions to the tailoring of quality improvement to the health care setting.

13. Michael P. Sipiora and Frank Lehner, *Work, Identity, Coaching.* See also http://www.psychoguys.com for more information on the narrative methods of staff development.

14. Committee on Quality of Health Care in America, Institute of Medicine, *Crossing the Quality Chasm,* 6.

15. Sayantani DasGupta, Dodi Meyer, Ayexa Calero-Breckheimer, Alex Costley, Sobeida Guillen, "Teaching Cultural Competency through Narrative Medicine: Community as Classroom, Classroom as Community," manuscript in preparation.

16. Eileen Moroney, "Home Is Where the Residents Visit."

17. For definitions and conceptual frameworks of cultural competence, see Terry Cross and M. Isaacs, *Toward a Culturally Competent System of Care;* Melissa Walsh, *Teaching Diversity and Cross-Cultural Competence in Health Care;* Michael Whitcomb, ed., "Cultural Competence in Medical Education and Practice."

18. See Richard Horton, *Health Wars,* especially chapter 17, "The Health of Peoples," for a cogent discussion of these recent trends in international development.

19. Amartya Sen, *Development as Freedom.*

20. Adrea Mach, "Amartya Sen on Development and Health," 1.

21. Paul Farmer, *Pathologies of Power,* 164. Subsequent page references to this work appear in parentheses in the text.

22. See Michael Marmot, *The Status Syndrome: How Social Standing Affects Our Health and Longevity* for compilations of data suggesting correlations between health and social/economic/political standing in society.

23. Robert Pear, "Mother on Medicaid Overcharged for Pain Relief," *New York Times,* cited by David Morris in "Narrative, Ethics, and Pain," 205.

24. David Morris, "Narrative, Ethics, and Pain," 206.

25. Cathy Caruth, "Trauma and Experience: Introduction," in *Trauma,* edited by Caruth, 10.

26. George Mead, *Mind, Self, and Society,* 386. Cited in Micah Hester, *Community as Healing,* 50.

27. Phuong N. Pham, Harvey M. Weinstein, and Timothy Longman, "Trauma and PTSD Symptoms in Rwanda."

28. Roy Schafer, "Narrating, Attending, and Empathizing," 248.

29. Richard Zaner, *Conversations on the Edge,* 80–81.

30. David Morris, "Voice, Genre, and Moral Community," 39–40.

31. Richard Zaner, "Power and Hope in the Clinical Encounter: A Meditation on Vulnerability," 270.

32. Paul Farmer, *Pathologies of Power,* 157–58. Subsequent page references to this work appear in parentheses in the text.

33. Donald Moss, "Does It Matter What the Terrorists Meant?" in *Hating in the First-Person Plural*, edited by Donald Moss, 327. Subsequent page references to this work appear in parentheses in the text.

34. E. M. Forster, *Aspects of the Novel*, 169.

35. Adrea Mach, "Amartya Sen on Development and Health," 2.

▣ REFERENCES

Abbott, H. Porter. *The Cambridge Introduction to Narrative*. Cambridge: Cambridge University Press, 2002.

Alcorn, M. W., and M. Bracher. "Literature, Psychoanalysis, and the Re-formation of the Self: A New Direction for Reader-Response Theory." *PMLA* 100 (1985): 342–54.

Allen, Guy. "The 'Good-Enough' Teacher and the Authentic Student." In *A Pedagogy of Becoming*, edited by Jon Mills, 141–76. Amsterdam: Rodopi Press, 2002.

Anderson, Charles, ed. "Writing and Healing." Special issue of *Literature and Medicine* 19 (2000): 1–132.

Anderson, Charles, and Martha Montello. "The Reader's Response and Why It Matters in Biomedical Ethics." In *Stories Matter: The Role of Narrative in Medical Ethics*, edited by Rita Charon and Martha Montello, 85–94. New York: Routledge, 2003.

Aring, Charles. "Sympathy and Empathy." *Journal of the American Medical Association* 167 (1958): 448–52.

Aristotle. *Poetics*. In *Aristotle's Poetics: A Translation and Commentary for Students of Literature*, translated by Leon Golden and O. B. Hardison Jr. Englewood Cliffs, N.J.: Prentice-Hall, 1968.

Arras, John D., and Bonnie Steinbock, eds. *Ethical Issues in Modern Medicine*. 5th edition. London: Mayfield, 1999.

Ashley, Kathleen, Leigh Gilmore, and Gerald Peters, eds. *Autobiography and Postmodernism*. Amherst: University of Massachusetts Press, 1994.

Bal, Mieke. *Narratology: Introduction to the Theory of Narrative*, 2nd edition. Toronto: University of Toronto Press, 1997.

Balint, Michael. *The Doctor, His Patient, and the Illness*. London: Tavistock, 1957.

Banks, Joanne Trautmann, and Anne Hunsaker Hawkins, eds. "The Art of the Case History." Special issue of *Literature and Medicine* 13 (1992): 1–180.

Barker, Pat. *Regeneration*. New York: Penguin, 1993.

Barondess, Jeremiah. "Medicine and Professionalism." *Archives of Internal Medicine* 163 (2003): 145–49.

Barr, Marleen S., and Carl Freedman, eds. Special topic: "Science Fiction and Literary Studies: The Next Millennium." *PMLA* 119 (2004): 429–546.

Barry, Michael, Floyd Fowler, Albert G. Mulley Jr., et al. "Patient Reactions to a Program Designed to Facilitate Patient Participation in Treatment Decisions for Benign Prostatic Hyperplasia." *Medical Care* 33 (1995): 771–82.

Barthes, Roland. *Camera Lucida*. Translated by Richard Howard. New York: Hill and Wang, 1981.

————. *Image-Music-Text*. Translated by Stephen Heath. New York: Hill and Wang, 1988.

————. *The Pleasures of the Text*. Translated by Richard Miller. New York: Hill and Wang, 1975.

————. *S/Z*. Translated by Richard Miller. New York: Hill and Wang, 1974.

Bauby, Jean-Dominique. *The Diving Bell and the Butterfly: A Memoir of Life in Death*. New York: Vintage, 1998.

Bayliss, Richard. "Pain Narratives." In *Narrative Based Medicine: Dialogue and Discourse in Clinical Practice*, edited by Trisha Greenhalgh and Brian Hurwitz, 75–82. London: BMJ Books, 1998.

Beauchamp, Tom L., and James F. Childress. *The Principles of Biomedical Ethics*. 4th edition. New York: Oxford University Press, 1994.

Beauchamp, Tom L., and LeRoy Walter. *Contemporary Issues in Bioethics*. Belmont, Calif.: Wadsworth, 2003.

Beauvoir, Simone de. *The Second Sex*. Translated by H. M. Parshley. New York: Alfred A. Knopf, 1975.

————. *A Very Easy Death*. Translated by Patrick O'Brian. New York: Pantheon Books, 1965.

Beckman, Howard, and Richard Frankel. "The Effect of Physician Behavior on the Collection of Data." *Annals of Internal Medicine* 101 (1984): 692–96.

Beecher, Henry. "Ethics and Clinical Research." *New England Journal of Medicine* 74 (1966): 1354–60.

Beels, C. Christian. *"A Different Story . . .": The Rise of Narrative in Psychotherapy*. Phoenix, Ariz.: Zeig, Tucker and Theisen, 2001.

Benjamin, Walter. *Illuminations*. Translated by Harry Zohn, edited by Hannah Arendt. New York: Schocken Books, 1988.

Benner, Patricia, and J. Wrubel. *The Primacy of Caring*. Menlo Park, Calif.: Addison-Wesley, 1989.

Berger, John. *Ways of Seeing*. London: Penguin Books and British Broadcasting Corporation, 1972.

Berger, John, and Jean Mohr. *A Fortunate Man*. New York: Pantheon Books, 1967.

Bergson, Henri. *Time and Free Will: An Essay on the Immediate Data of Consciousness*. London: G. Allen, 1913.

Berland, Lauren, ed. *Compassion: The Culture and Politics of an Emotion*. New York: Routledge, 2004.

Berlinger, Nancy. "Broken Stories: Patients, Families, and Clinicians after Medical Error." *Literature and Medicine* 22 (2003): 230–40.

Berwick, Donald. *Escape Fire: Designs for the Future of Health Care*. San Francisco: Jossey-Bass, 2003.

Berwick, Donald M., A. Blanton Godfrey, and Jane Roessner. *Curing Health Care: New Strategies for Quality Improvement*. San Francisco: Jossey-Bass, 2002.

Bloom, Harold. *The Anxiety of Influence: A Theory of Poetry*. New York: Oxford University Press, 1997.

Bolton, Gillie. *The Therapeutic Potential of Creative Writing*. London: Jessica Kingsley, 2000.

Bonebakker, Virginia. "Literature and Medicine: Humanities at the Heart of Health Care: A Hospital-Based Reading and Discussion Program Developed by the Maine Humanities Council." *Academic Medicine* 78 (2003): 963–67.

Booth, Wayne. *The Company We Keep: An Ethics of Fiction*. Berkeley: University of California Press, 1988.

———. "The Ethics of Medicine, as Revealed in Literature." In *Stories Matter: The Role of Narrative in Medical Ethics*, edited by Rita Charon and Martha Montello, 10–20. New York: Routledge, 2002.

———. *The Rhetoric of Fiction*, 2nd edition. Chicago: University of Chicago Press, 1983.

Borkan, Jeffrey M., Shmuel Reis, D. Steinmetz, and Jack H. Medalie, eds. *Patients and Doctors: Life-Changing Stories from Primary Care*. Madison: University of Wisconsin Press, 1999.

Bosk, Charles. *Forgive and Remember: Managing Medical Failure*. 2nd edition. Chicago: University of Chicago Press, 2003.

Brady, D. W., G. Corbie-Smith, William T. Branch. "'What's Important to You?' The Use of Narratives to Promote Self-Reflection and to Understand the Experiences of Medical Residents." *Annals of Internal Medicine* 137 (2002): 220–23.

Branch, William T. *Office Practice of Medicine*. 3rd edition. Philadelphia: Saunders, 1994.

Branch, William T., R. J. Pels, Robert Lawrence, and Ronald Arky. "Becoming a Doctor: Critical-Incident Reports from Third-Year Medical Students." *New England Journal of Medicine* 329 (1993): 1130–32.

Brock, Dan. "The Ideal of Shared Decision-Making between Physicians and Patients." *Kennedy Institute Ethics Journal* 1 (1991): 28–47.

Brody, Howard. "Narrative Ethics and Institutional Impact." In *Stories Matter: The Role of Narrative in Medical Ethics*, edited by Rita Charon and Martha Montello, 149–53. New York: Routledge: 2003.

———. *Stories of Sickness*. New Haven: Yale University Press, 1987.

Brooches, Joseph. "Black Autobiography in Africa and America." *Black Academy Review* 2 (1971): 61–70.

Brooks, Cleanth. *The Well-Wrought Urn*. New York: Harcourt and Brace, 1947.

Brooks, Peter. *Psychoanalysis and Storytelling*. Oxford, UK: Blackwell, 1994.

———. *Reading for the Plot: Design and Intention in Narrative*. New York: Vintage Books, 1984.

Brown, Phil. *Perspectives in Medical Sociology*, 3rd edition. Long Grove, Ill.: Waveland Press, 2000.

Broyard, Anatole. *Intoxicated by My Illness, and Other Writings on Life and Death*. Edited by Alexandra Broyard. New York: Clarkson and Potter, 1992.

Bruner, Jerome. *Acts of Meaning*. Cambridge: Harvard University Press, 1990.

———. *Actual Minds, Possible Worlds*. Cambridge: Harvard University Press, 1986.

———. *Making Stories: Law, Literature, Life*. New York: Farrar, Straus and Giroux, 2002.

Bruss, Elizabeth. *Autobiographical Acts: The Changing Situation of a Literary Genre*. Baltimore: Johns Hopkins University Press, 1976.

Buber, Martin. *Between Man and Man*. Translated by Ronald Gregor Smith. London: Routledge and Kegan Paul, 1949.

———. *I and Thou*. 2nd edition. Translated by Ronald Gregor Smith. New York: Charles Scribner's Sons, 1958.

Burrell, David, and Stanley Hauerwas. "From System to Story: An Alternative Pattern for Rationality in Ethics." In *Knowledge, Value, and Belief*, edited by H. T. Engelhardt Jr. and Daniel Callahan, 125. Hastings-on-Hudson, N.Y.: Hastings Center, 1977.

Butler, Judith. *Bodies That Matter: On the Discursive Limits of "Sex."* New York: Routledge, 1993.

Butterfield, Stephen. *Black Autobiography in America*. Amherst: University of Massachusetts Press, 1974.

Cadava, Eduardo, Peter Connor, and Jean-Luc Nancy, eds. *Who Comes after the Subject?* New York: Routledge, 1991.

Cameron, Sharon. *Beautiful Work: A Meditation on Pain*. Durham: Duke University Press, 2000.

———. "The Practice of Attention: Simone Weil's Performance of Impersonality." *Critical Inquiry* 29 (2003): 216–52.

Campo, Rafael. *The Desire to Heal: A Doctor's Education in Empathy, Identity, and Poetry*. New York: W. W. Norton, 1997.

Carson, Ronald A, Chester R. Burns, and Thomas R. Cole, eds. *Practicing the Medical Humanities*. Hagerstown, Md.: University Publishing Group, 2003.

Caruth, Cathy. *Unclaimed Experience: Trauma, Narrative, and History*. Baltimore: Johns Hopkins University Press, 1996.

———, ed. *Trauma: Explorations in Memory*. Baltimore: Johns Hopkins University Press, 1995.

Cassell, Eric. *Doctoring: The Nature of Primary Care Medicine*. New York: Oxford and Milbank Memorial Fund, 1997.

———. "The Nature of Suffering and the Goals of Medicine." *New England Journal of Medicine* 306 (1982): 639–45.

———. *The Nature of Suffering and the Goals of Medicine*. 2nd edition. New York: Oxford University Press, 2004.

Chambers, Ross. *Story and Situation: Narrative Seduction and the Power of Fiction*. Minneapolis: University of Minnesota Press, 1984.

Chambers, Tod. *The Fiction of Bioethics: Cases as Literary Texts*. New York: Routledge, 1999.

Chambers, Tod, and Kathryn Montgomery. "Plot: Framing Contingency and Choice in Bioethics." In *Stories Matter: The Role of Narrative in Medical Ethics*, edited by Rita Charon and Martha Montello, 77–84. New York: Routledge, 2002.

Charon, Rita. "The Life-Long Error, or John Marcher the Proleptic." In *Margin of Error: Mistakes in Ethics Practice and Clinical Medicine*, edited by Laurie Zoloth and Susan B. Rubin, 37–57. Hagerstown, Md.: University Publishing Group, 2000.

———. "Medical Interpretation: Implications of Literary Theory of Narrative for Clinical Work." *Journal of Narrative and Life History* 3 (1993): 79–97.

———. "Medicine, the Novel, and the Passage of Time." *Annals of Internal Medicine* 132 (2000): 63–68.

———. "Narrative and Medicine." *New England Journal of Medicine* 350 (2004): 862–64.

———. "Narrative Medicine: A Model for Empathy, Reflection, Profession, and Trust." *Journal of the American Medical Association* 286 (2001): 1897–902.

———. "The Narrative Road to Empathy." In *Empathy and the Practice of Medicine: Beyond Pills and the Scalpel*, edited by Howard Spiro et al., 147–59. New Haven: Yale University Press, 1993.

———. "The Seasons of the Patient-Physician Relationship." *Clinics in Geriatric Medicine* 16 (2000): 37–50.

———. "To Build a Case: Medical Histories as Traditions in Conflict." *Literature and Medicine* 11 (1992): 115–32.

Charon, Rita, and Joanne Trautmann Banks, Julia Connelly, Anne Hunsaker Hawkins, Kathryn Montgomery Hunter, Anne Hudson Jones, Martha Montello, and Suzanne Poirier. "Literature and Medicine: Contributions to Clinical Practice." *Annals of Internal Medicine* 122 (1995): 599–606.

Charon, Rita, and Martha Montello, eds. *Stories Matter: The Role of Narrative in Medical Ethics*. New York: Routledge, 2002.

Chatman, Seymour. *Story and Discourse: Narrative Structure in Fiction and Film*. Ithaca: Cornell University Press, 1978.

Childress, Marcia Day. "Of Symbols and Silence: Using Narrative and Its Interpretation to Foster Physician Understanding." In *Stories Matter: The Role of Narrative in Medical Ethics*, edited by Rita Charon and Martha Montello, 119–25. New York: Routledge, 2002.

Close, William T. *A Doctor's Life: Unique Stories*. Marbleton, Wyo.: Meadowlark Springs Productions, 2001.

Cohn, Dorrit. *The Distinction of Fiction*. Baltimore: Johns Hopkins University Press, 1999.

Coles, Robert. *The Call of Stories: Teaching and the Moral Imagination*. Boston: Houghton Mifflin, 1989.

———. "Medical Ethics and Living a Life." *New England Journal of Medicine* 301 (1979): 444–46.

Committee on Quality of Health Care in America, Institute of Medicine. *Crossing the Quality Chasm: A New Health System for the 21st Century*. Washington, D.C.: National Academy Press, 2001.

———. *To Err Is Human: Building a Safer Health System*. Washington, D.C.: National Academy Press, 2000.

Connelly, Julia E. "Being in the Present Moment: Developing the Capacity for Mindfulness in Medicine." *Academic Medicine* 74 (1999): 420–24.

———. "In the Absence of Narrative." In *Stories Matter: The Role of Narrative in Medical Ethics*, edited by Rita Charon and Martha Montello, 138–40. New York: Routledge, 2002.

Conrad, Joseph. *Great Short Works of Joseph Conrad*. New York: Harper and Row, 1966.

Conway, Kathlyn. *Ordinary Life: A Memoir of Illness*. New York: W. H. Freeman, 1996.

Cooper-Patrick, Lisa, Joseph J. Gallo, Junius J. Gonzales, Hong Thi Vu, Neil R. Powe, Christine Nelson, and Daniel E. Ford. "Race, Gender, and Partnership in the Patient-Physician Relationship." *Journal of the American Medical Association* 282 (1999): 583–89.

Coulehan, Jack. "Empathy." In *Teaching Literature and Medicine*, edited by V. Gilchrist and Delese Wear, 128–44. Kansas City, Mo.: Society of Teachers of Family Medicine, 1995.

———. "The First Patient: Reflections and Stories about the Anatomy Cadaver." *Teaching and Learning in Medicine* 7 (1995): 61–66.

Coulehan, Jack, and Marian Block. *The Medical Interview: A Primer for Students of the Art*. Philadelphia: F. A. Davis, 1987.

Coulter, Harris L. *Divided Legacy: A History of the Schism in Medical Thought*, vol. 1. Washington, D.C.: Weehawken, 1975.

Couser, G. Thomas. *Recovering Bodies: Illness, Disability, and Life Writing*. Madison: University of Wisconsin Press, 1997.

———. *Vulnerable Subjects: Ethics and Life-Writing*. Ithaca: Cornell University Press, 2004.

Couser, Thomas G., and Joseph Fichtelberg, eds. *True Relations: Essays on Autobiography and the Postmodern*. Westport, Conn.: Greenwood Press, 1998.

Cousins, Norman. *Anatomy of an Illness as Perceived by the Patient: Reflections on Healing and Regeneration*. Toronto and New York: Bantam, 1979.

Crawford, T. Hugh. "The Politics of Narrative Form." *Literature and Medicine* 11 (1992): 147–62.

Crookshank, F. G. "The Importance of a Theory of Signs and a Critique of Language in the Study of Medicine." In *The Meaning of Meaning*, C. K. Odgen and I. A. Richards, Supplement 2, 337–55. New York: Harcourt, Brace and World, 1923.

Cross, Terry, and M. Isaacs. *Toward a Culturally Competent System of Care*. Washington, D.C.: Georgetown University Child Development Center, 1989.

Culler, Jonathan. "Omniscience." *Narrative* 12 (2004): 22–34.

———. *Structuralist Poetics: Structuralism, Linguistics, and the Study of Literature.* Ithaca: Cornell University Press, 1975.

Currie, Mark. *Postmodern Narrative Theory.* New York: St. Martin's Press, 1998.

Damasio, Antonio R. *Descartes' Error: Emotion, Reason, and the Human Brain.* New York: G. P. Putnam, 1994.

———. *The Feeling of What Happens: Body and Emotion in the Making of Consciousness.* New York: Harcourt Brace, 1999.

———. *Looking for Spinoza: Joy, Sorrow, and the Feeling Brain.* Orlando, Fla.: Harcourt, 2003.

Dan, B. B., and Rosemary Young. *A Piece of My Mind: A Collection of Essays from the Journal of the American Medical Association.* New York: Ballantine, 1990.

Danto, Arthur. *Narration and Knowledge.* New York: Columbia University Press, 1985.

DasGupta, Sayantani, and Rita Charon. "Personal Illness Narratives: Using Reflective Writing to Teach Empathy." *Academic Medicine* 79 (2004): 351–56.

Davis, Cortney, and Judy Schaeffer, eds. *Between the Heartbeats: Poetry and Prose by Nurses.* Iowa City: University of Iowa Press, 1995.

———, eds. *Intensive Care: More Poetry and Prose by Nurses.* Iowa City: University of Iowa Press, 2003.

De Lauretis, Teresa. "Statement Due." *Critical Inquiry* 30 (2004): 365–68.

Delbanco, Thomas L. "Enriching the Doctor-Patient Relationship by Inviting the Patient's Perspective." *Annals of Internal Medicine* 116 (1992): 414–18.

Deleuze, Gilles. *Negotiations.* Translated by Martin Joughin. New York: Columbia University Press, 1990.

De Man, Paul. *Allegories of Reading: Figural Language in Rousseau, Nietzsche, Rilke, and Proust.* New Haven: Yale University Press, 1979.

———. "Autobiography as De-Facement." *MLN* 94 (1979): 919–30.

———. *Blindness and Insight: Essays in the Rhetoric of Contemporary Criticism.* Minneapolis: University of Minnesota Press, 1983.

De Moor, Katrien. "The Doctor's Role of Witness and Companion: Medical and Literary Ethics of Care in AIDS Physicians' Memoirs." *Literature and Medicine* 22 (2003): 208–29.

Dennett, Daniel. *Kinds of Minds: Toward an Understanding of Consciousness.* New York: Basic Books, 1996.

Derrida, Jacques. "La différance." In *Théorie d'Ensemble.* Paris: Seuil, 1968.

———. *Of Grammatology.* Translated by Gayatri Chakravorty Spivak. Baltimore: Johns Hopkins University Press, 1997.

———. *Writing and Difference.* Translated by Alan Bass. Chicago: University of Chicago Press, 1978.

DeSalvo, Louise. *Breathless: An Asthma Journal.* Boston: Beacon Press, 1997.

Donaldson, Molla S., and Julie J. Mohr. *Exploring Innovation and Quality Improvement in Health Care Micro-Systems: A Cross-Case Analysis.* Washington, D.C.: Institute of Medicine, National Academy Press, 2000.

Donne, John. *Devotions upon Emergent Occasions.* Ann Arbor: University of Michigan Press, 1959.

Downing, Christine. "Re-Visioning Autobiography: The Bequest of Freud and Jung." *Soundings* 60 (1977): 210–28.

Dubler, Nancy N., and Carol B. Liebman. *Bioethics Mediation: A Guide to Shaping Shared Solutions.* New York: United Hospital Fund of New York, 2004.

Dubose, Edwin R., Ronald P. Hamel, Laurence J. O'Connell, eds. *A Matter of Principles? Ferment in U.S. Bioethics.* Valley Forge, Penn.: Trinity Press International, 1994.

Duplessis, Rachel Blau. *Writing beyond the Ending: Narrative Strategies of Twentieth-Century Women Writers*. Bloomington: Indiana University Press, 1985.

Eakin, Paul John. *Fictions in Autobiography: Studies in the Art of Self-Invention*. Princeton: Princeton University Press, 1985.

————. *How Our Lives Become Stories: Making Selves*. Ithaca: Cornell University Press, 1999.

————. *Touching the World: Reference in Autobiography*. Princeton: Princeton University Press, 1992.

Edelman, Gerald M. *Bright Air, Brilliant Fire: On the Matter of the Mind*. New York: Basic Books, 1992.

Edson, Margaret. *Wit*. New York: Faber and Faber, 1993.

Ehrenreich, Barbara, and Deirdre English. *Witches, Midwives, and Nurses: A History of Women Healers*. 2nd edition. Old Westbury, N.Y.: Feminist Press, 1973.

Eliot, T. S. *Four Quartets*. London: Faber and Faber, 1959.

Elliott, Carl. *Better than Well: American Medicine Meets the American Dream*. New York: W. W. Norton, 2003.

Emanuel, Ezekiel, and Linda Emanuel. "Four Models of the Physician-Patient Relationship." *Journal of the American Medical Association* 2267 (1992): 2221–26.

Empson, William. *Seven Types of Ambiguity*. Harmondsworth, UK: Penguin, 1961.

Engel, George. "The Need for a New Medical Model: A Challenge for Biomedicine." *Science* 196 (1977): 129–36.

Engelhardt, H. Tristam, Jr. *The Foundations of Bioethics*. 2nd edition. New York: Oxford University Press, 1996.

Epstein, Ronald M. "Mindful Practice." *Journal of the American Medical Association* 282 (1999): 833–39.

Epston, David, and Michael White. *Experience, Contradiction, Narrative, and Imagination: Selected Papers of David Epston and Michael White, 1989–1991*. Adelaide, South Australia: Dulwich Centre, 1992.

Ernaux, Annie. *I Remain in Darkness*. Translated by Tanya Leslie. New York: Seven Stories Press, 1999.

Fadiman, Anne. *The Spirit Catches You and You Fall Down: A Hmong Child, Her American Doctors, and the Collision of Two Cultures*. New York: Farrar, Straus and Giroux, 1997.

Farber, Neil. "Love, Boundaries, and the Patient-Physician Relationship." *Archives of Internal Medicine* 157 (1997): 2291–94.

Farmer, Paul. *Pathologies of Power: Health, Human Rights, and the New War on the Poor*. Berkeley: University of California Press, 2003.

Felman, Shoshana, ed. *Literature and Psychoanalysis: The Question of Reading, Otherwise*. Baltimore: Johns Hopkins University Press, 1982.

Felman, Shoshana, and Dori Laub. *Testimony: Crises of Witnessing in Literature, Psychoanalysis, and History*. New York: Routledge, 1992.

Felski, Rita. *Literature after Feminism*. Chicago: University of Chicago, 2003.

Fireman, Gary D., Ted E. McVay Jr., and Owen J. Flanagan, eds. *Narrative and Consciousness: Literature, Psychology, and the Brain*. New York: Oxford University Press, 2003.

Fish, Stanley. *Is There a Text in This Class? The Authority of Interpretive Communities*. Cambridge: Harvard University Press, 1980.

Fleischman, Avrom. *Figures of Autobiography: The Language of Self-Writing in Victorian and Modern England*. Berkeley: University of California Press, 1983.

Fludernik, Monika. "The Diachronization of Narratology." *Narrative* 11 (2003): 331–48.

Forster, E. M. *Aspects of the Novel*. San Diego: Harcourt Brace Jovanovich, 1985.

Foucault, Michel. "What Is an Author?" In *Textual Strategies: Perspectives in Post-*

Structuralist Criticism, edited and translated by Josue Harari, 141–60. Ithaca: Cornell University Press, 1979.

Frank, Arthur W. "Asking the Right Question about Pain: Narrative and Phronesis." *Literature and Medicine* 23 (2004): 209–25.

———. *The Renewal of Generosity: Illness, Medicine, and How to Live.* Chicago: University of Chicago Press, 2004.

———. *The Wounded Storyteller: Body, Illness, and Ethics.* Chicago: University of Chicago Press, 1995.

Frankel, Richard M., Timothy E. Quill, and Susan H. McDaniel, eds. *The Biopsychosocial Approach: Past, Present, Future.* Rochester, N.Y.: University of Rochester Press, 2003.

Freedman, Benjamin. *Duty and Healing: Foundations of a Jewish Bioethic.* New York: Routledge, 1999.

Freud, Sigmund. "Creative Writers and Daydreaming." In *Standard Edition of the Complete Psychological Works of Sigmund Freud,* vol. 9, edited by James Strachey, 141–53. London: Hogarth Press, 1959.

———. "The Ego and the Id." In *Standard Edition of the Complete Psychological Works of Sigmund Freud,* vol. 19, edited by James Strachey, 3–66. London: Hogarth Press, 1961.

———. "Mourning and Melancholia." In *Standard Edition of the Complete Psychological Works of Sigmund Freud,* vol. 14, edited by James Strachey, 237–58. London: Hogarth Press, 1957.

———. "The Unconscious." In *Standard Edition of the Complete Psychological Works of Sigmund Freud,* vol. 14, edited by James Strachey, 161–215. London: Hogarth Press, 1957.

Gawande, Atul. *Complications: A Surgeon's Notes on an Imperfect Science.* New York: Picador, 2003.

Geller, Matthew. *Difficulty Swallowing: A Medical Chronicle.* New York: Works Press, 1981.

Genette, Gérard. *Narrative Discourse: An Essay in Method.* Translated by Jane Levin. Ithaca: Cornell University Press, 1980.

Gerrig, Richard. *Experiencing Narrative Worlds: On the Psychological Activities of Reading.* New Haven: Yale University Press, 1993.

Giglio, Richard, B. Spears, David Rumpf, and Nancy Eddy. "Encouraging Behavior Changes by Use of Client-Held Health Records." *Medical Care* 16 (1978): 757–64.

Gilbert, Pamela K. *Disease, Desire, and the Body in Victorian Women's Popular Novels.* Cambridge: Cambridge University Press, 1997.

Gilbert, Sandra. *Wrongful Death: A Medical Tragedy.* New York: W. W. Norton, 1995.

Gilbert, Sandra, and Susan Gubar. *The Madwoman in the Attic: The Woman Writer and the Nineteenth-Century Literary Imagination.* 2nd edition. New Haven: Yale University Press, 2000.

Gilman, Sander. "Collaboration, the Economy, and the Future of the Humanities." *Critical Inquiry* 30 (2004): 384–90.

Goleman, Daniel. *The Meditative Mind: The Varieties of Meditative Experience.* New York: G. P. Putnam's Sons, 1988.

Golodetz, Arnold, Johanna Ruess, and Raymond L. Milhous. "The Right to Know: Giving the Patient His Medical Record." *Archives of Physical Medicine and Rehabilitation* 57 (1976): 78–81.

Good, Byron. *Medicine, Rationality, and Experience: An Anthropological Perspective.* Cambridge: Cambridge University Press, 1994.

Good, Byron, and Mary-Jo DelVecchio Good. "In the Subjunctive Mood: Epilepsy Narratives in Turkey." *Social Science and Medicine* 38 (1994): 835–42.

Grealy, Lucy. *Autobiography of a Face.* New York: HarperCollins, 1994.

Greenhalgh, Trisha, and Brian Hurwitz, eds. *Narrative Based Medicine: Dialogue and Discourse in Clinical Practice*. London: BMJ Books, 1998.

Gregory, Marshall. "Ethical Engagements over Time: Reading and Rereading *David Copperfield* and *Wuthering Heights*." *Narrative* 12 (2004): 281–305.

Griffin, Fred L. "The Fortunate Physician: Learning from Our Patients." *Literature and Medicine* 23 (2004): 280–303.

Groopman, Jerome. *The Measure of Our Days: A Spiritual Exploration of Illness*. New York: Penguin, 1998.

Grosz, Elizabeth. *Volatile Bodies: Toward a Corporeal Feminism*. Bloomington: Indiana University Press, 1994.

Gusdorf, Georges. "Conditions and Limits of Autobiography." In *Autobiography: Essays Theoretical and Critical*, translated and edited by James Olney, 28–48. Princeton: Princeton University Press, 1980. Originally published as "Conditions et limites de l'autobiographie." In *Formen der Selbstdarstellung: Analekten zu einer Geschichte des literarishcen Selbstportraits*, edited by Gunther Reichenkron and Erich Haase. Berlin: Duncker and Humblot, 1956.

Guyot, Felix. *Yoga: The Silence of Health*. Berlin: Schocken Books, 1937.

Hafferty, Fred. "Beyond Curriculum Reform: Confronting Medicine's Hidden Curriculum." *Academic Medicine* 73 (1998): 403–7.

Halpern, Jodi. *From Detached Concern to Empathy: Humanizing Medical Practice*. New York: Oxford University Press, 2001.

Harper, Ralph. *On Presence: Variations and Reflections*. Philadelphia: Trinity Press International, 1991.

Hartman, Geoffrey H. *A Critic's Journey: Literary Reflections, 1958–1998*. New Haven: Yale University Press, 1999.

———. "Judging Paul de Man." In *Minor Prophesies: The Literary Essay in the Culture Wars*. Cambridge: Harvard University Press, 1991.

———. "Narrative and Beyond." *Literature and Medicine* 23 (2004): 334–45.

———. "On Traumatic Knowledge and Literary Studies." *New Literary History* 26 (1995): 537–63.

———. *Scars of the Spirit: The Struggle against Inauthenticity*. New York: Palgrave/Macmillan, 2002.

Hatem, David, and Emily Ferrara. "Becoming a Doctor: Fostering Humane Caregivers through Creative Writing." *Patient Education and Counseling* 45 (2001): 13–22.

Hauerwas, Stanley, and L. Gregory Jones, eds. *Why Narrative? Readings in Narrative Theology*. Eugene, Oreg.: Wipf and Stock, 1997.

Hawkins, Anne Hunsaker. *Reconstructing Illness: Studies in Pathography*. 2nd edition. West Lafayette, Ind.: Purdue University Press, 1999.

Hawkins, Anne Hunsaker, and Marilyn Chandler McEntyre, eds. *Teaching Literature and Medicine*. New York: Modern Language Association, 2000.

Heller, Jean. "Syphilis Victims in US Study Went Untreated for 40 Years." *New York Times*, July 26, 1972, A1, A8.

Heller, Joseph. *Catch-22*. New York: Dell, 1970.

Henderson, Cary Smith, Ruth D. Henderson, Jackie Henderson Main, and Nancy Andrews. *Partial View: An Alzheimer's Journal*. Dallas: Southern Methodist University Press, 1998.

Herman, David. *Narratologies: New Perspectives in Narrative Analysis*. Columbus: Ohio State University Press, 1999.

———. "Story Logic in Conversational and Literary Narratives." *Narrative* 9 (2001): 130–37.

———. *Story Logic: Problems and Possibilities of Narrative*. Lincoln: University of Nebraska Press, 2002.

Hester, Micah. *Community as Healing*. Landham, Md.: Rowman and Littlefield, 2001.

Hilfiker, David. "Facing Our Mistakes." *New England Journal of Medicine* 310 (1984): 118–22.

———. *Healing Our Wounds: A Physician Looks at His Work*. New York: Pantheon, 1985.

Hirsch, E. D. *Validity in Interpretation*. New Haven: Yale University Press, 1967.

Holland, Norman. *The Dynamics of Literary Response*. New York: Columbia University Press, 1989.

———. *5 Readers Reading*. New Haven: Yale University Press, 1975.

Holman, Halsted, and Kate Lorig. "Patients as Partners in Managing Chronic Disease: Partnership Is a Prerequisite for Effective and Efficient Health Care." *BMJ* 7234 (2000): 526–27.

Holmes, Helen B., and Laura M. Purdy, eds. *Feminist Perspectives in Medical Ethics*. Bloomington: Indiana University Press, 1992.

Horace. *Ars Poetica*. Translated by Burton Raffel. Albany: State University of New York Press, 1974.

Horowitz, C. R., Anthony Suchman, William T. Branch, and Richard M. Frankel. "What Do Doctors Find Meaningful about Their Work?" *Annals of Internal Medicine* 138 (2003): 772–75.

Horton, Richard. *Health Wars: On the Global Front Lines of Modern Medicine*. New York: New York Review of Books, 2003.

Hudson, Robert. *Disease and Its Control: The Shaping of Modern Thought*. Westport, Conn.: Greenwood Press, 1983.

Hull, John. *Touching the Rock: An Experience of Blindness*. New York: Vintage Books, 1990.

Hunter, Kathryn Montgomery. *Doctors' Stories: The Narrative Structure of Medical Knowledge*. Princeton: Princeton University Press, 1991.

Hunter, Kathryn Montgomery, Rita Charon, and John L. Coulehan. "The Study of Literature in Medical Education." *Academic Medicine* 70 (1995): 787–94.

Hurwitz, Brian, Trisha Greenhalgh, and Vieda Skultans, eds. *Narrative Research in Health and Illness*. London: BMJ Books, 2004.

Husserl, Edmund. *Cartesian Meditations: An Introduction to Phenomenology*. Translated by Dorion Cairns. The Hague: Martinus Nijhoff, 1929.

Inui, Thomas S. *A Flag in the Wind: Educating for Professionalism in Medicine*. Washington D.C.: Association of American Medical Colleges, 2003.

———. "What Are the Sciences of Relationship-Centered Primary Care?" *Journal of Family Practice* 42 (1996): 171–77.

Iser, Wolfgang. *The Implied Reader: Patterns of Communication in Prose Fiction from Bunyan to Beckett*. Baltimore: Johns Hopkins University Press, 1974.

———. *The Range of Interpretation*. New York: Columbia University Press, 2000.

James, Henry. "The Art of Fiction." In *Selected Literary Criticism*, edited by Morris Shapira, 49–67. Cambridge: Cambridge University Press, 1981.

———. *The Art of the Novel: Critical Prefaces*. Boston: Northeastern University Press, 1984.

———. *Autobiography*. Edited by Frederick Dupee. Princeton: Princeton University Press, 1983.

———. "The New Novel." In *Selected Literary Criticism*, edited by Morris Shapira, 49–67. Cambridge: Cambridge University Press, 1981.

———. *The New York Edition: The Novels and Tales of Henry James*. New York: Charles Scribner's Sons, 1909.

————. "The Novels of George Eliot." First printed in *Atlantic Monthly*, 1866. Reprinted in *Discussions of George Eliot*, edited by R. Stang. Boston: D. C. Heath, 1960.

Jameson, Fredric. "The End of Temporality." *Critical Inquiry* 29 (2003): 695–718.

Jay, Paul. *Being in the Text: Self-Representation from Wordsworth to Roland Barthes.* Ithaca: Cornell University Press, 1984.

Johnson, Barbara. *The Critical Difference: Essays in the Contemporary Rhetoric of Reading.* Baltimore: Johns Hopkins University Press, 1980.

Jones, Anne Hudson. "Literary Value: The Lesson of Medical Ethics." *Neohelicon* 14 (1987): 383–92.

————. "Literature and Medicine: Traditions and Innovations." In *The Body and the Text: Comparative Essays in Literature and Medicine*, edited by Bruce Clarke and Wendell Aycock , 11–23. Lubbock: Texas Tech University Press, 1990.

Jonsen, Albert R. *The Birth of Bioethics.* New York: Oxford University Press, 1998.

Jonsen, Albert R., and Stephen Toulmin. *The Abuse of Casuistry: A History of Moral Reasoning.* Los Angeles: University of California Press, 1988.

Joyce, James. "The Dead." In *Dubliners*, 175–224. New York: Viking Press, 1961.

Kafka, Franz. "A Country Doctor." In *The Complete Stories*, edited by Nahum N. Glatzer. New York: Schocken Books, 1976.

Kearney, Michael. *Mortally Wounded: Stories of Soul Pain, Death, and Healing.* New York: Simon and Schuster, 1996.

Kearns, Michael. *Rhetorical Narratology.* Lincoln: University of Nebraska Press, 1999.

Kerby, Anthony Paul. *Narrative and the Self.* Bloomington: Indiana University Press, 1991.

Kermode, Frank. *The Genesis of Secrecy: On the Interpretation of Narrative.* Cambridge: Harvard University Press, 1979.

————. *The Sense of an Ending: Studies in the Theory of Fiction.* London: Oxford University Press, 1968.

Klass, Perri. *A Not Entirely Benign Procedure: Four Years as a Medical Student.* New York: Putnam, 1987.

Klein, Joan. "Narrative Oncology: Medicine's Untold Stories." *Oncology Times*, February 25, 2003, 10,13.

Kleinfield, N. R. "Old Patients: Making Doctors Better: Myths Explode as Physicians Get to Know the Elderly." *New York Times*, July 17, 2004.

Kleinman, Arthur. *The Illness Narratives: Suffering, Healing, and the Human Condition.* New York: Basic Books, 1988.

Kleinman, Arthur, Veena Das, and Margaret Lock, eds. *Social Suffering.* Berkeley: University of California Press, 1997.

Konner, Melvin. *Medicine at the Crossroads: The Crisis in Health Care.* New York: Pantheon, 1993.

Koopman, Richelle J., Arch G. Mainous, Richard Baker, James M. Gill, and Gregory E. Gilbert. "Continuity of Care and Recognition of Diabetes, Hypertension, and Hypercholesterolemia." *Archives in Internal Medicine* 163 (2003): 1357–61.

Kreiswirth, Martin. "Trusting the Tale: The Narrativist Turn in the Human Sciences." *New Literary History* 23 (1992): 629–57.

Kroenke, Kurt. "Studying Symptoms: Sampling and Measurement Issues." *Annals of Internal Medicine* 134 (2001): 844–53.

LaCapra, Dominick. *Representing the Holocaust: History, Theory, Trauma.* Ithaca: Cornell University Press, 1994.

————. *Writing History, Writing Trauma.* Baltimore: Johns Hopkins University Press, 2000.

Laine, Christine, and Frank Davidoff. "Patient-Centered Medicine: A Professional Evolution." *Journal of the American Medical Association* 275 (1996): 152–56.

Lakoff, George, and Mark Johnson. *Metaphors We Live By*. Chicago: University of Chicago Press, 2003.

Lantos, John. "Reconsidereing Action: Day-to-Day Ethics in the Work of Medicine." In *Stories Matter: The Role of Narrative in Medical Ethics*, edited by Rita Charon and Martha Montello, 154–59. New York: Routledge, 2002.

Lanzmann, Claude. *Shoah: An Oral History of the Holocaust*. New York: Pantheon, 1985.

Laqueur, Thomas W. "Bodies, Details, and the Humanitarian Narrative." In *The New Cultural History*, edited by Lynn Hunt, 176–204. Berkeley: University of California Press, 1989.

Latour, Bruno. "Why Has Critique Run out of Steam? From Matters of Fact to Matters of Concern." *Critical Inquiry* 30 (2004): 225–48.

Laub, Dori. "Bearing Witness, or the Vicissitudes of Learning." In *Testimony: Crises of Witnessing in Literature, Psychoanalysis, and History*, edited by Shoshana Felman and Dori Laub, 57–74. New York: Routledge, 1992.

———. "An Event without a Witness: Truth, Testimony, and Survival." In *Testimony: Crises of Witnessing in Literature, Psychoanalysis, and History*, edited by Shoshana Felman and Dori Laub, 75–92. New York: Routledge, 1992.

Lazare, Aaron. "Shame and Humiliation in the Medical Encounter." *Archives of Internal Medicine* 147 (1987): 1653–58.

LeBaron, Charles. *Gentle Vengeance: An Account of the First Years at Harvard Medical School*. New York: Marek, 1981.

Leder, Drew. *The Absent Body*. Chicago: University of Chicago Press, 1990.

Lejeune, Philippe. *Le pacte autobiographique*. Paris: Seuil, 1975.

———. *On Autobiography*. In *Theory and History of Literature*, vol. 52, edited by Paul John Eakin, translated by Katherine Leary. Minneapolis: University of Minnesota Press, 1989.

Lentricchia, Frank, and Andrew DuBois, eds. *Close Reading: The Reader*. Durham: Duke University Press, 2003.

Lerner, Barron. *The Breast Cancer Wars: Hope, Fear, and the Pursuit of a Cure in Twentieth-Century America*. New York: Oxford University Press, 2001.

Lévinas, Emmanuel. *Time and the Other*. Translated by Richard A. Cohen. Pittsburgh: Duquesne University Press, 1987.

———. *Totality and Infinity*. Translated by Alphonso Lingis. Boston: M. Nijhoff, 1979.

Levinson, Wendy, Debra Roter, J. P. Mulhooly, V. T. Dull, and Richard M. Frankel. "Physician-Patient Communication: The Relationship with Malpractice Claims among Primary Care Physicians and Surgeons." *Journal of the American Medical Association* 227 (1997): 553–59.

Lewis, R. W. B. *The American Adam: Innocence, Tragedy, and Tradition in the Nineteenth Century*. Chicago: University of Chicago Press, 1955.

Lifton, Robert J. *The Genocidal Mentality: Nazi Holocaust and Nuclear Threat*. New York: Basic Books, 1990.

———. *The Nazi Doctors: Medical Killing and the Psychology of Genocide*. New York: Basic Books, 1986.

Lipkin, Mack, Jr., Samuel Putnam, and Aaron Lazare, eds. *The Medical Interview: Clinical Care, Education, and Research*. New York: Springer-Verlag, 1995.

Lorde, Audre. *The Cancer Journals*, special ed. San Francisco: Aunt Lute Books, 1997.

Lovrod, Marie. "'Art/i/fact' Rereading Culture and Subjectivity through Sexual Abuse Survivor Narratives." In *True Relations: Essays on Autobiography and the Postmodern*, edited by G. Thomas Couser and Joseph Fichtelberg, 23–32. Westport, Conn.: Greenwood Press, 1998.

Lown, Bernard. *The Lost Art of Healing: Practicing Compassion in Medicine.* New York: Ballantine, 1996.

Lubbock, Percy. *The Craft of Fiction.* New York: Jonathan Cape and Harrison Smith, 1931.

Ludmerer, Kenneth. *Time to Heal: American Medical Education from the Turn of the Century to the Era of Managed Care.* New York: Oxford University Press, 1999.

Lukács, Georg. *The Theory of the Novel: A Historico-Philosophical Essay on the Forms of Great Epic Literature.* Cambridge: MIT Press, 1971.

Mach, Adrea. "Amartya Sen on Development and Health." *To Our Health—The Internal Newsletter of the World Health Organisation.* (1997): http://www.who.int/infwhat52/to_our_health/amartya.html.

MacIntyre, Alasdair. *After Virtue: A Study in Moral Theory,* 2nd edition. Notre Dame, Ind.: Notre Dame University Press, 1984.

Mairs, Nancy. *Waist-High in the World: A Life among the Nondisabled.* Boston: Beacon, 1996.

Mancuso, James C., and Theodore Sarbin. "The Self-Narrative in the Enactment of Roles." In *Studies in Social Identity,* edited by Theodore Sarbin and Karl E. Scheibe, 233–53. New York: Praeger, 1983.

Mann, Thomas. *The Magic Mountain.* Translated by H. T. Lowe-Porter. New York: Vintage Books, 1969.

Marcel, Gabriel. *Mystery of Being,* 2 vols. South Bend, Ind.: Gateway Editions, 1978.

———. *The Philosophy of Existence.* London: Harvill Press, 1948.

Marmot, Michael. *The Status Syndrome: How Social Standing Affects Our Health and Longevity.* New York: Times Books/Henry Holt, 2004.

Marshall, Patricia, and John O'Keefe. "Medical Students' First-Person Narratives of a Patient's Story of AIDS." *Social Science and Medicine* 40 (1995): 67–76.

Martensen, Robert. "Thought Styles among the Medical Humanities: Past, Present, and Near-Term Future." In *Practicing the Medical Humanities: Engaging Physicians and Patients,* edited by Ronald Carson, Chester Burns, and Thomas Cole, 99–122. Hagerstown, Md.: University Publishing Group, 2003.

Martin, Wallace. *Recent Theories of Narrative.* Ithaca: Cornell University Press, 1986.

Mates, Susan. *The Good Doctor.* Iowa City: University of Iowa Press, 1994.

Mattingly, Cheryl. *Healing Dramas and Clinical Plots: The Narrative Structure of Experience.* Cambridge: Cambridge University Press, 1998.

Mattingly, Cheryl, and Linda C. Garro. *Narrative and the Cultural Construction of Illness and Healing.* Berkeley: University of California Press, 2000.

Mayfield, James F. "Memory and Imagination in William Maxwell's *So Long, See You Tomorrow.*" *Critique* 24, no. 1 (1982): 21–37.

McCann, Richard. "The Resurrectionist." In *The Best American Essays of 2000,* edited by Alan Lightman, 101–9. Boston: Houghton Mifflin, 2002.

Mead, George. *Mind, Self, and Society.* Edited by Charles W. Morris. Chicago: University of Chicago Press, 1962.

Mechanic, David. *Medical Sociology,* 2nd edition. New York: Free Press, 1978.

Mehlman, Jeffrey. *A Structural Study of Autobiography: Proust, Leiris, Sartre, Lévi-Strauss.* Ithaca: Cornell University Press, 1974.

Meier, Diane, and Anthony Beck. "The Inner Life of Physicians and the Care of the Seriously Ill." *Journal of the American Medical Association* 286 (2001): 3007–14.

Metzl, Jonathan. *Prozac on the Couch: Prescribing Gender in the Era of Wonder Drugs.* Durham, N.C.: Duke University Press, 2003.

Michaels, Walter Benn. *The Shape of the Signifier: 1967 to the End of History*. Princeton: Princeton University Press, 2004.

Middlebrook, Christina. *Seeing the Crab: A Memoir of Dying*. New York: Basic Books, 1996.

Miller, J. Hillis. *The Ethics of Reading: Kant, de Man, Eliot, Trollope, James, and Benjamin*. New York: Columbia University Press, 1987.

Miller, Patricia A., Sigrid McCabe, Shelly Dubin, Barry Gurland, and Mathew Maurer. "Infusing a Geriatric Intern Program with Narrative Medicine: The Columbia Cooperative Aging Program." *Journal of the American Geriatrics Society*, Supplement, Annual Scientific Meeting Abstract Book, 52 (2004): 115.

Mishler, Elliot G. *The Discourse of Medicine: Dialectics of Medical Interviews*. Norwood, N.J.: Ablex Press, 1984.

———. *Research Interviewing: Context and Narrative*. Cambridge: Harvard University Press, 1986.

Mitchell, W. J. T. "The Commitment to Form; or, Still Crazy after All These Years." *PMLA* 118 (2003): 321–25.

———. The Future of Criticism—A Critical Inquiry Symposium. *Critical Inquiry* 30 (2004): 324–479.

———, ed. *On Narrative*. Chicago: University of Chicago Press, 1981.

———, ed. *The Politics of Interpretation*. Chicago: University of Chicago Press, 1983.

Moi, Toril. *Sexual/Textual Politics: Feminist Literary Theory*. 2nd edition. New York: Routledge, 2002.

———, ed. *What Is a Woman? and Other Essays*. New York: Oxford University Press, 2001.

Montello, Martha. "Narrative Competence." In *Stories and Their Limits*, edited by Hilde Nelson, 185–97. New York: Routledge, 1997.

Morantz-Sanchez, Regina. *Sympathy and Science: Women Physicians in American Medicine*. New York: Oxford University Press, 1985.

Moroney, Eileen. "Home Is Where the Residents Visit." *P & S Journal* 22, no.2 (2002): 23–26.

Morris, David. "How to Speak Postmodern: Medicine, Illness, and Cultural Change." *Hastings Center Report* 30 (2000): 7–17.

———. *Illness and Culture in the Postmodern Age*. Berkeley: University of California Press, 1998.

———. "Narrative, Ethics, and Pain: Thinking with Stories." In *Stories Matter: The Role of Narrative in Medical Ethics*, edited by Rita Charon and Martha Montello, 196–218. New York: Routledge, 2002.

———. "Voice, Genre, and Moral Community." In *Social Suffering*, edited by Arthur Kleinman, Veena Das, and Margaret Lock. Berkeley: University of California Press, 1997.

Morrissey, Charles T. "On Oral History Interviewing." In *The Oral History Reader*, edited by Robert Perks and Alistair Thomson, 107–13. London and New York: Routledge, 1998.

Moss, Donald. *Hating in the First Person Plural: Psychoanalytic Essays on Racism, Homophobia, Misogyny, and Terror*. New York: Other Press, 2003.

Mullan, Fitzhugh. *White Coat, Clenched Fist: The Political Education of an American Physician*. New York: Macmillan, 1976.

Murdoch, Iris. *The Sovereignty of Good*. London and New York: Routledge, 2001.

Murphy, Robert F. *The Body Silent: The Different World of the Disabled*. New York: W. W. Norton, 1990.

Nafisi, Azar. *Reading Lolita in Tehran: A Memoir in Books*. New York: Random House, 2003.

Nalbantian, Suzanne. *Aesthetic Autobiography: From Life to Art in Marcel Proust, James Joyce, Virginia Woolf, and Anaïs Nin*. New York: St. Martin's Press, 1994.

Nelson, Hilde Lindemann, ed. *Stories and Their Limits: Narrative Approaches to Bioethics*. New York: Routledge, 1997.

Nelson, Katherine. "Narrative and the Emergence of a Consciousness of Self." In *Narrative and Consciousness: Literature, Psychology, and the Brain*, edited by Gary D. Fireman, Ted E. McVay Jr., and Owen J. Flanagan. New York: Oxford University Press, 2003.

———. *Narratives from the Crib*. Cambridge: Harvard University Press, 1989.

Neugeboren, Jay. *Open Heart: A Patient's Story of Life-Saving Medicine and Life-Giving Friendships*. New York: Houghton Mifflin, 2003.

Neuman, Shirley. "'An appearance walking in a forest the sexes burn': Autobiography and the Construction of the Feminine Body." In *Autobiography and Postmodernism*, edited by Kathleen Ashley, Leigh Gilmore, and Gerald Peters, 293–316. Amherst: University of Massachusetts Press, 1994.

Newton, Adam Zachary. *Narrative Ethics*. Cambridge: Harvard University Press, 1999.

Noddings, Nel. *Caring: A Feminist Approach to Ethics and Moral Education*. Berkeley: University of California Press, 1984.

Novack, Dennis, Anthony Suchman, William Clark, Ronald Epstein, Edith Najberg, and Craig Kaplan. "Calibrating the Physician: Personal Awareness and Effective Patient Care." *Journal of the American Medical Association* 278 (1997): 502–9.

Nuland, Sherwin. *How We Die: Reflections on Life's Final Chapter*. New York: Knopf, 1994.

Nussbaum, Martha. *Love's Knowledge: Essays on Philosophy and Literature*. New York: Oxford University Press, 1990.

O'Farrell, Mary Ann. "Self-Consciousness and the Psoriatic Personality: Considering Updike and Potter." *Literature and Medicine* 20 (2001): 133–50.

Olney, James. *Memory and Narrative: The Weave of Life-Writing*. Chicago: University of Chicago Press, 1998.

———. *Metaphors of Self: The Meaning of Autobiography*. Princeton: Princeton University Press, 1972.

———, ed. *Autobiography: Essays Theoretical and Critical*. Princeton: Princeton University Press, 1980.

———, ed. *Studies in Autobiography*. New York: Oxford University Press, 1988.

Ozick, Cynthia. *Metaphor and Memory: Essays*. New York: Knopf, 1989.

Pascal, Roy. *Design and Truth in Autobiography*. Cambridge: Harvard University Press, 1960.

Paulos, John Allen. *Once upon a Number: The Hidden Mathematical Logic of Stories*. New York: Basic Books, 1998.

Pellegrino, Edmund, and David Thomasma. *For the Patient's Good: The Restoration of Beneficence in Health Care*. New York: Oxford University Press, 1988.

Perks, Robert, and Alistair Thomson, eds. *The Oral History Reader*. London and New York: Routledge, 1998.

Pham, Phuong N., Harvey M. Weinstein, and Timothy Longman. "Trauma and PTSD Symptoms in Rwanda: Implications for Attitudes toward Justice and Reconciliation." *Journal of the American Medical Association* 292 (2004): 602–12.

Phelan, James. "Dual Focalization, Retrospective Fictional Autobiography, and the Ethics of *Lolita*." In *Narrative and Consciousness: Literature, Psychology, and the Brain*, edited by Gary D. Fireman, Ted E. McVay Jr., and Owen J. Flanagan. New York: Oxford University Press, 2003.

————. *Living to Tell about It: A Rhetoric and Ethics of Character Narration*. Ithaca: Cornell University Press, 2005.

————. *Narrative as Rhetoric: Technique, Audiences, Ethics, Ideology*. Columbus: Ohio State University Press, 1996.

Phillips, Susan S., and Patricia Benner, eds. *The Crisis of Care: Affirming and Restoring Caring Practices in the Helping Professions*. Washington, D.C.: Georgetown University Press, 1994.

Poirier, Suzanne, William Ahrens, and Daniel Brauner. "Songs of Innocence and Experience: Students' Poems about their Medical Education." *Academic Medicine* 73 (1998): 473–78.

Poirier, Suzanne, and Daniel J. Brauner. "The Voices of the Medical Record." *Theoretical Medicine* 11 (1990): 29–39.

Poses, Roy M., and A. M. Isen. "Qualitative Research in Medicine and Health Care: Questions and Controversy." *Journal of General Internal Medicine* 13 (1998): 32–38.

Poulet, Georges. "Criticism and the Experience of Interiority." In *Reader-Response Criticism: From Formalism to Post-Structuralism*, edited by Jane Tompkins. Baltimore: Johns Hopkins University Press, 1980.

————. "Phenomenology of Reading." *New Literary History* 1 (1969): 53–67.

Price, Reynolds. *A Whole New Life: An Illness and a Healing*. New York: Atheneum, 1994.

Prince, Gerald. *A Dictionary of Narratology*, rev. ed. Lincoln: University of Nebraska Press, 2003.

Proust, Marcel. *A la recerce du temps perdu*. 3 vols. Paris: R. Laffont, 1987.

Quill, Timothy. *Death and Dignity: Making Choices and Taking Charge*. New York: W. W. Norton, 1993.

Reifler, Douglas "'I Actually Don't Mind the Bone Saw': Narratives of Gross Anatomy." *Literature and Medicine* 15 (1996): 183–99.

Reiser, Stanley Joel. "Creating Form out of Mass: The Development of the Medical Record." In *Transformation and Tradition in the Sciences: Essays in Honor of I. Bernard Cohen*, edited by Everett Mendelsohn, 303–16. Cambridge: Cambridge University Press, 1984.

Remen, Rachel. *Kitchen Table Wisdom: Stories That Heal*. New York: Berkley, 1997.

————. *My Grandfather's Blessings: Stories of Strength, Refuge, and Belonging*. New York: Riverhead Books, 2000.

Renza, Louis. "The Veto of the Imagination: A Theory of Autobiography." In *Autobiography: Essays Theoretical and Critical*, translated and edited by James Olney, 268–95. Princeton: Princeton University Press, 1980.

Reverby, Susan. *Ordered to Care: The Dilemma of American Nursing, 1850–1945*. New York: Cambridge University Press, 1987.

Reynolds, P. P. "Reaffirming Professionalism through the Education Community." *Annals of Internal Medicine* 120 (1994): 609–14.

Richards, I. A., and C. K. Ogden. *The Meaning of Meaning: A Study of the Influence of Language upon Thought and of the Science of Symbolism*. New York: Harcourt, Brace and World, 1923.

Richardson, Brian. *Narrative Dynamics*. Columbus: Ohio State University Press, 2002.

Ricoeur, Paul. *Time and Narrative*. 3 vols. Translated by Kathleen McLaughlin and David Pellauer. Chicago: University of Chicago Press, 1984–88.

Rimmon-Kenan, Shlomith. *Narrative Fiction: Contemporary Poetics*. 2nd edition. London: Routledge, 2002.

————. "The Story of 'I': Illness and Narrative Identity." *Narrative* 10 (2002): 9–27.

————, ed. *Discourse in Psychoanalysis and Literature*. London: Methuen, 1987.

Risdon, Cathy, and Laura Edey. "Human Doctoring: Bringing Authenticity to Our Care." *Academic Medicine* 74 (1999): 896–99.

Rosenblatt, Louise M. *Literature as Exploration*. New York: Modern Language Association, 1995.

Rothman, David. *Strangers at the Bedside: A History of How Law and Bioethics Transformed Medical Decision-Making*. New York: Basic Books, 1991.

Rothman, Sheila, and David Rothman. *The Pursuit of Perfection: The Promise and Perils of Medical Enhancement*. New York: Pantheon, 2003.

Royle, Nicholas. *The Uncanny*. New York: Routledge, 2003.

Russell, Diana. *The Secret Trauma: Incest in the Lives of Girls and Women*. New York: Basic Books, 1986.

Ryan, Marie-Laure. *Narrative as Virtual Reality: Immersion and Interactivity in Literature and Electronic Media*. Baltimore: Johns Hopkins University Press, 2004.

Sacks, Oliver. *The Man Who Mistook His Wife for a Hat and Other Clinical Tales*. New York: Summit Books, 1985.

Sarbin, Theodore R., ed. *Narrative Psychology: The Storied Nature of Human Conduct*. New York: Praeger, 1986.

Sarbin, Theodore R., and Karl E. Scheibe, eds. *Studies in Social Identity*. New York: Praeger, 1983.

Sartre, Jean Paul. *What Is Literature? and Other Essays*. Translated by Bernard Frechtman. Cambridge: Harvard University Press, 1988.

Savett, Laurence A. *The Human Side of Medicine: Learning What It's Like to Be a Patient and What It's Like to Be a Physician*. Westport, Conn.: Auburn House, 2002.

Schafer, Roy. *The Analytic Attitude*. New York: Basic Books, 1983.

————. "Generative Empathy in the Treatment Situation." *Psychoanalytic Quarterly* 28 (1959): 343–73.

————. "Narrating, Attending, and Empathizing." *Literature and Medicine* 23 (2004): 241–51.

————. *Retelling a Life: Narration and Dialogue in Psychoanalysis*. New York: Basic Books, 1992.

Scheier, Michael F., and Charles S. Carver. "Effects of Optimism on Psychological and Physical Well-Being: Theoretical Overview and Empirical Update." *Cognitive Therapy and Research* 16 (1992): 201–28.

Scheier, Michael F., Karen A. Matthews, June F. Owens, Richard Schulz, Michael W. Bridges, George J. Magovern, and Charles S. Carver. "Optimism and Rehospitalization after Coronary Artery Bypass Graft Surgery." *Archives of Internal Medicine* 159 (1999): 829–35.

Schnell, Lisa. "Learning How to Tell." *Literature and Medicine* 23 (2004): 265–79.

Schön, Donald. *The Reflective Practitioner*. Boston: MIT Press, 1986.

Schweickart, Patricinio. "Reading Ourselves: Toward a Feminist Theory of Reading." In *Speaking of Gender*, edited by Elaine Showalter, 17–44. New York: Routledge, 1989.

Searles, John. *Strange but True*. New York: Morrow, 2004.

Seeley, Karen M. *Cultural Psychotherapy: Working with Culture in the Clinical Encounter*. Northvale, N.J.: Jason Aronson, 2000.

Selwyn, Peter. *Surviving the Fall: The Personal Journey of an AIDS Doctor*. New Haven: Yale University Press, 1998.

Sen, Amartya. *Development as Freedom*. New York: Oxford University Press, 1999.

Shelley, Percy Bysshe. "Defence of Poetry." In *The Critical Tradition: Classic Texts and*

Contemporary Trends, edited by David H. Richter, 323–40. New York: Bedford Books, 1989.

Shem, Sam. *The House of God*. New York: Dell, 1978.

Sidney, Philip. "An Apology for Poetry" In *The Critical Tradition: Classic Texts and Contemporary Trends*, edited by David H. Richter, 134–59. New York: Bedford Books, 1989.

Siebers, Tobin. *The Ethics of Criticism*. Ithaca: Cornell University Press, 1988.

Sipiora, Michael P., and Frank Lehner. *Work, Identity, Coaching: Welcome to Your Success Story!* Pittsburgh: PsychoGuys, 2004.

Sisson, Larry. "The Art and Illusion of Spiritual Autobiography." In *True Relations: Essays on Autobiography and the Postmodern*, edited by G. Thomas Couser and Joseph Fichtelberg. Westport, Conn.: Greenwood Press, 1998.

Skott, C. "Caring Narratives and the Strategy of Presence: Narrative Communication in Nursing Practice and Research." *Nursing Science Quarterly* 14 (2001): 249–54.

Skura, Meredith. *The Literary Use of the Psychoanalytic Process*. New Haven: Yale University Press, 1981.

Smith, Barbara Herrnstein. "Narrative Versions, Narrative Theories." In *On Narrative*, edited by W. J. T. Mitchell, 209–32. Chicago: University of Chicago Press, 1981.

Smith, Paul. *Discerning the Subject*. In *Theory and History of Literature*, vol. 55, edited by Wald Godzich and Jochen Schulte-Sasse. Minneapolis: University of Minnesota Press, 1988.

Smith, Robert C. *The Patient's Story: Integrated Patient-Doctor Interviewing*. Boston: Little, Brown, 1996.

Smith, Sidonie. *Subjectivity, Identity, and the Body: Women's Autobiographical Practices in the Twentieth Century*. Bloomington: Indiana University Press, 1993.

Smith, Sidonie, and Julia Watson. *Reading Autobiography: A Guide for Interpreting Life Narratives*. Minneapolis: University of Minnesota Press, 2001.

Solomon, Andrew. *The Noonday Demon: An Atlas of Depression*. New York: Touchstone, 2001.

Sontag, Susan. *Illness as Metaphor*. New York: Vintage, 1979.

———. *On Photography*. New York: Picador, 2001.

———. *Regarding the Pain of Others*. New York: Farrar Straus and Giroux, 2002.

Spacks, Patricia Meyer. "Reflecting Women." *Yale Review* 63 (1973): 26–42.

———. "Women's Stories, Women's Selves." *Hudson Review* 30 (1977): 29–46.

Spengemann, William. *The Forms of Autobiography: Episodes in the History of a Literary Genre*. New Haven: Yale University Press, 1980.

Sprinker, Michael. "Fictions of the Self: The End of Autobiography." In *Autobiography: Essays Theoretical and Critical*, translated and edited by James Olney, 321–42. Princeton: Princeton University Press, 1980.

Stafford, Jean. "The Interior Castle." In *The Interior Castle*, 194–217. New York: Harcourt, Brace, 1953.

Stanley, Patricia. "The Patient's Voice: A Cry in Solitude or a Call for Community." *Literature and Medicine* 23 (2004): 346–63.

Stewart, Moira. "Towards a Global Definition of Patient Centred Care." *BMJ* 322 (2001): 444.

Stewart, Moira, Judith B. Brown, Wayne W. Weston, Ian R. McWhinney, Carol L. McWilliams, and Thomas Freeman. *Patient-Centered Medicine: Transforming the Clinical Method*. Abingdon, UK: Radcliffe Medical Press, 2003.

Stewart, Moira, and Debra Roter, eds. *Communicating with Medical Patients*. Newbury Park, Calif.: Sage, 1989.

Stoeckle, John, ed. *Encounters between Patients and Doctors—An Anthology.* Cambridge: MIT Press, 1987.

Stone, John. *In the Country of Hearts: Journeys in the Art of Medicine.* New York: Delacorte Press, 1990.

Sturrock, John. "The New Model Autobiographer." *New Literary History* 9 (1977): 51–63.

Styron, William. *Darkness Visible: A Memoir of Madness.* New York: Vintage, 1992.

Suchman, Anthony L., Penelope R. Williamson, Debra K. Litzelman, Richard M. Frankel, David L. Mossbanger, Thomas S. Inui, and the Relationship-Centered Care Initiative Discovery Team. "Toward an Informal Curriculum That Teaches Professionalism: Transforming the Social Environment of a Medical School." *Journal of General Internal Medicine* 19 (2004): 501–4.

Sullivan, Mark D. "Pain in Language: From Sentience to Sapience." *Pain Forum* 4 (1995): 3014.

Swenson, Melinda M., and Sharon L. Sims. "Toward a Narrative-Centered Curriculum for Nurse Practitioners." *Journal of Nursing Education* 39 (2000): 109–15.

Taylor, Charles. *Sources of the Self: The Making of the Modern Identity.* Cambridge: Harvard University Press, 1989.

Todorov, Tzvetan. *Littérature et Signification.* Paris: Larousse, 1967.

Tolstoy, Leo. "The Death of Ivan Ilych." In *The Death of Ivan Ilych and Other Stories,* translated by Aylmer Maude, 95–156. New York: Signet, 1960.

Tompkins, Jane, ed. *Reader-Response Criticism: From Formalism to Post-Structuralism.* Baltimore: Johns Hopkins University Press, 1980.

Trautmann, Joanne. *Healing Arts in Dialogue: Medicine and Literature.* Carbondale: Southern Illinois University Press, 1981.

Tresolini, C. P., and the Pew-Fetzer Task Force. *Health Professions Education and Relationship-Centered Care.* San Francisco: Pew Health Professions Commission, 1994.

Trillin, Alice. "Of Dragons and Garden Peas: A Cancer Patient Talks to Doctors." *New England Journal of Medicine* 304 (1981): 699–701.

Trilling, Lionel. *The Liberal Imagination: Essays on Literature and Society.* New York: Viking Press, 1950.

———. "On the Teaching of Modern Literature." In *Beyond Culture: Essays on Literature and Learning.* New York: Harcourt Brace Jovanovich, 1965.

———. Preface to the *Experience of Literature.* New York: Harcourt Brace Jovanovich, 1967.

Tronto, Joan. *Moral Boundaries: A Political Argument for an Ethic of Care.* New York: Routledge, 1993.

Turner, Victor. *The Ritual Process: Structure and Anti-Structure.* Chicago: Aldine Books, 1995.

Updike, John. *Self-Consciousness: Memoirs.* New York: Knopf, 1989.

Verghese, Abraham. *My Own Country: A Doctor's Story.* New York: Vintage/Random House, 1995.

Vidal, Fernando. "Brains, Bodies, Selves, and Science: Anthropologies of Identity and the Resurrection of the Body." *Critical Inquiry* 28 (2002): 930–74.

Waitzkin, Howard. *At the Front Lines of Medicine: How the Health Care System Alienates Doctors and Mistreats Patients and What We Can Do about It.* Lanham, Md.: Rowman and Littlefield, 2001.

Walker, Mary Urban. *Moral Understandings: A Feminist Study in Ethics.* New York: Routledge, 1998.

Walsh, Melissa. *Teaching Diversity and Cross-Cultural Competence in Health Care: A Trainer's Guide.* San Francisco: Perspectives of Differences Diversity Training and Consultation for Health Professionals (PODSDT), 2003.

Wear, Delese, Martin Kohn, and Susan Stocker, eds. *Literature and Medicine: A Claim for a Discipline*. McLean, Va.: Society for Health and Human Values, 1987.

Weil, Simone. *Gravity and Grace*. Translated by Arthur Wills. New York: Putnam, 1952.

———. *Waiting for God*. Translated by Emma Craufurd. New York: Perennial Classics, 2001.

Weine, Stefan M. "The Witnessing Imagination: Social Trauma, Creative Artists, and Witnessing Professionals." *Literature and Medicine* 15 (1996): 167–82.

Weinstein, Arnold, ed. "Contagion and Infection." Special issue of *Literature and Medicine* 22 (2003): 1–115.

Welty, Eudora. *One Writer's Beginnings*. Cambridge: Harvard University Press, 1984.

Whitcomb, Michael, ed. "Cultural Competency in Medical Education." Special issue of *Academic Medicine* 77 (2002): 191–228.

White, Hayden. *Tropics of Discourse: Essays in Cultural Criticism*. Baltimore: Johns Hopkins University Press, 1978.

White, James Boyd. *When Words Lose Their Meaning: Constitutions and Reconstitutions of Language, Character, and Community*. Chicago: University of Chicago Press, 1984.

White, Michael, and David Epston. *Narrative Means to Therapeutic Ends*. New York: Norton, 1990.

Williams, Bernard. *Moral Luck: Philosophical Papers, 1973–1980*. Cambridge: Cambridge University Press, 1981.

Williams, William Carlos. *The Autobiography of William Carlos Williams*. New York: New Directions Books, 1967.

———. "Old Doc Rivers." In *Make Light of It: Collected Stories*, 77–105. New York, Random House, 1950.

Winckler, Martin. *The Case of Dr. Sachs*. Translated by Linda Asher. New York: Seven Stories Press, 2000.

Winnicott, D. W. *Playing and Reality*. London: Tavistock, 1971.

Woolf, Virginia. *The Second Common Reader*. New York: Harcourt Brace Jovanovich, 1932.

Zaner, Richard M. *Conversations on the Edge: Narratives of Ethics and Illness*. Washington, D.C.: Georgetown University Press, 2004.

———. *Ethics and the Clinical Encounter*. Englewood Cliffs, N.J.: Prentice Hall, 1988.

———. "Power and Hope in the Clinical Encounter: A Meditation on Vulnerability." *Medicine, Health Care, and Philosophy* 3 (2000): 265–75.

———. "Sisyphus without Knees: Exploring Self-Other Relationships through Illness and Disability." *Literature and Medicine* 22 (2003): 188–207.

Žižek, Slavoj. "The Ongoing 'Soft Revolution.'" *Critical Inquiry* 30 (2004): 292–323.

▣ INDEX

Lightning Source UK Ltd.
Milton Keynes UK
14 May 2010

154168UK00001B/35/P

9 780195 340228